AN INTRODUCTION TO HUMAN SERVICES

AN INTRODUCTION TO HUMAN SERVICES

EIGHTH EDITION

Marianne Woodside
University of Tennessee

Tricia McClam
University of Tennessee

The authors contributed equally
to the writing of this text.

CENGAGE
Learning®

Australia • Brazil • Mexico • Singapore • United Kingdom • United States

CENGAGE
Learning®

An Introduction to Human Services,
Eighth Edition
Marianne Woodside and Tricia McClam

Product Director: Jon-David Hague

Product Manager: Julie Martinez

Content Developer: Amy Hill

Product Assistant: Kyra Kane

Media Developer: Audrey Espey

Outsource Development Manager: Jeremy Judson

Outsource Development: Coordinator: Joshua Taylor

Vice President, Marketing for Softside: Kimberly Russell

Associate Marketing Manager: Shanna Shelton

Manufacturing Planner: Judy Inouye

Senior Rights Acquisitions Specialist: Dean Dauphinais

Art and Cover Direction, Production Management, and Composition: PreMediaGlobal

eBook Project Manager: Holly Klaft

Cover Image: Crowd (© danishkhan/ iStockphoto)

For product information and technology assistance, contact us at **Cengage Learning Customer & Sales Support, 1-800-354-9706**.

For permission to use material from this text or product, submit all requests online at **www.cengage.com/permissions**. Further permissions questions can be e-mailed to **permissionrequest@cengage.com**.

Library of Congress Control Number: 2013946687

Student Edition:

ISBN-13: 978-1-285-74990-7

ISBN-10: 1-285-74990-1

Cengage Learning
200 First Stamford Place, 4th Floor
Stamford, CT 06902
USA

Cengage Learning is a leading provider of customized learning solutions with office locations around the globe, including Singapore, the United Kingdom, Australia, Mexico, Brazil, and Japan. Locate your local office at **www.cengage.com/global**.

Cengage Learning products are represented in Canada by Nelson Education, Ltd.

To learn more about Cengage Learning Solutions, visit **www.cengage.com**.

Purchase any of our products at your local college store or at our preferred online store **www.cengagebrain.com**.

Printed in the United States of America
3 4 5 6 7 17 16 15

CONTENTS

PREFACE

In writing the first seven editions of this book, our goal was to offer students and human service educators a textbook choice devoted entirely to human services—not psychology, sociology, or social work. We addressed the definition of the term *human services* in its broadest sense and described a variety of clients, the generalist human service professional, and the interaction between helper and client. We approached human services as a profession that continues to grow and develop. Our goals remain the same for this eighth edition of *An Introduction to Human Services*, but we have revised the book in ways that we believe improve it.

Our revisions are based upon the feedback we received from faculty and students during the review process. Many other revisions resulted from our own research and teaching; they document the changing face of the environment in which human services are delivered. Finally, we were guided by the changes that are occurring in our world, such as the shifting demographics, the periods of economic turmoil, the emergence of new client groups, the increasing importance of the global community, and ever-developing technologies. Throughout the text we emphasize and address the cultural dimensions of human services and clients.

Part I describes human services. The focus of Chapter 1 continues to be the principles that define human services. We revised the case of Almeada and baby Anne to better represent the human service delivery system and climate that exists today. Chapter 2 combines a history of helping with an update on current challenges facing the helping professions, a combination that allows thoughtful integration of human services into a long-standing historical context with developments to the present time. Unfortunately, many of the current challenges remain unresolved at this writing. Chapter 3 examines the influences on human services today: technology, the international dimension, the changing workforce, and diversity. This chapter reflects the impact that these influences continue to have on human services. Chapter 4 concludes Part I by introducing three models that contribute to our understanding of human services. Updated case studies illustrate each model, and a final case study helps students integrate the three models. The human service model is expanded to include a strengths perspective, an approach that we believe captures the spirit and commitment of human services.

Part II focuses on the participants in the delivery of human services—the helper and the client—and includes new information about client populations. Chapter 5 adds a new discussion about wellness and strengths-based helping and the feminist perspective. Chapter 6 explores the identity of the human service professional.

Part III addresses the delivery of human services. Chapter 7 introduces the helping process. Motivational interviewing, crisis intervention, and resolution-focused brief therapy illustrate the helping strategies used by human service professionals. These three approaches to helping seem particularly relevant today in light of the incidence of natural disasters and traumatic events, and the challenges the economic downturn presents. Chapter 8 reviews the environment in which human service delivery occurs and presents practical information about organizations, missions, and job descriptions. This emphasis on the agency setting includes a description of the day-to-day challenges of human service delivery. Chapter 9 continues to focus on the ethical issues that permeate human service work.

FEATURES

Two unique features of the textbook remain. The first is that the textbook continues to be introductory rather than encyclopedic. It presents the basic information that future helping professionals need to know about the human service field and provides the foundation for the further study of helping techniques, different client populations, emerging human problems, and the ethical dilemmas that inevitably occur. We believe the inclusion of resources for further study is also necessary given how rapidly changes are occurring in our world. We hope the resources here will be useful tools to help students expand their worldview, appreciate different cultural perspectives, and reflect on the knowledge and skills they are acquiring.

What students think and how they learn are important to us. Our own students tell us how much they like case studies, films, DVDs, and other materials that make concepts and events come alive for them. This information has led to a revision of *Introduction to Human Services: Cases and Applications*. It is a companion text that provides the case studies, practitioner voices, and application opportunities that make introductory concepts meaningful. Its chapters parallel those in this text so content is reinforced.

We think this eighth edition retains the best of previous editions, such as the international focus, the resources, and the examples and vignettes. Video resources available on the book's CourseMate will facilitate the mastery of important human service concepts and skills. We hope to hear from you about your experiences with this edition.

THE EIGHTH EDITION

We would like to highlight salient features and revisions to this text that we believe will enhance student learning about human services and human service delivery. Every chapter of *An Introduction to the Human Services* has been revised and updated with a new chapter structure, the latest information, new case examples, and more. The chapter structure includes Self-Assessment sections at the end of each chapter to help students measure their comprehension after reading. A "Want to Know More?" section, also at the end of each chapter, provides students with resources for further study. We revised the content and format of the Web exploration boxes to help students find the most current sites that describe the topics relevant to the text material. Finally, the revised Key Terms and References sections ensure that students are learning from the most current material in the discipline.

New case examples have been added to several chapters, and many that appeared in previous editions have been updated with relevant new information. Case studies were revised to reflect the current context in which human service occurs. For example, the case of Susan and Ted is written in clearer language to make the case easier to follow. The case describes problems so complex that use of all three models of service delivery must be integrated to address all of their problems. The case represents what we now know about mental health and substance abuse issues, as well as the influence of the economic downturn. The first-person accounts introduce how individuals deliver services. In Chapter 3, Cathy Hamlin writes about what she learned during her human service work in Angola. Allison Anders, also in Chapter 3, shares information about her work with Burundian refugee children and parents in a city school setting. In Chapter 6, Amanda Nalls describes her experience as a military personnel officer in Iraq, and Ellen Carruth recounts her experience working with the persistently mentally ill.

Additional revisions focus on four dimensions of human services: multicultural, current trends and issues, service delivery, and development of the profession. The changes of each of the four dimensions are integrated into the text and cases to present a holistic picture of a dynamic field.

In this edition there is a continued emphasis on the multicultural dimensions of human service delivery. This includes additions to Almeada's case, introduction to World Bank efforts to advocate for gender equity in developing countries, and information about Native American traditional healing as a form of helping interventions. Many of the cases in the text were revised to capture the multicultural characteristics of helpers, clients, and the helping process. We provide concrete strategies for developing a cultural competence and working with clients from other cultures.

Current trends and events also framed revisions to each chapter. Human service delivery exists within a political, economic, and social context that is continually changing. For example, to capture these new trends, we moved the managed care section from Chapter 3, "Human Services Today," to Chapter 2, "A History of Human Services," reflecting the acceptance of managed care in service delivery. We revised our discussion of welfare reform, added a section on political partisanship, discussed the influence of President Obama and his administration on the delivery of human services, expanded our description of homelessness, and integrated the influence of the economic downturn into text and cases. We described the changing workplace and outlined how these changes create challenges for human service agencies and clients served.

A number of changes relate to service delivery. We included a section on evidence-based practice and how it influences human service work, expanded the focus on strengths-based practice (as a part of the human service model), highlighted the importance of outreach, and provided additional information about issues of children and youth and military veterans and their families. Attention to wraparound services updates service delivery strategies. We also revised the various perspectives in which students might view clients. To do so, we revised the concept of lifespan development, in particular adult development, and we broadened considerations of client issues and challenges beyond a problems perspective. In addition, a wellness model and a feminist perspective add ways of viewing clients and their needs.

Finally, there is information in the text reflecting professional changes such as the new effort to credential human service professionals. In addition, we focused on helping students gain a clearer view of the roles and responsibilities of the human service professional. First, we describe how values and personal characteristics of the helper influence the helping process. Second, we simplified the discussion of the typology of helping, placing helpers into three categories: specialists, professionals, and nonprofessionals. Third, we described the role of the generalist helper and integrated this description with the *Occupational Outlook Handbook*. Fourth, we expanded the section on nonprofessional helpers and categorized them into community caretakers, natural helpers, self-help groups, and volunteers. This range more accurately reflects the nonprofessional helper at work today. We expanded roles and responsibilities to include grant writing and evidence-based practice, again mirroring current human service work. We added the role of the cultural broker. We believe this is an advocacy role all human service professionals assume with the clients, families, and groups they serve.

Although not new, we continue to offer with this eighth edition video resources to accompany the text. In the previous edition, we offered a DVD; the videos are now located on the book's CourseMate, found at www.cengagebrain.com. This video product is one we are especially excited about, and we believe it is the next step in making introductory human service concepts real for students. We provide segments for each chapter. These segments vary from vignettes about clients and helping strategies to professionals and some of their challenges. For example, Katharine discusses her work with Burundian refugees to illustrate the relevance of international human services introduced in Chapter 3. Chapter 8 includes a discussion of referral; on the video, Joel and Susan demonstrate how referral actually occurs. We believe these segments and others will illustrate and reinforce some of the important human service concepts you will read about in each chapter.

FINAL WORDS

We approach each new addition with curiosity and enthusiasm. After several revisions, we find the research and writing provide us with a measure of how quickly the field of human services changes and evolves. There are some bedrock principles such as values and history that guide our practice. But, as sure as those principles are, changing contexts and client needs challenge us to learn and develop new ways to approach defining human service and describing clients, helpers, and the helping process. We hope that the eighth edition of *An Introduction to*

Human Services provides you with a foundation from which to understand and practice in the helping professions.

ANCILLARIES

The eighth edition of *An Introduction to the Human Services* includes the videos that bring the topics in the book to life, helping students to better grasp the work of the human service professional. The segments are available online through the new CourseMate Web site for *An Introduction to the Human Services*, which brings course concepts to life with interactive learning, study, and exam preparation tools that support the printed textbook. Students and instructors can access an integrated eBook, glossary, quizzes, videos and more in the CourseMate for *An Introduction to the Human Services*. CourseMate is accessible to students when they receive a printed access card bundled with their text or when they go to CengageBrain.com to register or purchase access. In addition, the revised *Cases and Applications* text provides students with a series of cases in a workbook format, asking them to engage in critical thinking and case evaluation.

A suite of instructor's resources are available to help faculty prepare for the course. These include chapter objectives, summaries, and outlines; an expanded test bank; and critical thinking questions that assist in reading, reviewing, and applying concepts. For additional assessment support we provide web quizzes for each chapter. These resources as well as PowerPoint Lecture slides can be downloaded from the Instructor Companion site.

ACKNOWLEDGMENTS

Many friends and colleagues have contributed both to our growth as human service educators and to the writing of the eighth edition. We are particularly grateful to our colleagues at the National Organization for Human Services and the Council for Standards in Human Service Education for their support, feedback, and contributions throughout the years. We would especially like to thank our students and the students in other programs throughout the country who use our book, for we have learned much from them about human services. Introductory students continue to be a favorite group for us to teach because of their enthusiasm and interest in the helping professions.

Our families have encouraged us during this endeavor, and we are grateful for their patience and support. The reviewers whose constructive comments helped us improve the manuscript include Sylvia Bane Malta, St. Charles Community College; Maxwell Kwenda, Cameron University; Iris Wilkinson, Washburn University; Denise Hamilton, Wheelock College; Rena Bushman, Empire State College and SUNY; Justine Pawlukewicz, City University of New York.

We would also like to thank the staff at Cengage for all their work with this manuscript. This includes our editor, Jon-David Hague; Amy Hill, developmental editor; and Amelia Blevins, editorial assistant. Our thanks also to Julie Martinez and Kailash Rawat.

Marianne Woodside
Tricia McClam

ABOUT THE AUTHORS

MARIANNE WOODSIDE   TRICIA McCLAM

Involvement in human services as practitioners and instructors for the past 35 years brings us a commitment to and understanding of human services. From our years as practitioners in public schools and in rehabilitation settings, we gained an understanding of helpers' commitment to their clients, their work, and their professions. For the past twenty years we conducted in-depth interviews with practitioners and clients in an effort to better understand the methods of delivering services, the interaction between clients and human service professionals, and the changing context of service delivery.

Defining Human Services

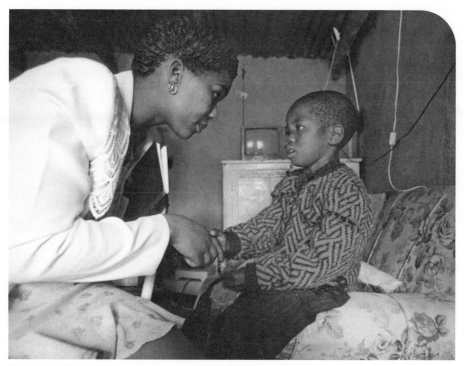

© Louise Gubb/Corbis Saba

Questions to Consider

- What are the perspectives for defining human services?
- How has human services evolved in the last 75 years? What factors influenced its development?
- How has society responded to the needs of people throughout history?
- What are the current trends in human service delivery? What is projected for the future?
- What model is most often used in human service delivery? How is it influenced by other models?

Human services may be a question mark to you as you begin this book. It is a difficult concept to define. Some think of it as the professional activities of helpers who try to meet the needs of people. Others think of local and state agencies that are named *department of human services*. Still others consider human services a **profession** for which a person receives special education and training. We present human services as a professional approach to helping individuals, families, and communities address their unique needs.

Part I is titled "Defining Human Services." If you think of human services as a puzzle, the chapters in this part will provide you with the pieces necessary to understand this complex concept. Each piece will give you a different perspective from which to consider human services. Chapter 1 introduces Almeada, a client who needs help from the human service delivery system. Through Almeada's experience, this chapter examines both scholarly and professional definitions.

Chapter 2 provides a historical overview of helping, the development of human services as a profession, and emerging 21st-century issues. Chapter 3 describes current influences on human service delivery and considers the future of such services. Chapter 4 describes three models of service delivery and includes a case study to illustrate each one.

AN INTRODUCTION TO HUMAN SERVICES

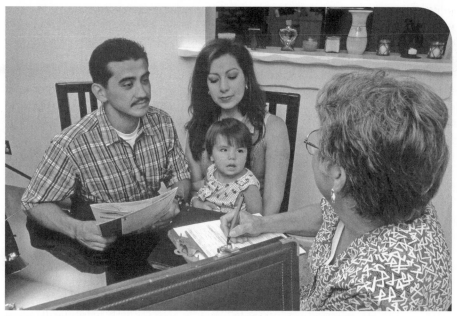

Tony Freeman/PhotoEdit

After reading this chapter, you will be able to:

- Identify the themes and purposes of human services.
- Define problems in living and provide an illustration of how individuals experience these problems.
- Compare the differences in the functions of social care, social control, and rehabilitation.
- Identify four tasks that human service professionals perform during the helping process.
- List abilities of human service professionals that enhance the helping relationship.
- Name three characteristics of human service teams.
- List the characteristics of the generalist human service professional working in today's delivery system.

One of the first questions you will probably ask as you pick up this book is, "What is human services?" This question has come up often in the last several decades as the field has changed and restructured. The purpose of this chapter is to help you gain an understanding of the term. The definition of *human services* is derived from six perspectives: (1) the themes and purposes of human services, (2) the interdisciplinary nature of human services, (3) the helping relationship, (4) management principles, (5) professional roles, and (6) professional activities. Understanding and integrating these diverse perspectives will help you formulate a definition of human services. Underlying all six aspects is the work of a human services professional addressing the unique needs of individuals, families, and communities.

This chapter introduces the themes and purposes of human services as described by scholars and prominent leaders in the field. The six themes presented summarize the principles that guide the delivery of human services. A case study of Almeada, a young mother who is living in a large city with her baby daughter, Anne, illustrates these concepts. We also describe the interdisciplinary nature of human services and the relationship between client and helper. Important ideas to consider here are the nature of the client, the client's environment, and the interaction between the client and the helper.

Another important and defining characteristic of the human service delivery system focuses on how human service professionals approach their work. We look at the management principles used by human service providers as they continually work to improve services to clients. The fifth perspective on human services introduces roles of professionals. Finally, a description of the professional activities of human service helpers illustrates their commitment to helping the client by providing needed services within a supportive environment.

Together, the six perspectives presented in this chapter will help clarify what human services is. They will also provide a basic understanding that serves as a framework for the remainder of the book.

Before you begin your exploration of the nature of human services, take a moment to become acquainted with the videos that accompany this text. Visit this text's website at www.cengagebrain.com, then choose Chapter 1, then Videos. In the first segment, Porche introduces the video program and describes how it will help you learn more about human services. In the second segment, several human service professionals introduce themselves and the work they do. You will see them in several of the video segments that follow.

THEMES AND PURPOSES OF HUMAN SERVICES

The first perspective from which human services can be defined is a scholarly one. Scholars approach the definition of human services by describing the themes and purposes that guide human services; these themes and purposes have emerged over the past five decades. Those presented in this section represent the ideas of a range of scholars writing in the field today and include concerns with problems in living, the increase in problems in our modern world, the need for self-sufficiency, and the goals of social care, social control, and rehabilitation. A case study of Almeada and her daughter, Anne, illustrates these themes.

PROBLEMS IN LIVING

Human beings are not always able to meet their own needs. Human services has developed in response to the need of individuals, groups, or communities for assistance to live better lives. Examples of such people are often publicized in the media: the very young; older adults; people with limited physical or mental capabilities; victims of crimes, disasters, or abuse; immigrants; people with acquired immunodeficiency syndrome (AIDS); veterans, and many others. Assisting individuals is an example of the helping interaction. Families and groups also receive the attention of human service professionals, as do communities and larger geographic areas.

Anne, a one-year-old child, lives with her mother, Almeada, in a housing project in Chicago. Their home is a dirty, rat-infested, one-room apartment that offers little beyond protection from the weather. Almeada, 17 years old, works six days a week for a local clothing manufacturer for minimum wage. She spends day after day in a large, hot, noisy warehouse, sewing sleeves in dresses and shirts. Almeada feels lucky to have this job, since the plant downsized twice. Most of her friends who work do so in the fast-food industry or in local supermarkets in the area.

This summer, Luis, a 10-year-old neighbor, watches baby Anne from 7:30 a.m. until 5:30 p.m. Luis takes Anne to the playground each day and watches her while he plays with his friends. When she needs a nap, he puts her down to sleep on the only grassy spot. He changes her once a day at noon and feeds her a bottle of watered juice, a bottle of watered milk, and cut-up hot dogs. The playground is located in a rough neighborhood and is the hangout for one of the many street gangs in the area. Almeada leaves the house at 7:30 a.m. and does not return until 6:00 p.m. During the hours that Luis is not watching Anne, she is alone in her bed in the apartment. Almeada stays in touch with Luis by cell to keep track of baby Anne. For her the phone is the first bill she pays. It is the key to her support system and care of baby Anne.

Almeada knows that she needs help for herself and Anne. Before she moved from her old neighborhood, Almeada had been seeing a case manager, Barbara LaRosa. She plans to call Ms. LaRosa tomorrow from work and hopes Ms. LaRosa will be able to give her some ideas about where to go for help in this new part of the city. Almeada also visited a faith healer living near her parent's home. The healer, Ms. Morales, a *curandera*, combined prayers and an herbal treatment to calm Almeada and reduce her stress.

Baby Anne cannot take care of herself. She is one of the many individuals who require human services just to have the necessities of life. Anne lacks adequate food, housing, and developmental opportunities. She is in danger because she does not receive appropriate supervision during the day. There is also some question as to whether Almeada can take care of herself properly. She is only 17, works long hours for little pay, and has the major responsibility of raising a child, although she is little more than a child herself.

Human services recognizes problems such as Almeada's as **problems in living**. As part of this recognition, the focus is not on the past but rather on improving the present and changing the future. Doing so involves directing attention to the client, the environment, and the interaction between the two. Individuals grow and develop through the life cycle, encountering problems in living such as adolescent rebellion, parenthood, mid-life crises, caring for aging parents, and death and dying. Many difficulties in living arise in connection with families and communities; these may involve relating to children, spouses, and parents; maintaining progress in education; adapting to a new culture and language; sustaining performance at work; and assuming responsibility for the very young or the very old. An important aspect of problems in living is the difficulty individuals encounter in interacting with their environments. If unemployment is high, finding work is not easy; if friends or relatives abuse drugs and alcohol, abstaining is difficult; if parents and peers do not value education, choosing to stay in school is problematic; if the family is living in a new country and culture, adjustment is difficult; if a natural or human disaster occurs, recovery is not easy. Human services addresses problems in living, with a focus on both the individual or group and the situation or event. These problems occur throughout the life span. This dual focus on the client and the environment strengthens the nature of the help offered and provided.

Anne's mother, Almeada Estrada, was 16 years old when Anne was born. Almeada received her early schooling in Chicago but quit attending school regularly when she was in the fifth grade. She was held back in the first grade and again in the third grade because she had not mastered basic math and reading skills. Her parents, immigrants to the United States, did not think education was important; in fact, they spoke little English themselves and did not require that Almeada attend school at all. They were both alcoholics, continually unemployed, and dependent on Almeada to structure their family life.

By the time Almeada was 10, she had discovered that life was more pleasant away from home. After school, she would spend long hours playing with her friends on the streets; nights, she would spend with girlfriends. She became sexually active at the age of 12 under pressure from her friends, who ridiculed her until she became "one of the gang." At the time she became sexually active, she knew about AIDS but did not understand it as a problem for her.

Between the ages of 12 and 16, Almeada was in constant turmoil, wondering how and where to live her life. She received advice as well as pressure from parents, friends, and teachers to do what they wanted. Occasionally, she was asked to join special programs at school, but her parents would not give their permission. No one was particularly interested in what she wanted to do. She was entangled in a troublesome adolescent rebellion in which she rejected parents and teachers and accepted peers as models. Relating to peers brought unwelcome pressure to go along with the norms of the group. But she was part of a group, and that support extended beyond face-to-face contact to texting and talking by phone. This way of communicating put her further from her parents' reach.

In responding to the needs of clients, human service professionals are encountering an increasing number of problems to be solved, a rise that many experts attribute partly to a changing culture and lifestyle. This broad increase in problems is another theme in human services.

THE GROWING NUMBER OF PROBLEMS IN THE MODERN WORLD

Human services has emerged in response to the growth in human problems in our modern world. A growing number of people feel alienated and isolated from their neighborhoods and communities. No longer can they count on family and neighbors to share everyday joys and sorrows and assist in times of trouble and crisis. Households are in constant transition, as people leave family and friends to seek new job opportunities. Schools, religious organizations, and recreation centers still provide meeting places, but because of the constant turnover, newcomers are welcoming newcomers. Stress is a hallmark of today's world. We worry about how to feed, clothe, and shelter children, families, adults, and the elderly. Illiteracy, a lack of employable skills, and unemployment rates or low-wage employment add to people's feelings of helplessness and hopelessness, particularly in a technological age.

The lifestyles that were once ensured with a good education and a robust economy are no longer guaranteed. The current economic downturn or recession that began in 2008 exacerbated the difficulties individuals experienced. The number of individuals experiencing difficulties related to the economic situation increased markedly. For example, people may be trained for jobs that are being phased out or no longer exist. In addition, new technology may also cause many to lose their jobs. Many individuals and families lost their homes and their ability to afford alternative housing. Access to quality health care declined.

The world appears smaller as we have increased our capability for global communication. As more information is available, more choices appear possible. At the same time, the problems of overpopulation, malnutrition, urbanization, the environment of the planet, natural disasters, and, as stated earlier, the economic downturn are new sources of worry. There is also threat of nuclear war, terrorism, civil wars and genocide, and religious and social conflict. The media bring vivid pictures of all these problems into the home through television, radio, and the Internet. Electronic communication and social media increases communications, including those related to global issues.

> For the past two years, Almeada has felt the weight of daily problems in living. When she was 16, she discovered she was pregnant, and she received this information with mixed feelings. She was familiar with the problems of pregnancy because many of her friends had been pregnant. They often discussed choices, but to Almeada there was only one choice: to have the baby and take care of it. She tried to seek help from a reproductive health agency but was frightened when she had to walk through a picket line of abortion protesters to get there. After her first and only visit, the agency requested she call them when she arrived so one of the staff could meet her outside and escort her into the building.
>
> Of course, she could not expect much support from her parents, who were the only family she had ever known. She could not expect help from the father of her unborn baby or any of the other males in her life; most were just passing through the neighborhood. She was not sure where she would live or how she would support herself, but she knew that she would make it.

Almeada lives in a complex world with little support. An effective human service delivery system will teach her to use the skills she needs to manage her own life and survive the difficult challenges that face her. This **self-sufficiency** is another theme of human services.

SELF-SUFFICIENCY

For many human service professionals, the key to successful service delivery is providing clients, or consumers of human services, the opportunity and support to be self-sufficient. Economic self-sufficiency strengthens an individual's self-esteem. This economic stability is even more difficult to achieve in today's environment.

When these individuals are able to contribute financially to meeting their own basic needs for food, clothing, and shelter, they gain a certain degree of independence and feeling of competence, but they may still need some assistance. One important facet of moving clients to self-sufficiency is to empower them to make decisions and assume responsibility for their actions. Human services is committed to giving individuals and groups sufficient assistance to allow them to help

---

BOX 1.1   INTERNATIONAL FOCUS: *TEEN PREGNANCY*

Teen pregnancy rates in the United States were once the highest among developed countries. These rates have fallen steadily during the past decade for all racial and ethnic groups, including non-Hispanic White teens, Black non-Hispanic teens, and Hispanic teens. Even so, of the one million teens who become pregnant each year, approximately 80% are unintended. Whether planned or unplanned, teen mothers are more disadvantaged than are other teens and have children who face negative health, cognitive, and behavior outcomes. *Healthy People 2020*, a federal initiative to improve health in the United States, includes a goal to reduce teen pregnancy among 15- to 17-year-old and 18- to 19-year-old adolescent females.

In developed countries adolescent or teen pregnancy generally refers to girls younger than 18 years of age, most of whom are not married, and is considered a social issue. By contrast, teens in developing countries are often married, and the pregnancy may be accepted and welcomed. Unfortunately, in combination with malnutrition and poor health care, the pregnancy may lead to medical problems.

Sub-Saharan Africa has the highest incidence of teenage pregnancy in the world with 143 pregnancies per 1,000 girls aged 15–19 years. Generally speaking, women in Africa marry at much younger ages than women elsewhere and have pregnancies earlier in life. Of the 10 countries identified by Save the Children as places where motherhood carries the most risk for mother and baby, nine were in sub-Saharan Africa.

The situation in South Asia is similar: Early age at marriage means high adolescent pregnancy rates. This is truer in rural areas where knowledge and use of contraceptive methods is low. Some areas such as Indonesia and Malaysia are experiencing a decrease in the rate of early marriage and pregnancy, yet the rate remains high when compared with the rest of Asia.

In some areas of the world, little information is available on sexual behavior. This is the case in the Pacific Islands although teen pregnancy is considered an emerging problem.

Regardless of location or society, there are some common outcomes of teenage pregnancy. One is the higher incidence of premature birth and low birth weight. For the baby, other problems may include developmental disabilities, behavioral issues, and poor academic performance. Daughters are more likely to become teen mothers, and sons are more likely to serve time in prison. Outcomes for the mother are lack of education, poverty, and a second child within 24 months.

themselves. Clients are encouraged to be independent and gain control of their lives as soon as they are able. They gain belief in themselves or in the efficacy to make the changes needed to become self-sufficient.

> It was difficult for Almeada to become economically self-sufficient when she was 16, barely educated, and pregnant. She had little parental guidance or support and few skills. She was forced to move back home to live with her parents and seek the little help they could give her. In fact, she began taking care of them again. She got a job as a cashier at the local grocery store. Almeada saved a few dollars a week and bought groceries for the family with the rest. Her parents tried to borrow money from her to buy alcohol; they took her money if she brought it home.
>
> In the early days of her pregnancy, Almeada's life became routine. She worked from 8 a.m. to 5 p.m., walked home, prepared dinner, and visited with her friends later at night. Her advancing pregnancy changed her relationships with some of her friends because she did not have the stamina or the desire to share their evening activities. Even as her life changed, she was determined that no one would interfere with it; she did not want help. Almeada wanted to make her own decisions. Despite that fiercely independent attitude, she would soon need assistance.

Almeada was somewhat self-sufficient because she was working and her parents provided housing. As her pregnancy advanced, however, she had to quit work and rely on others. She also needed prenatal care, parenting skills, and an opportunity to assess her decision to keep the baby. Although economic self-sufficiency is a key for many clients, it would clearly be only a beginning for Almeada. Almeada would be hindered by her lack of education and skills. And the difficult economic environment would heighten her difficulties.

INTERNET EXERCISE

See this text's website at *www.cengagebrain.com* for video exercises. Choose Chapter 1, then Videos.

Listen to Blair, a human service professional, discuss Almeada and baby Anne, and answer the following questions:

1. *Why are Almeada and baby Anne considered vulnerable?*
2. *What is the value of viewing Almeada and baby Anne in a holistic way?*
3. *How does considering Almeada's strengths support the helping process?*
4. *What challenges will the helping professional face when working with Almeada and her baby?*

SOCIAL CARE, SOCIAL CONTROL, AND REHABILITATION

Early in the history of human services, scholars described the three distinct functions of human services: social care, social control, and rehabilitation (Neugeboren, 1991). **Social care** is assisting clients in meeting their social needs, with the focus on those who cannot care for themselves. The elderly, children, people with mental disabilities or mental illness, and victims of crime, disasters, or crises are populations who might need social care.

Social control differs from social care in two fundamental ways: who receives the services and under what conditions they receive them. Social care is given to those who cannot provide for themselves (either temporarily or in the long term). In contrast, most recipients of social control are able to care for themselves but have either failed to do so or have done so in a manner that violates society's norms for appropriate behavior. Often society, rather than the individual, determines who receives services that represent social control. The purpose of such services is to restrict or monitor clients' independence for a time because the clients have violated laws of the community. Children, youth, and adults in the criminal justice system are examples of clients of social control.

Rehabilitation is the task of returning an individual to a prior level of functioning. What creates the need for rehabilitation? An individual who was once able to live independently becomes unable to function socially, physically, or psychologically. The inability to function can be caused by a crisis, a reversal of economic or social circumstances, an accident, or other circumstances. Rehabilitative services, which are designed to enable the individual to function near or at a prior level of independence, can have a short- or long-term focus. Veterans, people with physical disabilities, and victims of psychological trauma are among those who receive rehabilitative human services.

In actuality, separating these three functions of human services is often difficult. Many clients have multiple problems, so social care, social control, and rehabilitation may be occurring at the same time.

Almeada finally became involved in the human service system in mid-autumn, when she was seven months pregnant. She refused to go to school. Her parents let her continue to work at the neighborhood store—in fact, they encouraged her to. Life was easier for them when she was available to translate for them and help with their daily living needs. Her friends often missed school as well, so she saw them everyday when they came to the grocery store to do their shopping. At evening, they all gathered at a shop in the neighborhood.

Two new programs were started at Almeada's school to provide more comprehensive support to many of its students. One program—Students, Parents Are Receiving KARE (SPARK)—targeted students who had irregular attendance, low math and reading scores, no discipline record, and no positive teacher reports. In the fall, the school officials noted that Almeada, who qualified for this new program, had not returned to school after the summer vacation. The second program—Students, Parents Each Are Special (SPEAS)—provided health care and other services to teen mothers. The case manager of SPARK, Barbara LaRosa, visited the most recent address on the school records and found Almeada's father at home. He was in a drunken stupor and was unable to give Ms. LaRosa information about Almeada. When she talked to the neighbors, they suggested she try the grocery store where Almeada worked. Ms. LaRosa found Almeada in the middle of her daily shift and made an appointment to pick her up after work and take her home.

In the next few months, Barbara LaRosa provided social care for Almeada and then for her baby, Anne. She connected with her by phone and text and tried to check in with her at least three times a week. The school offered Almeada several options for continuing her education: She could receive homebound instruction until and after the baby was born; she could come back to school; or she could attend a special night school for potential dropouts who work during the day. Ms. LaRosa also referred Almeada to the SPEAS program. Almeada attended a prenatal care class taught by a local teacher one night a week at the school. Because of Almeada's youth and lack of parental support, Ms. LaRosa discussed with Almeada the options of keeping the baby or placing it for adoption. She also took Almeada to the health clinic located in the school to further discuss these options. Almeada remained sure that she wanted to keep her child. Ms. LaRosa introduced Almeada to the welfare staffer who was available on school grounds one day a week. Almeada rejected welfare as an option.

Once the baby was born, Almeada needed rehabilitative assistance but, instead, returned to work immediately. She expected her parents to care for Anne while she was gone, but her parents refused to babysit. Almeada was afraid that one day they might harm Anne out of their own frustrations. Her parents could not stand to have the baby in the home because they had to compete with her for attention. Instead of receiving rehabilitative services, Almeada moved to a new neighborhood, rented a one-room apartment, and found a new job working in a garment factory six days a week. In her new neighborhood, Almeada again had neither human service support nor social support.

The story of Almeada's struggles and need for assistance is just one of many about individuals who cannot meet their own needs without assistance from others. A common element seen in all human services is that these services help individuals, families, and groups with their problems. There would be little need for these services if people did not need assistance and support from others. The term *human services* encompasses the variety of helping services that address the range of problems that people experience (Table 1.1).

The themes and purposes of human services—problems in living, the growing number of problems, self-sufficiency, and social care, social control, and rehabilitation—contribute to a definition of human services. Examining the contributions of different disciplines also helps define human services.

TABLE 1.1   SUMMARY POINTS: ALMEADA'S CASE

- Both Almeada and baby Anne experience problems in living because their needs for adequate food, housing, and education are not met.

- Almeada's world is complex, and she had little support during her pregnancy and after Anne's birth.

- Self-sufficiency was easier for Almeada when she was working, but her needs soon outgrew her resources.

- Social care provided Almeada with several choices to continue her education.

- Social control was not part of Almeada's case history because she maintained her independence throughout the pregnancy.

- Following Anne's birth, Almeada returned to work, moved, and found a new job rather than receive rehabilitative services.

THE INTERDISCIPLINARY NATURE OF HUMAN SERVICES

The study of human service delivery, an understanding of the professionals who deliver services, and familiarity with the clients who are recipients of services requires the integration of knowledge from a wide variety of academic disciplines. These disciplines include but are not limited to sociology, psychology, and anthropology.

Each discipline brings a unique perspective to the understanding of the nature of the individual, families, and groups of people. In addition, they focus upon the context of the environment in which "daily living" occurs and the interaction between the two.

> While Barbara LaRosa was working with Almeada, she knew that it was important to understand as best as she could about Almeada and her environment. The program in which Ms. LaRosa received her training required her to take a large number of social science courses. According to her instructors, in order to understand the complexities of human behavior within the social environment, the study of sociology, psychology, and anthropology is helpful.

Sociology, as a discipline, examines the ways in which human societies influence the people who live in these societies. In other words, sociology assesses the individual and the broader culture and tries to account for and understand the differences within human culture. Sociology helps human service professionals understand elements of life that affect living, such as family structure, family roles, gender, race, and poverty.

According to the American Psychological Association, "Psychology is the study of the mind and behavior. The discipline embraces all aspects of the human experience—from the functions of the brain to the actions of nations, from child development to care for the aged. In every conceivable setting from scientific research centers to mental health care services, 'the understanding of behavior' is the enterprise of psychologists" (American Psychological Association, 2010). Many individuals believe that psychology helps explain "what makes people tick." Numerous theories examine how people think, feel, and behave and explore why they think, feel, and behave in the ways in which they do. These theories analyze behavior and mental processes from the physiological, behavioral, cognitive, and psychodynamic perspectives. As they study psychology, students use these theories to develop a better understanding of people.

Anthropology studies the cultural, physical, and social development of humans and the variation in their customs and beliefs. A critical component of the study of anthropology is fieldwork. Anthropologists often live at the site they are studying as they try to learn about human groups and the role of culture in the lives of the individuals within these groups.

Today anthropologists study culture in its broadest sense. Not only are they studying about such groups who live in remote areas of the globe, but they are also studying individuals in mainstream culture in diverse settings. Similar to the tasks of the organizational psychologist, anthropologists are working in the business environment and studying topics such as the culture of work, employee relations, and human resources. In other words, they are learning about employee problems on the job by learning about employee perceptions and behavior. Directly related to human services are projects that help bring more clarity about the clients served. For example, one project may focus on individuals with AIDS. Another may explore the life and problems of the homeless in contemporary society.

BOX 1.2   EXPLORING THE WEB FOR MORE INFORMATION

Check out the following sources on the Web to learn more about meeting Almeada's needs.

Annie E. Casey Foundation

Department of Health and Human Services

Latina teen pregnancy

Guttmacher Institute

As Barbara LaRosa tried to think about Almeada and her new life with baby Anne, she realized that the young woman's life would change as she moved away from her neighborhood, her friends, and her parents—and Ms. LaRosa was worried about her. For many years, Ms. LaRosa has been able to use the information she learned in school to understand her clients and the situations they faced. Almeada would be struggling to care for baby Anne and herself without a social support network or formal human services. In fact, Almeada would not even speak Spanish, the primary language spoken in the neighborhood. Even though Almeada was strong and determined, the difficult environment within which she was living would present challenges that would be difficult to meet without help.

The work of human service delivery is an interdisciplinary endeavor that requires knowledge of individuals, an understanding of society and its relationship to individual and family life, and a view of the culture in which people live. Helpers like Barbara LaRosa often work with clients who are very different from themselves. By integrating disciplines such as sociology, psychology, and anthropology, human service professionals can better understand the nature of their clients and their environments. This allows them to understand and relate to their clients more effectively.

Integrated into all three disciplines, psychology, sociology, and anthropology, is a multicultural perspective that provides the foundation for understanding the client. Assuming that all interactions are multicultural, psychology provides information about individuals, their cultural identity, and strengths and barriers these present. On the other hand, sociology looks at culture in terms of ways in which individuals think and act based upon cultural norms and rules. Finally, anthropology sees culture as multiethnic. What this means to the anthropologist is culture and its various subcultures represent complex dynamics, rather than simple ones, that describe the world in which clients live. Although understanding the culture of others is difficult and continuous, all three disciplines note the importance of cultural considerations.

THE RELATIONSHIP BETWEEN CLIENT AND HELPER

The delivery of human services involves both the client and the helper. The process of helping is client oriented as the helper focuses on assisting clients to meet their needs. To do this, the helper performs many roles and assumes a wide variety of responsibilities. As stated earlier, effective helpers are also sensitive to culture and religion. In the case of Almeada, for example, important influences on Almeada's perspective were the Latino culture and the Catholic Church in her neighborhood. Let us look at Almeada and her human service professional, Barbara LaRosa, to see the helping relationship in action with special attention to the cultural dimensions.

When Barbara LaRosa first approached Almeada, she talked at length with Almeada about her situation. Ms. LaRosa had contacted Almeada to learn whether she would come back to school and to help her with problems that were barriers to her school attendance. After they talked, it was obvious that Almeada faced many problems. Ms. LaRosa planned to work with Almeada, baby Anne, and Almeada's parents if they would accept the help. First, Ms. LaRosa wanted to introduce Almeada to services available at school, because Almeada and her parents were familiar with the school context.

During these early meetings, Ms. LaRosa asked Almeada to help her understand Almeada's world. They talked about how they were similar and how they were different. This consideration for Almeada's culture provided Almeada a sense of worth. She felt respected as Ms. LaRosa continually returned to ask Almeada about her point of view and her goals.

At one time, a helping professional in Barbara LaRosa's position would have focused on school-related issues; her work would have been "culture-free." Today, Ms. LaRosa's approach included assessing Almeada's needs in areas other than school and referring her to other services. She might have told Almeada about other human service agencies, but Almeada would have had to contact them on her own. Today, human service professionals assist the whole person and empower clients to help themselves. In addition, the focus on Almeada's culture helped Ms. LaRosa better understand Almeada's basic needs and goals.

In practical terms, Barbara LaRosa was not able to meet all Almeada's needs, but she did work actively to connect her with other human service agencies in and outside of the school setting. In fact, multiple services at school reflect a current trend in human services to integrate client services. Ms. LaRosa was providing assistance to Almeada and Anne, who need help with their social, psychological, and economic problems. She also was coordinating the care that Almeada and Anne received. Equally important, she considered Almeada an important part of the helping process as she increased her own understanding of the many dimensions of Almeada's culture.

As a human service professional, Barbara LaRosa has the skills to develop a relationship with Almeada. In this situation, much of Ms. LaRosa's success is dependent on her personal interaction with Almeada and her ability to use professional skills such as active listening, observation, and assessment to establish a relationship. One way she does this is to emphasize Almeada's strengths rather than her weaknesses or deficits. She is also able to apply her problem-solving skills to address the needs of Almeada and Anne. Using the problem-solving process, she initiates human service delivery by considering the relationship of her client with the environment and other professionals in the human service delivery system. Ms. LaRosa was also able to talk openly about culture and rely upon Almeada as the expert related to herself and her world. This increased the trust in their relationship and Almeada's belief that Ms. LaRosa wanted to help her reach her own goals for herself and baby Anne.

Barbara LaRosa, the human service professional who helped Almeada, was a very effective helper. First, although she was employed by the school system, she was able to work with other professionals to develop a plan of assistance for Almeada and Anne, using the existing human service organizations for their benefit. Second, she established a helping relationship with Almeada and worked to understand Almeada's perspective. Third, Ms. LaRosa had the ability to engage in problem solving with Almeada and to recommend alternatives. She took a special interest in Almeada, provided a structure for Almeada's service plan, and linked Almeada with other organizations. As she attended to Almeada's culture, Barbara LaRosa communicated to Almeada that she was an important person and one to be treated with respect and dignity.

THE CLIENT AND THE CLIENT'S ENVIRONMENT

Individuals who receive help do not exist in a vacuum; they are active participants in many different systems that influence their circumstances. Services to the client must be delivered with an understanding of the client's culture and with the client's participation. To be effective, the human service professional must ask the client questions about present conditions, current stresses and relationships, and everyday events. The helper listens to the client, always attempting to see a situation through the client's eyes. Questioning and listening should help the human service professional understand the client's world. The helper must show both a strong commitment to the client and concern for the client's well-being. The helper also assists the client in identifying personal strengths and limitations and developing new skills and abilities to enhance personal development.

Human service professionals also function as educators. As educators, these professionals help clients develop certain skills to increase their intellectual, emotional, and behavioral options. The client is a complex individual with many intellectual, emotional, and behavioral possibilities. Clients feel better about themselves when human service professionals treat them as thinking, feeling, and acting human beings who are capable of change. One way this happens is actively involving the client in setting goals: "What would you like to work on?" "Where would you like to be in one month or two months?" If the human service professional believes in and promotes change, then change will be easier for the client.

In many situations the human service professional helps the client learn how to use the problem-solving process. The purpose of performing the teaching role is to empower the client to solve future problems independently of the human service professional or agency. This leads to clients who begin to operate with increasing independence and self-esteem.

Almeada now lives in her new neighborhood with her daughter, Anne, and works six days a week in a garment factory. She knows she needs help. Because her major contact has been with human service professionals in another neighborhood, she does not really know who to call, so she calls her previous helper, Barbara LaRosa.

Ms. LaRosa is delighted to hear from Almeada again and is alarmed at her plight. Almeada talks of her current work and child-care situation in depressed and hopeless terms. Almeada seems to feel that she has limited options, especially since most of her neighbors speak little English, and Ms. LaRosa wants to refer Almeada to a source who can help increase those options. She tells Almeada that she will make a few phone calls and then call her back. Ms. LaRosa also wants to bolster Almeada's confidence in herself. As she gathers information about Almeada's move, her new employment, and her care of Anne, she praises Almeada's responsibility and maturity. She helps Almeada see how she has been a successful problem solver, reinforcing her strengths. She also praises Almeada's calling her and reaching out for help. Ms. LaRosa knows that any positive change Almeada can make will help solve the rest of her problems.

A function of the human service professional is to help clients develop their ability to assess fundamental needs and to focus on the problems early in the helping process. Abraham Maslow, a psychologist, described a hierarchy of human needs that begins with basic physical needs and rises through higher levels to address safety and security needs, social belonging needs, self needs, and finally self-actualization needs at the highest level. He stressed that addressing higher-level needs is difficult unless an individual's basic needs have been met (Maslow, 1971). In other words, if a child is hungry or very tired, or an adult is very scared, that child or that adult will have difficulty focusing on needs related to belonging or self-actualization. Clients are often so overwhelmed by their situations that they do not know how to identify what they need or where to begin to look for help or solutions. A good place to start is with the most basic needs, which are often the simplest to address and give the client satisfaction early in the helping process.

As an educator, the helper also teaches clients to recognize how their physical and interpersonal environments affect them. Clients are responsible for their own thoughts and behavior. Sometimes, however, clients are unable to make changes because their environments do not support such changes. Clients must be taught to determine the influence their environments have on their lives and to assess when and how their environments can be changed. Sometimes, such changes are very difficult or impossible.

In summary, an important conception of human services is the relationship between the helper and the client. The helper is committed to developing a relationship with the client that facilitates problem solving within the client's own environment. Many times the human service professional is also an educator who is teaching the client important skills that can be used long after the helping relationship has ended.

John Boykin/PhotoEdit, Inc.

MANAGEMENT PRINCIPLES IN HUMAN SERVICE DELIVERY

Understanding how services are delivered is an important part of defining human services. Three principles of management related to the delivery of services characterize the profession today: networking to develop a human service umbrella, forming teams and partnerships to provide service, and using **case management** to facilitate client growth. These management strategies help professionals provide more effective and efficient assistance to clients as well as enhance their own work environment.

NETWORKING TO DEVELOP A HUMAN SERVICE UMBRELLA

Human services is not a single service delivery system but a complex web of helping agencies and organizations whose primary goal is to assist people in need. It encompasses a variety of services that include but are not limited to child, youth, and family services; corrections; mental health; public health; crisis intervention; and education and employment (see Figure 1.1).

BOX 1.3   A PIONEER IN HUMAN SERVICES

Dr. Harold McPheeters, a psychiatrist by training, is considered a key figure in the development of human service education. After serving as an administrator in the department of mental health in two states, he joined the Southern Regional Education Board (SREB) in 1965 as director for the Commission on Mental Health and Human Services and director of health programs.

His work began with a planning grant to bring together mental health professionals and community college officials to explore the feasibility of educating mental health practitioners in two-year colleges. That grant provided the groundwork for 20 years of research and training in the mental health and human service field. Under Dr. McPheeters's leadership and with his support, efforts to define the concept of the generalist helper, provide support for training mental health and human service professionals, develop a certification program for human service professionals, and begin an approval process for training programs were completed. Before his retirement from the SREB in September 1987, Dr. McPheeters wrote (at our request) the following definition of human services, based on his 30 years of experience in the field. His definition integrates many of the ideas that have been presented.

I never came up with an absolute definition of human services. Originally, our work began with the associate degree programs that were training people to work in some aspect of mental health. However, it soon became apparent that the graduates of those programs and the graduates of other programs that were titled according to other human service fields, such as child care staff, youth service staff, and aging program professionals, were all finding employment in a variety of human service fields—not just in the narrow subspecialty areas of mental health, addiction, aging, and so on. So the terminology began to change to "human services" although no very precise definitions were applied.... Human services works with those same problems and people, but with a blend of primarily psychological and sociological theories and principles. Human services also has an eclectic approach to collaborating with whatever approaches (for example, medical) are needed to help people solve their problems. I suppose my definition would be something like this: Human services is the occupation/profession that uses a blend of primarily psychological and sociological theories and skills in preventing, detecting, and ameliorating psychosocially dysfunctioning people and in helping them attain the highest level of psychosocial functioning of which they are capable.

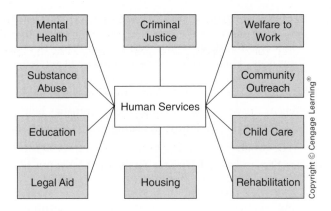

FIGURE I.I   HUMAN SERVICES NETWORK

Karin Eriksen (1981), a founding scholar in human service education, notes that "human services is often called the umbrella for our society's professions which are involved either directly or indirectly in promoting and reinforcing satisfying, healthy living and community cohesiveness" (p. 8). Going beyond the metaphor of the umbrella, Eriksen describes human services as a "bridge" between people and systems. One function of bridging is to narrow the gap between the services being offered and the needs of the individuals who are receiving those services.

Another bridging responsibility is to link human service agencies. Agencies and organizations share the common goal of assisting people in need. In the past, there has been little coordination, and the result has been overlapping professional responsibilities and competition for resources. Today, as service delivery philosophy changes and resources become scarce, agencies are limiting services, tightening eligibility criteria, and focusing on short-term interventions. Only increased communication, cooperation, and collaboration among helpers and agencies can promote effective service delivery. **Networking** is one way that service providers work together to serve clients.

> Barbara LaRosa wants to help Almeada in her new neighborhood, and she knows that finding a good entry into the system is critical. Ms. LaRosa worries that, without the right help, Almeada will be lost in the human service delivery system. She needs to find another professional who is familiar with Almeada's neighborhood human service system and knows the formal and informal linkages that need to be made to deliver multiple services. She is looking for a helper who will assist Almeada to move among the many agencies whose services she will require.
>
> Almeada needs the support of those who provide child care and teach parenting skills. In addition, she needs assistance in improving her work skills and health. Vocational development and public health services are rarely offered together. Coordination, monitoring, and evaluation are key services that are needed. Where will Barbara LaRosa locate such a professional?

For Almeada or any other client to assume the responsibility of negotiating, the networking would be difficult; human service professionals must build the bridges among agencies, organizations, and services. Working together to provide services for the good of the client is often called **teaming** and is another management tool used for delivering good-quality services to the client.

FORMING TEAMS AND PARTNERSHIPS TO PROVIDE SERVICES

Working as a team to provide services is part of the history of human services. Developers of the human service movement from early in its history stressed the importance of working with other professionals to assist the client in receiving services. More recently, the concept of working as a team has expanded, and "teaming" has become a common approach to organizing the work of an agency or organization.

> After talking to several child and youth services offices, Barbara LaRosa contacted Hernando Alvarez, a case manager in the child services division of the state department of human services. He recommended that Almeada call his office and schedule a meeting with an intake staff member. His office, just recently reorganized to be more customer oriented, was open for intake and service from 7 a.m. to 10 p.m. Mondays through Thursdays and on Saturdays from 8 a.m. until noon. These new hours are posted on their updated website. The agency also provides access to services through the online intake, outreach services, and social media. At first, Almeada would be assigned to a case manager who would not provide services but would coordinate them. In addition, four other professionals would help plan, implement, and evaluate work with Almeada. A backup case manager would also know Almeada's case in detail and be available to support her if her primary case manager was absent. Almeada would be able to reach members of the professional team by cell phone, office phone, texting, and social media.
>
> In fact, this particular team treats the entire human service delivery system as a larger team. They continually explore ways technology is changing and how they can use new ways of communicating to support their clients. They were early adopters of Facebook, using it to enhance communication. They cooperate with each organization, sharing problems and finding creative solutions that benefit clients. One warning that Mr. Alvarez gave was the uncertainty of the agency's funding because of the evaluation of their outcome efforts and the changes the agency was making to staff assignments and service delivery. He hoped that Almeada would not get lost in the possible changes. At the conclusion of her conversation with Mr. Alvarez, Ms. LaRosa felt she could make a good referral for Almeada, and she made a promise to herself to contact Hernando Alvarez in two months to check on her client's progress.

The primary beneficiary of teaming in a human service setting is the client. The team approach yields more efficient and more effective service. As suggested in the case of Almeada, many professionals, functioning as a group, are working together to provide creative, coordinated services. Such teams are able to evaluate their own performance and make changes to improve their service delivery. The bottom line is improving the delivery of services to clients.

Partnerships are also emerging as a way that organizations in the human service delivery system can work together to serve their clients more completely.

These partnerships are formed when two or more human service organizations agree to work together toward common goals. In addition, partnerships form with corporations, businesses, and government entities as those organizations outside the human service delivery system see benefits in supporting the social service sector. Partnering requires many of the same qualities as teaming: a high degree of cooperation, a commitment of time, and a high level of trust. When partnering is successful, there is mutual gain for each of the parties involved.

The concept of partnership has emerged as a way for human service organizations to relate to each other for several reasons. Many of them are financial. As the cost of service provision increases and available financial resources decrease, many organizations are finding that they can provide services more cost effectively when they work with other agencies. Partnerships have also been encouraged by the increasing pressure to be accountable for resources expended. Agencies find that combining their resources and expertise enables them to provide better services to their clients.

> Hernando Alvarez contacted Almeada the day after he talked with Barbara LaRosa. Rather than place the burden of contacting the state Department of Human Services (DHS) on Almeada, he went to see her at her workplace. This is part of the outreach service that is an important part of their service delivery. He explained that Ms. LaRosa had called him and that he was interested in working with Almeada to decide what services she needed and to help her find a way to access those services.
>
> Because the department had partnerships with many businesses and industries, Hernando Alvarez was able to schedule a time when he could meet with Almeada at her business site. Her employer had a small office for DHS staff and encouraged his employees to use the services the agency made available. Hernando knew that some services could be provided very quickly; others would evolve more slowly.

Hernando Alvarez and other DHS staff increased their ability to work effectively with clients through their partnership agreements with many local corporations and businesses. For DHS and other agencies, partnerships are usually established at the organizational level and are marked by a general statement of agreement that two or more organizations will work together. The text of the agreement contains language similar to the following: "This statement represents an acknowledgment by Organization A and Organization B of their mutual interest in forming a joint, long-term cooperative relationship whose purpose would be to encourage interaction between the two organizations." Later, the organizations work together to find specific projects and activities that would invite mutual support, and in Almeada's case, her employer encourages DHS to support his employees (Table 1.2).

Just as teaming and partnerships have emerged as powerful tools to improve the delivery of human services, another tool, the role and responsibility of case management, provides a way to expand services available to meet the needs of the multiproblem or long-term client.

TABLE 1.2   SUMMARY POINTS: ALMEADA'S CASE

- Integrating different social science perspectives helps human service professionals understand clients and their environments.

- Barbara LaRosa illustrates the importance of integrating and coordinating services as she teaches Almeada about problem solving and the influence of her environment on her life.

- Barbara LaRosa's networking skills are useful in locating a human service professional who is knowledgeable about services in Almeada's new neighborhood.

- Almeada benefits from the creative, coordinated services provided by Hernando Alvarez and his team.

- A case management approach to Almeada's situation involves both providing and coordinating services.

CASE MANAGEMENT

Case management is a service delivery strategy that is often necessary when several agencies or professionals are involved in providing services. When so many people are engaged in service delivery with the same client, the services may become fragmented, uncoordinated, or both, leaving the client dissatisfied and often with unresolved problems. Assuming case management responsibilities is one way to deliver multiple services in a more effective and efficient manner.

Several factors have created the need for case management services. One factor is the shift from large state-operated institutions to smaller, community-based facilities. This shift gives special importance to interorganizational coordination, a team approach, and helping professionals with a concern for the whole person because services are not being assessed or delivered in one comprehensive system. A second factor is the categorical public funding of the past, which resulted in highly complex, redundant, fragmented, and uncoordinated services. The resulting system is burdensome for people with complex problems who are least able to act as advocates for themselves. In many cases, multiproblem clients are assigned a different staff within a given agency for each service and different helpers in different agencies. Often there is no central staff member who knows and understands the client's total situation or who is responsible for planning and coordinating treatment strategies.

A third factor is the very nature of human service work today. Service providers increasingly find themselves with a dual role: providing direct services and coordinating services from other agencies and professionals. Helping professionals we know often talk about feeling like an air traffic controller or traffic cop, multitasking and juggling several cases simultaneously. This dual role can create problems in terms of time management, effective and efficient service delivery, and quality assurance. In addition, the dual role continues to expand as the clients experience the increasing pressures related to the economic downturn and a decrease in the support available.

The goal of case managers is to teach those who need assistance to manage their own lives but to support them when expertise is needed or a crisis occurs. In reality, the use of case management continues to expand into the many aspects of human service delivery. Long-term care involving work with individuals encountering problems associated with aging, mental illness, physical and mental disability, veteran's issues, immigration, and education uses case management as a method of coordinating and delivering services. A new use of case management is to link it with outreach functions to serve targeted populations, such as prenatal care for low-income, inner-city women, grandparents raising grandchildren, and substance abusers.

What exactly do case managers do? They gather information, make assessments, and monitor services. In addition, they arrange services from other agencies, provide advocacy service, and assume responsibility for allocating scarce resources and providing quality assurance. They also provide direct services. Many human service professionals believe that being a case manager means they will do whatever they must to help their clients.

The case management structure affects both coordination of services and client access to services. Given the fragmented state of service delivery and claims of coordination that are not borne out in practice, what is needed is interorganizational and interagency coordination that does not shuffle clients from one office to another. Exchanging resources rather than clients would ensure that clients do not get lost in the system or become frustrated with service delivery. Another necessary structural change is the establishment of a single point of access rather than entry points at each agency. Still another approach is to introduce clients to an array of community services. True coordination and integration allow clients to proceed through central intake, have their needs assessed, and be assigned to providers.

EVIDENCE-BASED PRACTICE

Evidence-based practice represents a growing trend in the human services to provide services to clients based upon knowledge about their effectiveness. The "father" of this approach to service delivery was Dr. Archie Cochrane, a physician in the United Kingdom, who promoted using evidence to guide medical practice (Cochrane, 1971). He had observed during his practice of medicine that there were not enough health care services to meet the public need. Because of this deficit in resources and his projection that the deficit would always exist, Dr. Cochrane suggested that decisions about what type of care to provide be based upon research findings.

Today evidence-based practice influences the development of interventions in human services. How do members of the human service profession implement evidence-based practice? First, helping professionals guide their service delivery using the results of quantitative or qualitative research. Sometimes, they use the conclusions or results of a meta-analysis or a collection of research studies focused on one topic, such as interventions that prevent child abuse. The heart of evidence-based practice integrates research, practitioner experience, and client input to create quality services (Rubin & Babbie, 2011). Examples of evidence-based practice might also include one of the following: successful ways to motivate children, youth, or adults to engage in the change process; strategies that encourage youth to complete probation; and intervention that effectively teaches teen parents positive parenting skills.

Providing evidence-based practice requires a new set of skills related to reading and understanding research studies. First, professionals must be able to evaluate reported research findings. This means understanding the variety of research designs and their strengths and limitations, looking for evidence of internal and external validity, and understanding the relevance of reported statistics. Second, professionals need to determine if there is enough evidence to suggest the effectiveness of certain programs, policies, or interventions. Third, professionals need to assess if the suggested programs, policies, or interventions will work in their settings with their populations.

The Substance Abuse and Mental Health Services Administration (SAMHSA) currently gathers data and provides mental health professionals with toolkits of evidence-based interventions (SAMHSA, 2010). These toolkits, as a part of the new science-to-services strategies, focus on illness management and recovery, assertive community treatment, family psychoeducation, supported employment, and dual diagnosis. Each toolkit describes a collection of strategies with documented effectiveness. For example, the dual diagnosis toolkit, officially known as *Co-occurring disorders: Integrated dual diagnosis treatment*, includes (a) individualized treatment depending upon stage of recovery, (b) education about illness, (c) case management, (d) help with housing, (e) money management, (f) relationship and social support, and (g) counseling designed especially for people with co-occurring disorders (SAMHSA, 2010). Evidence-based practice reflects a concern for accountability in the context of dwindling resources for serving those in need.

ROLES AND ACTIVITIES OF THE HUMAN SERVICE PROFESSIONAL

The human service professional provides services in a variety of settings. To respond to the many settings and the diversity of clients these settings represent, the helper needs a broad-based education and a willingness to adapt to changing roles and circumstances.

THE GENERALIST

The concept of the **generalist** is fundamental to human services. It describes the kinds of skills the professional has and the types of functions the professional performs. The term *generalist* has not always been associated with human services; the concept has evolved over the last few decades. Early in the history of human services, the term referred to a person who worked within a specific discipline, such as psychology or psychiatry. Professionals in these disciplines performed many functions: interviewing, diagnosis, therapy, and follow-up. As a generalist, the professional performed all the duties expected of a member of that particular profession.

As the role expanded, the term took on a new meaning, connected to a specific client group. Generalists performed duties and had the skills to work with only one group. For example, youth mental health professionals specialized in working with children. This would include working with individuals and with groups in educational, recreational, and counseling situations. Such helpers would also be familiar with social, biological, and developmental problems of children and adolescents; they would also understand the importance of working with the family.

A third emerging concept of the generalist is most representative of human services today. The human service generalist has the knowledge, values, and skills to perform several job functions in most human service settings. The generalist also understands how these functions fit with client and agency goals. For example, a helper trained to conduct interviews, write social histories, and define a treatment plan should be able to perform those responsibilities with the elderly, young children, or people with mental disabilities. This means the professional works with a variety of client groups across the life span and with clients facing varying issues and challenges.

The human service generalist works with the client using both micro and macro perspectives. The micro system is represented by the individuals in the client's environment and might include family, friends, teachers, coworkers, and individuals within the human service delivery system. The macro system is represented by the organizations, agencies, communities, and neighborhood locales with which the client interacts. For example, if the human service professional is working with the individual client using the micro perspective, then the professional is interviewing the client, establishing rapport, and engaging in planning and problem solving. Using the macro perspective, the same professional works with the client to understand his or her larger environment. This might include learning how to use the human service bureaucracy to convert needs into political action or to understand how school relates to the neighborhood. It is interesting to examine follow-up studies of graduates of human service programs to see the development of the generalist concept as well as the broadening definition of human services.

Early studies compiled by the Southern Regional Education Board indicated that graduates of human service programs were getting jobs in state hospitals, educational settings, mental health centers, children's agencies, and general hospitals. Three-fourths of the jobs were in mental health agencies. Although these graduates were performing a wide range of services, most were indirect services dealing with patients and other staff members. Their job functions were client advocacy, community consultation, and collecting basic research data—in other words, working from the macro perspective (Southern Regional Education Board, 1979).

Studies of graduates of human service programs since 1972 differ significantly from the earlier surveys. The results reflect a diversity of employment settings for graduates, including state hospitals, mental health centers, centers for the developmentally disabled, schools, child and family services centers, correctional facilities, nursing homes and other service facilities for the aging, abuse prevention and treatment centers, recreation centers, centers for people with physical disabilities, crisis intervention units, child- and elder-abuse prevention and treatment centers, group homes, and specialized fund-raising organizations. The job functions of these graduates include direct service activities, group and individual counseling, patient advocacy, interviewing, referral, gathering and recording information, treatment planning, discharge, follow-up, grant writing, fund-raising, and administration. These responsibilities reflect work within both the micro and the macro perspectives.

Future job opportunities for human service graduates are expected to be excellent and will continue to reflect the generic nature of helping. For example, the expanding elderly population, which will be discussed in Chapter 3, will require an increased human service network.

ACTIVITIES OF THE HUMAN SERVICE PROFESSIONAL

The professional activities of the human service helper are often discussed in the professional literature and are defined by the helper's relationship with clients and other professionals, academic training, ethical standards, continuing education, measured competence, and certification. Human service professionals often work with individuals who have few material possessions and little emotional support and who need many professional services and much professional care. The human service professional is often the first to provide support when the client enters the system. Clients become involved with helpers because they hope for a better existence. They view human service professionals as important people with special information and skills to help them identify and work toward their goals.

A human service professional's activities include academic training founded on a systematic body of knowledge. Academic preparation for human services takes either two or four years, depending on the training program. This intense training, academically and experientially based, focuses on the acquisition of knowledge and skills pertinent to **human service systems**, professionals, and clients. The training is also systematic. It begins with the study of introductory concepts of human services, then explores types of clients, problems, and methods of addressing those problems, and culminates in supervised field experiences. The body of knowledge on which the training is based is interdisciplinary, drawn from other helping fields including psychology, criminology, rehabilitation, counseling, and social work. This includes an emphasis on advocacy and social justice, a multicultural perspective, and a teamwork approach to service delivery. Human service field practice is unique in its diversity of settings and populations; however, the basic helping skills and methods of addressing client needs are both unique to human services and borrowed from other helping professions. Trained as generalists, human service professionals are thus taught knowledge and skills that can be transferred to diverse settings and populations. Even the guiding theories and principles include knowledge and values from disciplines such as psychology, sociology, biology, and anthropology. Practitioners need such a multidimensional approach to deal with the complex individuals and environments they encounter.

The good relationship the human service professional has with other social service professionals is a measure of the status of human services. Other helpers work with human service professionals side by side in a professional setting. For some, this professional is the one individual who is specifically designated to focus on the client's mental health and to coordinate social care.

In a nursing home, for example, the human service professional admits the client, takes a social history, monitors and facilitates the client's adjustment, coordinates services with family needs, counsels the client during troubled times, and

---

| BOX 1.4 | CLASSIFIED ADS |

Adult Case Manager:
Provide support for severely and persistently mentally ill adults.

Intensive Focus Specialist:
Creative, energetic individual needed to provide assessment, referral, and counseling in the public schools and utilize prevention theory to develop and implement program activities. Knowledge of adventure-based strategies required and ropes-course experience preferred.

Housing Counselor:
Bachelor's degree in human services or related field, or high school diploma or GED with supportive residential experience required. Must be able to provide 24-hour awake supervision and assistance to SPMI individuals performing daily living skills in a supportive-living facility.

---

attends treatment team meetings with the staff to discuss the client's admission, progress, and discharge. Other professionals, including physical therapists, physicians, nurses, and pharmacists, focus on the client's physical health. These professionals look to the human service helpers to address the client's mental health needs, which may involve support or referral to a specialist. In other settings, the human service professional is one of many mental health staff. In a mental health institution, for example, psychiatrists, psychiatric nurses, psychiatric social workers, psychologists, human service professionals, and psychiatric technicians all focus on the mental health of the client. Each of these professionals has a particular function within this setting, and each relies on the others to perform their appropriate tasks effectively. For clients and other social service providers, the work of human service professionals is essential.

Ethical standards also define professional human service activities. Human service professionals are committed to the ethical treatment of clients and the development of ethical relationships with coworkers, other professionals, and the system. Ethical standards guide this behavior. Because clients are the central focus in human services, their treatment and rights are of great concern, including issues of confidentiality and respect for the client's values, heritage, beliefs, and self-determination. Human service professionals are usually bound by two sets of ethical standards: those developed by human service professionals and educators, and those developed specifically for the populations they serve. See Chapter 9 for the ethical standards of human service professionals.

Another important professional activity of human service professionals is continuing education. A commitment to continued learning and development while working in the field is essential for such professionals. This continuing education takes many forms. According to follow-up studies of human service program graduates, many seek advanced degrees. More than half the graduates of two-year programs seek a bachelor's degree—most often in human services, psychology, sociology, criminal justice, or related fields. In addition, graduates of four-year human service programs seek master's degrees in social work, public health administration, nursing, counseling, educational psychology, rehabilitation, and related fields.

TABLE 1.3   SUMMARY POINTS: PROFESSIONAL ACTIVITIES

- Acquire the knowledge and skills that can be transferred across settings and populations.
- Establish good working relationships with other professionals.
- Abide by the ethical standards that guide professional behavior.
- Pursue continuing education opportunities to learn and develop as a professional.

Human service professionals also continue their education by belonging to professional organizations. Many of these organizations are related to the specific fields in which their members work or the specific population they serve. A final way human service professionals grow and develop is through in-service training. Many agencies sponsor seminars on current social or policy issues, on skill development, or on professional issues. Agencies that do not offer such seminars often encourage their staff to attend seminars sponsored by others.

A recent significant development in the professionalization of human service providers is certification that is offered by the Center for Credentialing and Education (CCE) (Center for Credentialing and Education, 2011). The National Organization for Human Services, in consultation with the Council for Standards for Human Service Education, worked with CCE to develop a process that leads to certification as a Human Services Board Certified Practitioner. Certification means that individuals have demonstrated that they meet established standards. The intent of this certification effort is to increase recognition of the unique and valued role of human service professionals. Additional information about certification is in Chapter 6.

In summary, human service professionals are concerned about and participate actively in training, ethical commitment, continuing education, and registration and certification. It is a relatively new occupation involved in professional activities of value to those who receive its service (Table 1.3).

KEY TERMS

case management	generalist	problems in living	social care
ethical standards	human service system	profession	social control
evidence-based practice	networking	rehabilitation	teaming
	partnerships	self-sufficiency	

THINGS TO REMEMBER

1. Human services has developed in response to the need of individuals or groups for assistance to live better lives.
2. Because human services recognizes client needs as problems in living, it does not focus on the past but seeks to improve the present and change the future.
3. Human services has emerged as a response to the increase in human problems in our modern world.

4. Human services provides three distinct functions: social care, social control, and rehabilitation.
5. Human services uses an interdisciplinary approach to understanding clients, helpers, and the context, including an understanding of the multicultural perspective.
6. Human services consists of those services that help people with their problems.
7. The relationship between client and helper is the foundation for human service delivery.
8. Certain management principles influence delivery and reflect the value of focusing on the client.
9. The interaction between the client and the human service system also defines human services.
10. The services provided are designed to improve an individual's well-being.
11. In the successful delivery of services, the client develops new insights, skills, and competencies.
12. The field of human services is respected by its clients and other helping professions.
13. Human service work is a profession committed to ethical standards, certification, and continuing education.

SELF-ASSESSMENT

- What are the perspectives that provide definitions of human services?
- Explain how the human service delivery system provides Almeada with social care, social control, and rehabilitation.
- List the reasons problems in living occur.
- Why is it important to understand the client and the client's environment?
- Why is the multicultural perspective important?
- How does networking help human service delivery?
- How does each of the principles of management enhance the effectiveness of service delivery?
- Describe the professional activities of the human service helper.

WANT TO KNOW MORE?

There are several resources you can access to learn more about human services and some of the concepts introduced in this chapter. Check them out!

Additional Resources: Focus on Poverty

Brush, L. D. (2011). *Poverty, battered women and work in U.S. policy*. New York, NY: Oxford Press. The author presents the story of the intersection of poverty, domestic violence, and welfare to work policies. She documents women's lives using first-person interview accounts, government records, and policies.

Corbett, S., Fikkert, B., & Platt, D. (2012). *When helping hurts: How to alleviate poverty without hurting the poor*. Chicago: Moody. The authors address faith-based efforts to eradicate poverty and make the case that individuals are helped from the "inside out" rather than the "outside in."

Dail, P. vW. (2011). *Women and poverty in 21st century America*. Jefferson, NC: Mcfarland.

Women tell their stories within their experiences of welfare to work and describe their lives as they relate to raising children, health care, crime, and employment. The focus is describing problems in living and ways in which current welfare policy fails to address issues of everyday life.

Ehrenreich, B. (2002). *Nickel and dimed: On (not) getting by in America*. New York: Owl Books. Essayist Barbara Ehrenreich explores how women in the labor market survive as low-wage earners by looking for a job and a place to live, working, and trying to make ends meet. She tries waitressing in the Florida Keys, working as both a cleaning woman and a nursing home assistant in Maine, and clerking at Walmart in Minnesota.

Novograntz, J. (2009). *The blue sweater: Bridging the gap between rich and poor in an interconnected world.* New York: Rodale.

The author recounts her work in microfinance in Africa, India, and Pakistan fighting global poverty.

Polak, P. (2008). *Out of poverty: What works when traditional approaches fail.* San Francisco: Berrett-Koehler.

The author examines three myths related to eradicating poverty. He challenges our policies that public programs offering financial assistance, national economic growth, and successes of the corporate world will reduce poverty. He presents alternatives that have had successfully addressed issues of poverty.

Singer, P. (2009). *The life you can save: Acting now to end world poverty.* New York: Random House.

The author focuses on two questions: Why people in affluent countries should donate money to fight global poverty and how much each should give. He highlights the successes of microfinance and charitable giving.

Smith, S. C. (2005). *Ending global poverty: A guide to what works.* New York: Palgrave Macmillan. Grass-roots programs and organizations help people in urban slums and rural areas break free of poverty. The author examines innovative and effective programs, describes how companies and foreign investors can help, and offers tools, guidelines, and suggestions.

Slumdog Millionaire (2008). This Academy Award-winning movie directed by Danny Boyle is the story of an orphan in Mumbai, India, who raised himself in various slums and crime-ridden neighborhoods. He becomes a contestant on the Indian version of "Who Wants to Be a Millionaire?" Events of his life are shown after he is arrested for cheating and during interrogation by the police.

Case Study

Case studies are another way to learn about human services. If you would like to know more about the application of the concepts discussed in Chapter 1, read the case of Ruth, a widow and a stepmother, and Beth, her stepdaughter in Chapter 1 of *Introduction to Human Services: Cases and Applications*, the companion text to

Introduction to Human Services. When Beth's father dies, she and Ruth must grapple with a number of issues that many older adults face as they age, lose a spouse, and develop medical problems. The case illustrates many of the important concepts introduced in Chapter 1 and their applicability to an aging population.

References

American Psychological Association. (2010). *About APA.* Retrieved from http://www.apa.org/about/

Center for Credentialing and Certification (2011). *Human services board-practitioner application packet.* Retrieved from http://www.cce-global.org/credentials-offered/hsbcp

Cochrane, A. (1971). *Effectiveness and efficiency: Random reflections of health services* (2nd ed.). London: Nuffield Provincial Hospitals Trust.

Eriksen, K. (1981). *Human services today.* Reston, VA: Reston Publishing.

Healthy People 2020 (2013). Retrieved from http://www.healthypeople.gov

Maslow, A. (1971). *The further reaches of human nature.* New York: Viking Press.

Neugeboren, B. (1991). *Organization, policy, and practice in the human services.* New York: Longman.

Rubin, A., & Babbie, E. R. (2011). *Research methods for social work.* Pacific Grove, CA: Brooks Cole/Cengage.

Save the Children. (2013). *Surviving the first day: State of the world's mothers 2013.* Retrieved from http://www.savethechildren.org.uk/sites/default/files/images/State_of_World_Mothers_2013.pdf

Southern Regional Education Board. (1979). *Staff roles for mental health personnel: A history and a rationale.* Atlanta, GA: Author.

SAMHSA. (2010). SAMHSA offers new evidence-based behavioral health practice tool kit series. Retrieved from http://www.samhsa.gov/newsroom/advisories/1004145809.aspx

2   A HISTORY OF HELPING

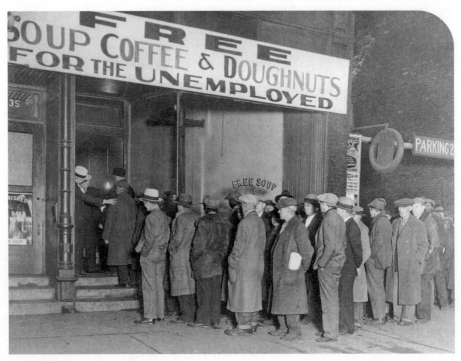

Bettmann/Corbis

After reading this chapter, you will be able to:

- Trace the historical development of helping.
- Describe the evolution of human needs since the Middle Ages.
- Illustrate three 19th-century philosophies about human needs and how those beliefs shaped human service delivery.
- Identify the significant legislation that supported the development of human services in the 20th century.
- Trace U.S. government involvement in human services in the 20th century.
- Summarize the impact of 21st-century legislation on human services.

Chapter 2 presents an overview of the history of helping to provide insight into the emergence and growth of services to people in need. History in this chapter traces how beliefs change over time. It describes who is "less fortunate" and examines the different categorizations of less fortunate people throughout history. The categories familiar to us today—the poor, people with mental impairments, and criminals—have not always been used. What is central to a definition of *less fortunate*, both then and now, is consideration of the "have-nots" in society, who meets their needs, and how those needs are met. In addition, we examine the emergence and growth of human services. This chapter assists us further in defining human services.

EARLY HISTORY: A SUMMARY

Until the Middle Ages, people believed that mental illness was caused by evil spirits, and early forms of treatment focused on ridding the body of these demons. One treatment used was trephining the skull (using a crude saw to remove circular disks of bone). This hole in the head allowed evil spirits to escape. Another popular method of treatment was exorcizing evil spirits through religious rites. People with mental illness were feared because their supposed possession by spirits was perceived as a link with the supernatural. Other attempts to control the demons included chaining, beating, starving, and bleeding the unfortunate human host (National Institute of Mental Health, 1971).

Hippocrates, a physician in the 3rd century BC, was one of the few professionals who used the scientific approach to explain and treat problem behavior and mental illness. He believed that problem behavior was a function of natural illness and that mental disorders had natural causes such as brain disease, heredity, or head injuries. In other words, evil spirits were not probable causes of mental illness. Hippocrates was also able to distinguish between different types of mental problems; among his most significant contributions were labels for illnesses, such as *melancholia* and *epilepsy*, which are still used in mental health today. His work marks the beginning of the medical model of service delivery.

Until the 1500s, the Catholic Church was chiefly responsible for providing human services. Religious figures such as St. Thomas Aquinas and St. Francis of Assisi are considered by some to be the first human service professionals. Under the Church's guidance, many institutions were founded for the poor, orphans, the elderly, and people with disabilities. At this time, deviant behavior was perceived

EARLY HISTORY: A SUMMARY TIMELINE

Early History	Mental illness, evil spirits
200 BC	Hippocrates defines mental illness
1500s AD	St. Thomas, St. Francis—first human service workers
1500–1600s	England protects mentally impaired
1601	First Elizabethan Poor Law
1700s	Almshouses established
1792	Pinel's humane treatment of the mentally ill

as a sickness, and **asylums** were established to house those who were so labeled. After 1500 AD, the power of the Church declined and that of government increased, producing conflict between church and state.

In addition to services provided by the Church, the needy in England also received attention from the government. In fact, the English Crown's right and duty to protect people with mental impairments had existed from the 13th century. For people with mental impairments, two categories were established: (a) natural fools or idiots and (b) those who were *non compos mentis*. *Idiots* became the preferred term for the first category, which included people with retarded intellectual development whose condition was permanent, present at birth, or both. The second category, *non compos mentis*, was the umbrella term for all other mental disabilities. By the 15th century, the term *lunatic* had replaced *non compos mentis*.

Diagnoses of mental illness were determined by inquisitions (unrelated to those established by the Catholic Church), which were conducted by a government official and a jury of at least 12 men (Neugebauer, 1979). The following questions were asked in the investigation:

- Was the person an idiot or a lunatic?
- When, how, and in what manner was the individual lucid?
- What lands and other property did the individual own?

The Crown's rights and duties were determined by these diagnoses. It was the king's duty to protect an idiot's lands and property and to provide the individual with the necessities of life; and the king was entitled to all the revenues from those lands.

Before the Middle Ages, feudal lords had assumed responsibility for much of the care of poor and sick people who lived on their lands. During the Middle Ages, needy people received aid from human service institutions such as orphanages, the Church, and, late in this period, the government. Several types of institutions provided services during the Middle Ages.

One important source of aid to the needy was hospitals. Not only did they provide medical assistance to the ill, but they also fed and housed tired travelers, orphans, the elderly, and the poor. A second type of institution, the insane asylum, was established in Europe during the 15th and 16th centuries. These institutions represented some concern for the care and housing of people with mental illness, but the patients did not receive effective treatment, and their living conditions were poor. The following excerpt describes the conditions at London's Bethlehem Hospital, an institution typical of the asylums established during that time:

> London's Bethlehem Hospital, better known as Bedlam, founded in the thirteenth century as a priory, converted in the fourteenth century into a hospital, given by Henry VIII to the City of London in 1547 as Britain's first insane asylum, became, within a few decades, little more than a dungeon. Women were chained by the ankles to one long wall. Men were liable to be attached by the neck to a vertical bar. One man was kept that way, even in the eighteenth century, for twelve years. (Friedrich, 1976, p. 49)

Relief for the poor was the responsibility of the Church during the Middle Ages. Church authorities at the diocese or parish level administered relief to feed and protect the poor within their districts. The money available for their care was sufficient to meet the needs in these local districts. In ministering to the poor, the Church served in the capacity of a public institution, and the tithe was considered a public tax. The care of the poor by the Church altered as the nature and incidence of poverty changed with the socioeconomic conditions. Specifically, the decline of feudalism, the growth of commerce, and the beginning of industrialization made it necessary to find new ways of assisting those in need. The poor, the unemployed, the disabled, widows, dependent children, the elderly, and people with mental disabilities and mental illnesses who were previously cared for on the feudal estates by the feudal lords now had no place to go. Most wandered around, often settling in cities that were ill equipped to handle them.

A new type of economy and the employment needs of the industrial revolution also affected a number of poor people. The growth of commerce encouraged the development of a money economy, based on capital investments, credit, interest, rent, and wages. This system was very different from the rural economy, which depended on the bartering of goods and services. As the poor could no longer survive by bartering and had little money, they often could not afford food, housing, and clothing. In England, the pressures of the poor in the cities created the need for a large-scale attack on poverty and prompted the passage of the Elizabethan Poor Law of 1601. This legislation was critical in the history of human services. It guided social welfare practices in England and the United States for the next 350 years by specifying who was to provide what services to those in need. For example, parents were legally responsible for their children and grandchildren, and

TABLE 2.1   SUMMARY POINTS: EARLY METHODS OF TREATMENT

- Trephining the skull involved using a crude saw to remove circular disks of bone.
- Exorcizing evil spirits was a religious rite to rid the body of their presence.
- Hippocrates believed that mental illness was a disease.
- Institutions were founded for the poor, orphans, the elderly, and people with disabilities.
- Asylums housed those with deviant behavior.
- Inquisitions determined diagnosis of mental illness as *non compos mentis* or idiocy.
- Poor relief was the responsibility of the Catholic Church during the Middle Ages.
- The Elizabethan Poor Law was passed to mount a large-scale attack on poverty.

BOX 2.1   ELIZABETHAN POOR LAWS

The Elizabethan Poor Laws were passed as a response to the increasing number of poor people in Great Britain. Few of the poor had the skills to earn a living wage, and as their numbers increased, pauperism became a national problem. The Poor Law of 1601 provided a clear definition of the poor and articulated services that they were to receive. It also defined what punishment those who refused to work would receive. This legislation is the foundation for the current social welfare system existing today in Great Britain. The following describes the law:

Poor Law of 1601

By this act two or more "substantial householders" were to be yearly nominated by the justices of the peace to serve as overseers of the poor in each parish. The overseers were to raise weekly or otherwise, by taxation of every inhabitant, such competent sums of money as they shall think fit, (a) for setting to work the children of all such whose parents shall not be thought able to keep and maintain them; (b) for setting to work all such persons, married and unmarried, having no means to maintain them, and who use no ordinary and daily trade of life to get their living by; (c) for providing a convenient stock of flax, hemp, wool, thread, iron, and other ware and stuff to set the poor on work; (d) for the necessary relief of the lame, old, impotent, blind, and such other among them being poor and not able to work.

Children whose parents cannot maintain them are to be apprenticed till the age of four-and-twenty years in the case of boys and twenty-one years or the time of marriage in the case of girls. The overseers may, with the leave of the Lord of the Manor, erect houses for the impotent poor on any waste or common … in many parishes of this land, especially in country towns; but many of those parishes turneth forth their poor, yea and their lusty laborers that will not work, or for any misdemeanor want work, to beg, filch, and steal for their maintenance, so that the country is pitifully pestered with them; yea, and the maimed soldiers that have ventured their lives and lost their limbs on our behalf are also thus requited.… So they are turned forth to travel in idleness (the highway to hell) … until the law bring them unto the fearful end of hanging.

Source: Excerpt from *The New Encyclopedia of Social Reform*, by W. Bliss, pp. 918–920. Copyright © 1908 Funk and Wagnalls.

---

children were responsible for the support of parents and grandparents. More significant, however, was the acknowledgment in the legislation that the state had a responsibility to relieve need and suffering and that the disadvantaged not only deserved assistance but also had a legal right to it.

The law included three main features. The first was compulsory taxation to raise funds to help the needy. The administration of this money resembled the Church's system developed during feudal times. Second, dependents were classified according to their ability to work: children, the able-bodied, and the "impotent poor" (adults unable to work). Relief was provided to each group: dependent children were apprenticed or indentured; the able-bodied worked or were punished; and the lame, the blind, and other poor people unable to work received home or institutional relief. Third, the responsibility for the sick, the poor, and others in need rested first with the family. If the family could not provide assistance, the government was responsible for doing so.

By the end of the 18th century, a dramatic change in the care of people with mental illness occurred. A move toward more humane treatment of those in mental institutions began in 1792 when Philippe Pinel unchained 50 maniacs at Bicétre

TABLE 2.2   SUMMARY POINTS: ELIZABETHAN POOR LAW OF 1601

- Law passed as the number of poor increased
- Compulsory taxation to raise funds to help the needy
- Classification of dependents according to ability to work: children, the able-bodied, and the "impotent poor"
- Responsibility for those in need was first with the family and then with the government

Hospital in Paris (see Chapter 4). This period is often called the first revolution in mental health. For those in mental institutions, this period meant improved diets, regular exercise, religious observance, and the development of the mind. As you will read later in this chapter, in the United States these efforts were led by Benjamin Rush. Unfortunately, the rise in moral treatment lasted only until the mid-19th century because of limited resources, overcrowding, and the passage of time (Macht, 1990).

HUMAN SERVICES IN THE UNITED STATES: COLONIAL AMERICA

As we examine the history of human services in the United States, we see the influence of the English approach to human services discussed in the preceding section. During the years of colonization, public relief was supported by individuals and groups who donated resources and labor to institutions such as schools and hospitals or directly to needy people. Much assistance took the form of neighborly kindness or mutual aid. As the populations of the cities in the colonies grew, so did the number of indigents, idlers, criminals, orphans, and others who needed assistance. The colonists used the Elizabethan Poor Laws as a model of how to meet the needs of those individuals.

The four principles that formed the basis of the local practice of poor relief in the colonies can be traced directly to the Elizabethan Poor Law of 1601. The first principle defined **poor relief** as a public responsibility. The second principle, the question of legal residence, therefore became a practical one, as services were provided at the local or parish level. The third principle spelled out the responsibility family members had to needy individuals; public aid was denied to those who had parents, grandparents, adult children, or grandchildren. Finally, legislation combined concerns about children and work by declaring that the children of paupers were to be apprenticed to farmers and artisans who agreed to care for them.

HUMAN SERVICES IN THE UNITED STATES: COLONIAL AMERICA TIMELINE

1600s	Recognition of the needs of the poor
1600–1700s	Almshouses established
1773	State hospital opens in Williamsburg, Virginia
1792	Philippe Pinel advocates more humane treatment
1800s	District workhouses established

Like England, the colonies responded to the needy by developing institutions. The first almshouse was built in Massachusetts in 1662 for dependents such as people with mental illness, the elderly, children, the able-bodied poor, those with physical disabilities, and criminals. **Almshouses** were not developed systematically, but over the next 150 years they were established throughout the colonies as the need arose. The numbers of these houses made it increasingly obvious that there were large groups of needy individuals the towns could not support. With this realization began the trend for larger governmental units to accept the responsibility for the "state poor." By the early 1800s, a system of district workhouses had been developed. Besides the almshouses, there were very few specialized formal institutions. Criminals were held in jail until trial and, if found guilty, were fined, whipped, or executed. Poor strangers or vagrants were simply told to leave town. People with mental illness had no special facilities before the American Revolution; their care was the responsibility of their families. Those without relatives to care for them were placed in almshouses. Those with mental illness were often locked up by their families in an attic or cellar or left to wander about the countryside.

Benjamin Franklin was instrumental in establishing one of the few formal institutions for people with mental disturbances, a section of the Pennsylvania Hospital. Another facility devoted exclusively to those with mental disturbances was a state hospital at Williamsburg, Virginia, which opened in 1773. Little attention was given to the treatment of mental disease because it was viewed as an economic and social problem rather than a medical one. Determining insanity was the responsibility of officials such as governors and church wardens, not members of the medical profession.

Providing services for those in need continued to be a concern for reformers and federal and state leaders. Widespread change in the 19th century required a different approach to providing services.

THE 19TH CENTURY: A TIME OF CHANGE

Large-scale immigration, rapid industrialization, and widespread urbanization led to many societal changes during the colonial years. These changes brought more poverty and more outlays for relief of the poor. During the Middle Ages, need was believed to arise from misfortune, for which society should assume responsibility. Belief in the right to public assistance was established and endorsed by the Elizabethan Poor Laws, which placed the responsibility on the government. In the early years in the United States, colonists used the English system as a model for their philosophy toward, and services for, the poor and needy. By the early 1800s, however, the philosophy in the United States had changed.

Destitution was viewed as the fault of the individual, and public aid was thought to cause and encourage poverty. This punitive attitude toward the poor—the belief that to be poor was a crime—was manifested in the Poor Law Reform Bill of 1834. Its purpose was to limit the expansion of services provided to the poor or the have-nots. This bill introduced the concept of "less eligibility," stating that assistance to any person in need must be lower than the lowest working wage paid. The social philosophies of individualism, the work ethic, economic laissez-faire, and Social Darwinism promoted further changes in attitudes toward the poor and the needy.

The 19th Century: A Time of Change Timeline

1800s	Rapid industrialization
1813	Practice of probation begins
1810s	Benjamin Rush influences mental health care
1820s	Rise of the philosophy of individualism
1840s	Dorothea Dix teaches prisoners
1850s	Rise of the philosophy of Social Darwinism
1854	Care of mentally ill becomes state responsibility
1880s	Philanthropy emerges
1889	Opening of Hull House

SOCIAL PHILOSOPHIES

During the 19th century, those espousing the philosophy of **individualism** viewed America as the land of opportunity. Hard work was the road to success, and that road could be traveled by anyone. The individual was held solely responsible for any failure. Similarly, proponents of the work ethic emphasized the importance of hard work and thrift for financial success and viewed poverty as a sign of spiritual weakness. Wealth was virtuous, and hard work represented the road to salvation.

Laissez-faire was an economic concept that focused on societal or governmental responsibility. The original French phrase means "leave alone," and this concept encouraged a social attitude of "live and let live." The most desirable government, then, was the one that governed least—negating society's responsibility to help its less fortunate citizens. Those adhering to this philosophy opposed the provision of any human services as a right of the individual.

Social Darwinism, in combination with laissez-faire and the work ethic, created a climate for the reform that was to follow. An outgrowth of Charles Darwin's theory of evolution, it was used to explain social and economic phenomena. According to those who interpreted Darwin in social terms, the natural order of life was that the fittest would survive, creating a society of perfect people. Those who were unfit would not be able to meet their own needs and would not survive. Supporters of Social Darwinism called for the repeal of poor laws and state-supported human services that facilitated the survival of the "unfit," as they believed that all change must be natural. Any attempt to help the less fortunate would be against progress, which depended on "natural selection." This belief was especially popular between 1870 and 1880. In reality, it often served as a rationalization for unscrupulous business practices. Furthermore, it encouraged the belief that nothing could be done about the situation of the working class and the poor, who faced long work hours, low wages, child labor, and unhealthy working conditions.

These prevailing philosophies discouraged the provision of human services and limited services to those who desperately needed assistance. The private sector became very important in filling the need. Wealthy individuals were instrumental in organizing and reforming institutions. Mental hospitals, almshouses, workhouses, penitentiaries, and institutions for unwed mothers and delinquent youths appeared. Philanthropic societies were formed to support these institutions. By the middle of the 19th century, public and private sectors were working side by side. As welfare problems grew, the private sector was unable to meet increasing needs. In spite of the prevailing philosophies, there was growing demand for public agencies to assume more responsibility for the poor and needy.

By the 1850s, specialized institutions had been established for persons with mental illness, juvenile delinquents, the hearing and visually impaired (then referred to as "the deaf and blind"), and criminals. These institutions were established primarily in the belief that reform, rehabilitation, and education were possible. Institutions could improve society by protecting individuals from negative environmental influences.

In summary, the 19th century was a time of dramatic change in the way society viewed its responsibilities toward the poor and needy. Government relinquished some of its role in providing services, and the private sector assumed more responsibility. Unfortunately, the problems of those in need multiplied, and gradually the government began to increase its assistance again. Institutions also developed in response to the needs of specific populations. Probation, mental health, and child welfare provide examples of how 19th-century attitudes affected the delivery of human services to specific populations.

INTERNET EXERCISE

See this text's website at *www.cengagebrain.com* for video exercises. Choose Chapter 2, then Videos.

Reform of the government's health care policy for those without access to care remains a controversial subject. Many opinions or positions on the health care issue are reminiscent of the three 19th-century social philosophies that are discussed in Chapter 2. Listen to these three speakers explain what they believe about health care reform, and then respond to the following questions.

1. *Identify the philosophy that most closely resembles each speaker's position on health care.*
2. *How did you know which philosophy was used to describe the speaker's beliefs about health care reform?*

PROBATION

In the United States, the earliest practice similar to **probation** as we know it today occurred in 1813, when Judge Peter O. Thatcher of Boston began placing youthful offenders under the supervision of officials such as sheriffs and constables. In 1841, the concept of "friendly supervision" was introduced by John Augustus, a shoemaker. He helped alcoholics and other unfortunates by bailing them out, sometimes paying their fines, and then providing friendly supervision as they adjusted to a new life. The most well-known organization to provide assistance to ex-convicts was the Salvation Army, created in England in the late 19th century by William Booth. Its members believed in taking a more sympathetic approach to the problems and circumstances of those in need. For example, members of its Prison Gate Brigade met prisoners upon their release and provided whatever assistance they could, including a home, food, and employment (Irvine, 2002).

TABLE 2.3 SUMMARY POINTS: SOCIAL PHILOSOPHIES OF THE 19TH CENTURY

- **Individualism**—hard work was the road to success and poverty was a sign of spiritual weakness.
- **Laissez-faire**—an economic concept that focused on societal, rather than individual, responsibility.
- **Social Darwinism**—any attempts to help the less fortunate would impede progress and facilitate the survival of the "unfit."

TREATMENT OF PEOPLE WITH MENTAL ILLNESS

Patients in the early asylums were mostly suffering from psychoses or severe mental disabilities. Treatment was medically oriented, and many patients were treated as if they had a physical illness. The beginnings of reform in the late 1700s can be attributed to Dr. Benjamin Rush at the Pennsylvania Hospital in Philadelphia. Dr. Rush, who is considered the "father of American psychiatry," fought the superstition and ignorance surrounding mental illness and elevated the study of mental illness to a scientific level. Before his study, mental patients lived in atrocious conditions and were treated with brutality and cruelty; customary treatment methods were bleeding, restraint, and cold showers. Dr. Rush introduced occupational therapy, amusements, and exercise for patients.

Dorothea Dix was another pioneer who fought to improve conditions and services for people with mental illness during the 19th century. She became involved in social reform when, in 1841, she accepted an offer to teach a Sunday school class of 20 female prisoners in the jail at East Cambridge, Massachusetts. She was appalled at the conditions she found in the jail: overcrowding, filthy quarters, and little or no heat. What alarmed her most was the crowding together of criminals and the mentally ill. She began a personal investigation of all the jails and almshouses in Massachusetts and made careful, systematic records of what she saw. Backed by a group of broad-minded, public-spirited citizens, Dix launched a whole new career as a moral reformer, calling for more enlightened treatment of those with mental illness. Controversy and outrage engulfed her, but those who checked her accounts found them to be factual (Marshall, 1937).

Dix encouraged the national government to assume additional responsibility for the care and treatment of people with mental illness. Using such methods as fact gathering, preparing memoranda and bills, and rallying public opinion, she began her campaign in Massachusetts, where the number of dependent insane was twice the total capacity of the state's three mental institutions (Trattner, 1999). The years between 1843 and 1853 are sometimes called her "decade of victory," because Dix was personally responsible for founding state hospitals in nine states.

By 1854, the U.S. Congress had declared the financial care of people with mental illness the responsibility of the states. This responsibility included paying for construction of proper facilities and needed treatment. In reality, however, the state systems were custodial warehouses, characterized by inadequate doctor–patient ratios, untrained personnel, overcrowding, and lack of public interest.

By the late 19th century, states began to separate people with mental illness and those with developmental disabilities. There was an attempt to upgrade research, treatment, and physical facilities, and the hospitals eventually provided aftercare and outpatient clinics. The medically oriented approach continued to prevail in institutions, and mental disorders were defined and classified into two groups: those caused by organic brain disturbance and those with no apparent physical cause (psychogenetic).

CHILD WELFARE

The first juvenile reformatory in America, the House of Refuge for Juvenile Delinquents in New York City, was supported by state funds. Massachusetts and Ohio quickly followed by establishing juvenile facilities. After the 1830s, the number of such institutions multiplied, as the public demanded the removal of children from almshouses. Unfortunately, juvenile institutions were not always an improvement, and overcrowded conditions and poor care prompted the establishment of a system that placed children in private homes.

Other forms of child welfare were the provision of mothers' or widows' pensions, the creation of juvenile courts and probation systems, the passage of compulsory school attendance laws, and crusades against child labor. There were several reasons for these actions. Many people believed that children were the most vulnerable and deserving group in society, and it was difficult to argue that the children were responsible for their own conditions. Children also constituted one of the largest groups of the neglected and needy.

REFORM MOVEMENTS

By the latter half of the 19th century, two population shifts were affecting the provision of services to people in need: immigration from abroad and migration from rural to urban areas. In 1860, one-sixth of Americans lived in the cities; by 1900, this figure was one-third; and by 1920, one-half (Trattner, 1999). Between 1860 and 1900, approximately 14 million immigrants from abroad settled in cities, creating an urban population that consisted primarily of former farmers and immigrants. Most were unskilled or semiskilled workers in search of employment. This population explosion in the urban areas created many problems for the urban governments. Two responses to these problems were the organized charity movement and the settlement house movement.

THE ORGANIZED CHARITY MOVEMENT   The goal of the organized charity movement was to eliminate difficulties such as fraud or duplication in the provision of services. According to the movement, the best way to deal with poverty was through personal contact or "friendly visiting" between the rich and the poor. Influenced by laissez-faire, individualism, and Puritanism, the movement soon shifted to reform, seeking better conditions in institutions, promoting better sanitation and health regulations, developing parks and recreation areas, and writing and enforcing housing codes.

BOX 2.2   International Focus: *Mental Health in Developing Countries*

All countries have systems of economics, religion, education, and law that have developed over time. Colonization by Western European countries interrupted the evolution of these systems in many developing countries, as Western traditions supplanted earlier systems, including mental health care systems.

Examples of developing countries using European systems of institutionalization or custodial care can be found in Southeast Asia in the early 1800s. In Singapore and Penang, lunatic asylums and hospitals for the mentally ill were modeled after European facilities. No better than warehouses for people with mental illness, these institutions also housed criminals, vagrants, and other social undesirables. With little hope of better care, many stayed for the remainder of their lives. By the end of the 19th century, the practice of institutionalization had expanded into India and Indonesia. Since such custodial care facilities did little to better the lives of people with mental illness, a negative perception of institutionalization still influences the attitudes of people in Southeast Asia today.

Today the World Health Organization (WHO) has launched a strong mental health agenda for low- and middle-income populations. The WHO stresses that it is not possible to have health without having mental health. They outline the barriers to providing mental health to those in developing countries. More about the WHO efforts can be explored by searching the WHO website and using the key words "mental health."

Mental disorders may be a source of fear, not only to family members and friends but also to administrators, health workers, and politicians. The belief that these conditions are caused by the supernatural continues to be widespread; it can lead to a person's rejection by or isolation from family members and community, skepticism among the public about treatment programs, and regressive attitudes regarding the development of mental health services. Institutionalization remains a dominant form of treatment.

The Charity Organization Society, a forerunner of the Community Chest and the United Way, is an example of society's response to the expanding urban population. Members of the Charity Organization Society believed that giving handouts of money and food actually encouraged people to remain poor and to beg for services. They supported the systematic distribution of alms only to the poor who needed them, thus helping the deserving poor while discouraging begging. They hoped to encourage thrift and independence among the poor. Eventually, this group evolved into a clearinghouse for all the city's charitable organizations, similar to the United Way of today.

The Settlement House Movement   The development of the **settlement house** movement was, in large part, a reaction to the inability of the organized charity movement to improve the living and working conditions of the poor. The leaders of the settlement house movement, unlike the leaders of the organized charity movement, did not support the laissez-faire philosophy. They wanted reform that included adequate housing, better schools, the abolition of child labor, and an end to the sweatshops. They thought that the best way to achieve this reform was not through alms or friendly visiting but through "social engineering." Human service professionals and reformers were "engineers"; they must participate in the system all the time, not only when something was wrong. Individual workers and reformers were perceived as members of an active and attentive movement that intervened at the neighborhood level. The settlement house is an example of social engineering in practice.

Typically, a settlement house was a large house in a slum area. It served as a community center, sponsoring such activities as recreation; classes in English, cooking, and citizenship; vocational training; and child care. Key elements to the success of a settlement house were the commitment of the workers and the location of the house. Social engineering could not be accomplished from afar; workers lived in the house or in the community in which they served. The house was part of the community.

Perhaps the best example of a settlement house is Hull House in Chicago, founded by Jane Addams in 1889. Addams was inspired by Toynbee Hall, a pioneer English settlement house she visited while in England in the 1880s. Upon returning from Europe, she and her college friend, Ellen Starr, moved to the poor section of Chicago and began raising money to support what was to become Hull House, located in the middle of the immigrant section of the city. Addams and Starr moved in and invited their immigrant neighbors to read Italian novels and see slides of Italian art. The women came and brought their children; the presence of children necessitated a nursery. Soon a boys' club was established, and then a men's club. Over the years, more than 50 services were available at Hull House.

These movements are important because they illustrate the continual struggle during the 19th century to assist those in need. Generally, the assistance took two forms: provision of services and advocacy of reform. It was difficult to blame all the problems of urban poverty on the individual. The settlement house movement, in particular, introduced a new philosophy of helping that recognized the impact of societal forces on the lives of individuals. This new philosophy continued to develop in the 20th century.

EARLY 20TH CENTURY: NEW DIRECTIONS

The beginning of the 20th century marked a change in the country's response to individuals in need. During this period of social reform, the first seeds of the mental health movement were formed, and federal legislation provided broad government support for many Americans.

The early 1900s, sometimes called the *sociological era*, continued the period of social reform. During this time, two significant events or changes affected the history of helping and human services. The first was the development of a new profession. Settlement house and Charity Organization Society workers became known as **social workers**. The basis for the new profession was the belief that such people needed specific skills, knowledge, and understanding to work effectively with the poor. Good intentions were admirable but not sufficient to provide assistance. During this time, social diagnosis, or casework, evolved as the method of practice. Mary Richmond, the author of *Social Diagnosis* (1917), identified this process as one of investigation, diagnosis, prognosis, and treatment. Her book is regarded as the first treatise on social casework theory and method (Zimbalist, 1977). The development of the social work profession is significant; it represents the beginning of the professionalization of human services. Later in this century, the fields of welfare, mental health, child guidance, and probation also became professionalized.

During the early 20th century, a reexamination of the causes of poverty also took place. A group of writers called "muckrakers" actively criticized the wealthy, accusing them of moral decay, cheating, and bribery. (The term was first used by President Theodore Roosevelt in criticizing sensationalist, untruthful writers.) Muckrakers such as Lincoln Steffens and Upton Sinclair exposed unfair business, government, and labor practices. They supported the idea that poverty was caused by social and economic conditions, not by the individual, and proposed that poverty was a condition that prevented people from reaching their potential. They claimed that because poverty and need resulted from societal shortcomings, improvements in housing and working conditions could help eliminate poverty.

Early 20th Century: New Directions Timeline

Early 1900s	Beginning of social work profession
1909	National Committee for Mental Hygiene founded
1910s	Muckrakers publicized social ills
1920–1930s	Free clinics for mentally ill opened
1935	Social Security Act passed
1945	Beers published *A Mind That Found Itself*
1955	Joint Commission on Mental Illness and Health met

SEEDS OF THE MENTAL HEALTH MOVEMENT

Clifford Beers, a victim of mental illness, was confined for three years in public and private mental institutions, where he experienced deprivation and cruelty. To publicize the plight of those with mental illness, he wrote about his collapse and treatment in *A Mind That Found Itself* (1945). In 1908, he founded the Connecticut Society for Mental Hygiene, considered by many to be the beginning of the organized mental health movement in America. By the following year, this pioneer state society had written a prospectus that included the following guidelines (Beers, 1945, p. 395):

> I "After all, what the insane most need is a friend!" By coordinating the friendly impulses of those who, if they but knew how, would gladly help the insane, the Society for Mental Hygiene can prove itself that friend.
>   II It is the aim of the Society for Mental Hygiene to become a permanent agency for education and reform in the field of nervous and mental diseases; an agency for education always, for reform as long as radical changes may be needed.
>   III The chief object of the Society for Mental Hygiene shall be the improvement of conditions among those actually insane and confined, and the protection of the mental health of the public at large.

Beers also proposed a national society, the National Committee for Mental Hygiene, which was formed in 1909. This group later changed its name to the National Association for Mental Health and is known today as the Mental Health Association. Its aim is to improve mental hospitals, arouse public concern, and prevent disease. By providing education on causes, diagnosis, prevention, and treatment, this organization furthered the development of the mental health movement.

BOX 2.3   An Asylum in 1902

After fifteen interminable hours the straitjacket was removed. Whereas just prior to its putting on I had been in a vigorous enough condition to offer stout resistance when wantonly assaulted, now, on coming out of it, I was helpless. When my arms were released from their constricted position, the pain was intense. Every joint had been racked. I had no control over the fingers of either hand, and could not have dressed myself had I been promised my freedom for doing so.

For more than the following week I suffered as already described, though of course with gradually decreasing intensity as my racked body became accustomed to the unnatural positions it was forced to take. This first experience occurred on the night of October 18th, 1902. I was subjected to the same unfair, unnecessary, and unscientific ordeal for twenty-one consecutive nights and parts of each of the corresponding twenty-one days. On more than one occasion, indeed, the attendant placed me in the straitjacket during the day for refusing to obey some trivial command. This, too, without an explicit order from the doctor in charge, through perhaps he acted under a general order.

During most of this time I was held also in seclusion in a padded cell. A padded cell is a vile hole. The side walls are padded as high as a man can reach, as is also the inside of the door. One of the worst features of such cells is the lack of ventilation, which deficiency of course aggravates their general unsanitary condition. The cell which I was forced to occupy was practically without heat, and as winter was coming on, I suffered intensely from the cold. Frequently it was so cold I could see my breath. Though my canvas jacket served to protect part of that body which it was at the same time racking, I was seldom comfortably warm; for, once uncovered, my arms being pinioned, I had no way of rearranging the blankets. What little sleep I managed to get I took lying on a hard mattress placed on the bare floor. The condition of the mattress I found in the cell was such that I objected to its further use, and the fact that another was supplied, at a time when few of my requests were being granted, proves its disgusting condition.

For this period of three weeks—from October 18th until November 8th, 1902, when I left this institution and was transferred to a state hospital—I was continuously either under lock and key (in the padded cell or some other room) or under the eye of an attendant. Over half the time I was in the snug, but cruel embrace of a straitjacket—about three hundred hours in all.

Source: Excerpt from *A Mind That Found Itself*, by Clifford W. Beers, pp. 133–134, 395. Copyright © 1907, renewed 1953 by the American Foundation of Mental Hygiene, Inc.

Services for people with mental illness continued to improve and expand. By the 1920s and 1930s, most large cities had free clinics for mental patients, where treatment and social services were provided. In fact, human services as we know it today began with the impact of World Wars I and II on the mental health field. By the end of World War II, the profession of clinical psychology was created, in part because the number of veterans who were hospitalized in Veterans Administration (VA) facilities for psychiatric evaluation had reached more than 40,000 (Cranston, 1986).

Until the 1930s, individual leaders such as Jane Addams, Clifford Beers, and the muckrakers spearheaded the development of services and the reform of conditions for the impoverished. As described previously, the development of professions that trained workers in social services also began. As important as these contributions were, they had little impact on poverty, mental illness, or other human service concerns on a large scale or at a national level. As a result, the federal government increased its financial commitment to those in need. Presidents of the United States assumed a leadership role in providing services.

Bettmann/CORBIS

INCREASED FEDERAL INVOLVEMENT

The Great Depression was marked by vast unemployment, failing business ventures, and the collapse of banks. The economic situation created a wave of panic and long-term psychological and economic depression for individuals who could see no end to financial hardship. President Franklin D. Roosevelt introduced New Deal legislation that fundamentally changed the federal government's role in providing human services, focusing on two goals. The first focus was to provide short-term aid to those who were unemployed. The Works Progress Administration (WPA) and the Civilian Conservation Corps (CCC) were but two of the work relief programs he initiated. The second focus was the enactment of the Social Security Act of 1935 as protection against future economic hardships.

The **Social Security** Act of 1935, the cornerstone of the present American social welfare system, was passed in response to the need for human services. This landmark piece of legislation was significant for several reasons. First, it translated into action the belief that Americans had the right to protection from economic instability. The federal government assumed responsibility for the economic security of all citizens, and thus began the American welfare state. Second, it expanded welfare activities and improved their standards by establishing a new alignment of responsibility in public welfare. The policy of federal aid or grants to states began, thus closing the door on three centuries of the "poor law" principle of local responsibility.

What the act actually did was to provide assistance in three areas: social insurance, public assistance, and health and welfare services. Social insurance programs included old-age, survivors, disability, and unemployment insurance, all of which supported an individual's right to benefits regardless of need. Public assistance provided federal funds to states to establish programs such as Aid to the Permanently

TABLE 2.4 SUMMARY POINTS: SOCIAL SECURITY ACT (1935)

- Social insurance programs (old-age, survivors, disability, and unemployment insurance) supported an individual's rights to benefits regardless of need.
- Public assistance helped states establish programs for the needy (e.g., AFDC, OAA, and Aid to the Blind).
- Health and welfare services provided programs for public health, vocational rehabilitation, and child welfare among others.

and Totally Disabled (APTD), **Aid to Families with Dependent Children** (**AFDC**), Aid to the Blind, and Old Age Assistance (OAA). Also available under this category were programs of general assistance to needy people who were not eligible under any other program. The third area, health and welfare services, focused on child welfare, vocational rehabilitation, public health, children with disabilities, and maternal and child health.

Of course, some pieces were missing from these new social welfare efforts. The Social Security Act did not provide for long-term hardships. Unemployment benefits were available for only a limited amount of time, and neither health insurance nor permanent physical disability insurance was provided. In spite of these limitations, the initiatives of the Social Security Act became well-established components of the social welfare system.

MID-20TH CENTURY: FOCUS ON MENTAL HEALTH

Forerunners of the mental health movement, such as Phillipe Pinel, Benjamin Rush, and Clifford Beers, all spoke eloquently about the needs of the mentally ill. The growth of mental health and human services continued during the middle years of the 20th century as the commitment to helping others increased. The social welfare system expanded to provide better service to the mentally ill, children, and the poor, to name a few.

An important step in the provision of services to those with mental illness was the passage of the National Mental Health Act of 1946 (Public Law 79–487). This act created a Mental Hygiene Division within the U.S. Public Health Service and a center for information and research, which later became the **National Institute of Mental Health** (NIMH). The Mental Hygiene Division emphasized preventive health measures. Its functions were to assist in the development of state and community health services; to study the causes, prevention, and treatment of mental illness; and to support training of psychiatrists, psychologists, social workers, and nurses. This agency played a critical role in developing the human services movement.

A second piece of legislation that helped set the stage for the emergence of human services was the Mental Health Study Act of 1955 (Public Law 84–82), which provided funding for a Joint Commission on Mental Illness and Health. The charge to the Commission was "to analyze and evaluate the needs and resources of the mentally ill in the United States and make recommendations for a national mental health program" (Albee, 1961, p. x). The Commission made recommendations for training, research, facilities, and programs.

MID-20TH CENTURY: FOCUS ON MENTAL HEALTH

1946	National Mental Health Act of 1946 created a Mental Hygiene Division to address preventive measures
1955	Mental Health Study Act acknowledged personnel shortage in mental health
1963	Community Mental Health Centers Act passed establishing National Institute of Mental Health
1965	President Lyndon Johnson declared "war on poverty"
1970s	National Organization for Human Service Educators and Council for Standards in Human Service Education established formal preparation of human service workers

Two of the Commission's recommendations directly affected the human service movement. First, the Commission concluded that the professional sector alone could not meet the health care needs of the majority of people if only traditional mental health professionals were used. According to the Commission,

> [a]ll mental health professions should recognize that nonmedical mental health workers with aptitude, sound training, practical experience, and demonstrable competence should be permitted to do general, short-term psychotherapy—namely, treating persons by objective, permissive, nondirective techniques of listening to their troubles and help-ing them resolve these troubles in an individually insightful and socially useful way. Such therapy, combining some elements of psychiatric treatment, client counseling, "someone to tell one's troubles to," and love for one's fellow man, obviously can be carried out in a variety of settings by institutions, groups, and individuals, but in all cases should be undertaken under the auspices of recognized mental health agencies. (Albee, 1961, p. x)

The Commission also recommended that "a national mental health program should set as an objective one fully staffed, full-time mental health clinic available to each 50,000 of population" (Albee, 1961, p. xiv). A major impact of the Mental Health Study Act on the human service movement was that it acknowledged the personnel shortage that existed, suggested a new type of mental health worker who could be trained in less time, and recommended a setting in which such new workers could be utilized effectively.

The Commission's recommendations were well received and quickly became law. The conditions that encouraged this immediate action were an awareness of the increasing numbers of people with mental health problems, the rising costs of institutional care, and the need for more effective use of personnel, treatment facili-ties, and treatment (James, 1981).

SERVING THOSE IN NEED

During the mid-20th century, under the leadership of Presidents Kennedy and Johnson, the government's commitment to mental health and the treatment of men-tal illness continued. Kennedy chose to focus on the problems of mental health and mental retardation, "because they are of such actual size and tragic impact and because their susceptibility to public action is so much greater than the attention they have received" (Kennedy, 1964). He called for a national plan to investigate causes, strengthen resources, and improve training and facilities. In a speech on proposed measures to combat mental illness and mental retardation, Kennedy stated:

> I have sent to the Congress today a series of proposals to help fight mental illness and mental retardation. These two afflictions have been long neglected. They occur more frequently, affect more people, require more prolonged treatment, cause more individual and family suffering than any other condition in American life. It has been tolerated too long. It has troubled our national conscience, but only as a problem unpleasant to mention, easy to postpone, and despairing of solution. (Kennedy, 1964, p. 51)

Funding for the recommendations of the Commission was provided by the Community Mental Health Centers Act of 1963, which directed NIMH to set up requirements and regulations for the establishment of **community mental health centers**. Additionally, grants were to be made available for activities such as staffing, planning, initial operations, consultation, and education services. The idea behind this act was to provide diverse services to the population, including inpatient and outpatient care, emergency services, assistance to the courts, and services for the mental health of children and the elderly. By 1975, Congress had authorized over 609 multiservice centers (James, 1981).

Another response to the personnel shortage was the Scheuer Subprofessional Career Act of 1966, administered by the Department of Labor. The philosophical basis for the act was that poor people and minority group members, if trained appropriately, could provide effective mental health services. Programs were developed to train such people to be teacher aides, child care workers, corrections officers, and mental health workers. Most of the education was essentially in-service training, but some programs had links to vocational schools or community colleges.

During Kennedy's years as president, he set the tone for increased emphasis on the eradication of poverty in the United States. His vision brought much hope to populations that had despaired of changing their situations without assistance. Following the assassination of Kennedy in 1963, Lyndon B. Johnson took the oath of office as president. Johnson assumed the legacy of Kennedy's commitment to the impoverished, but this was not a new role for him. Before his election to the vice presidency, he had spent 23 years as an advocate for those who had little hope for the future and no one to represent them.

Varying estimates are made of the number of poor people in America during the Johnson era. John K. Galbraith's (1976) well-known book, *The Affluent Society*, described a country in which people continuously improved their standard of living and the quality of their lives. Michael Harrington (1962) depicted the country very differently in *The Other America*. According to his research, 50 to 60 million Americans lived in poverty, a good many of them in isolated rural regions of the country, especially in the South and the Southeast, and others in large cities on the West and East Coasts. These poor people had few skills for employment, lived in substandard housing, and were malnourished and illiterate.

In 1964, Johnson ran for president on a platform addressing the social problems described by Harrington. He proposed a comprehensive network of social policies and program initiatives. The public response to positive government social intervention was overwhelming, and Johnson was reelected by a large majority. In his 1965 State of the Union address, he declared an "unconditional **war on poverty**" in order to create a "Great Society." Johnson believed the roots of poverty had to be attacked. Programs developed in the War on Poverty and Great Society initiatives included VISTA, the Neighborhood Youth Corps, the Job Corps, College Work Study, and Head Start. Their objective was to eradicate poverty by providing ways for the poor to improve their economic conditions. Many community action programs encouraged client participation in planning, delivering, and evaluating services.

Johnson also promoted the rights of the poor. For example, the Voting Rights Act of 1965 abolished the literacy tests that had been used to deny uneducated people the vote, and the Affirmative Action Order of 1968 and the Office of Economic Opportunity improved employment opportunities for minorities. Further evidence of the President's commitment were Medicare and Medicaid, amendments to the Social Security Act approved by President Johnson on July 30, 1965. **Medicare** (Title XVIII) provides health insurance for people over 65. **Medicaid** (Title XVIX) gives grants to the states to assist them in helping medically indigent citizens receive medical and hospital care.

THE HUMAN SERVICE MOVEMENT

Since the 1960s, the human service movement has experienced unprecedented growth, evidenced by the increase in the number of training programs, the increased size of the mental health delivery system, credentialing, and the development of the human service administration at the federal level. In 1966, the first human service program was established at Purdue University, a two-year associate degree program that focused on the training of entry-level mental health workers.

Originally, a new type of human service worker was envisioned that was a cross between the professional with an advanced degree and the volunteer. A major assumption about the new workers was that their firsthand work experiences, coupled with education and training, would enable them to establish greater rapport and credibility with their clients. In addition, their firsthand knowledge of the problems would give them greater understanding of clients and their difficulties. The initial intent was for these workers to perform innovative roles such as client advocacy and client–community liaison, but in reality they came to perform more traditional roles such as direct caregiving.

NIMH continued its involvement with the movement during the 1970s. The New Careers branch of NIMH was established to provide leadership in the development of entry-level programs for disadvantaged persons. There was much

TABLE 2.5   SUMMARY POINTS: HUMAN SERVICE MOVEMENT

- 1966—First human service program established at Purdue University
- 1975—Paraprofessional Manpower Branch defined training for human service workers
- 1970s—Mental health treatment shifted from institution to the community
- 1970s—Professional human service organizations established

concern in the existing mental health system about who the new paraprofessionals would be, what jobs they would perform, and whether they would perform adequately. It was the responsibility of this branch to address these questions.

In spite of the concern voiced by the other professionals in the mental health system, many of these newly trained human service workers were welcomed. During the 1970s, the number of clients served by the mental health system increased dramatically. New workers were needed, and the traditional ways of providing mental health services were not efficient or effective in meeting the changing needs. Highly skilled professionals with advanced degrees had been serving small numbers of clients. Human service workers could now provide the simpler direct-care services to greater numbers of clients while the highly skilled professionals worked with the more difficult problems and supervised the human service workers. **Deinstitutionalization,** a movement that began in the 1950s, called for transferring many institutionalized patients to the community for outpatient care. By the 1970s, a major segment of mental health treatment had shifted from the isolation of the institution to the complex environment of the community. As the concept of community mental health developed, different types of professional services were needed.

During this same time period, organizations emerged that signaled a move toward professionalism. Such organizations serve many purposes. They may regulate a profession or its workers, facilitate communication among its members, or foster excellence in research or service within the profession. Two organizations in particular were instrumental in the move toward a human service profession and recognition of human service workers as professionals: the National Organization for Human Services (NOHS) and the Council for Standards in Human Service Education (CSHSE). Both are active today and have been instrumental in working with the Center for Credentialing and Education (CCE), as discussed in Chapter 1, to establish a credential for human service practitioners, an important move toward increased professionalism. You can locate the organizations' websites using search terms such as National Organization for Human Services (NOHS) and the Council for Standards in Human Service Education (CSHSE). Read more about credentialing using the search term "Center for Credentialing and Education."

LATE 20TH CENTURY: ADDITIONAL DEVELOPMENTS IN SERVICE DELIVERY

The latter third of the 20th century was a time of change in human services. One way to examine the evolution of human services during this period is from the perspective of different presidential administrations. All administrations confronted human service challenges although their responses varied. You have read about the significant events of the Kennedy and Johnson administrations. The administrations that followed contributed to the development of the profession in other ways, some more than others.

Richard Nixon's election in 1968 signaled a more conservative approach to human services characterized by a decline in federal spending and a different approach to managing human resources. Nixon's **New Federalism** called for individuals to assume responsibility for their own situations. As power, resources, and influence began to flow back to the states and local communities, the emphasis was on the development of self-help programs and the provision of services by the private sector. The Supplemental Security Income (SSI) program, which provided additional financial support for people needing assistance, is one example. President Gerald Ford's administration continued the reduction of the federal government's involvement in human services by cutting more than $9.5 billion that had been appropriated by Congress. Among the programs he vetoed were proposed improvements in federal aid to education, in the school lunch program, and in health care.

Two major human service developments occurred during the Jimmy Carter administration. One was the creation of the Department of Health and Human Services. The use of the term *human services* denoted the wide variety of program services addressing human needs. The choice of the term clearly marks the point when human services became associated with a wide range of services, not restricted to those associated with mental health. The second major development was the appointment of the President's Commission on Mental Health, chaired by Rosalyn Carter. The commission discovered that between 10% and 15% of the population (20 to 32 million people) needed some form of mental health services at any one time, and that many people did not have access to good, affordable mental health care. A result was the Mental Health Systems Act, which promised comprehensiveness, flexibility, and innovation by emphasizing services for people with chronic mental illness and by emphasizing prevention. It also attempted to address the shortage of mental health personnel in underserved areas, requiring people who received federal money for their training to work in an area with a personnel shortage for a period as long as the time they received financial support.

DISMANTLING THE WELFARE SYSTEM

From the 1930s to the 1980s, the government's social policy was to assume responsibility for citizens who could not provide a reasonable quality of life for themselves. However, as you have just read, from the 1980s to the present, voters elected presidents who advocated substantial reduction of the federal budget and decreased federal government involvement in human services—a stark contrast to the policies of the previous administrations.

One of the first signs of retrenchment came from California. On June 7, 1978, California voters passed Proposition 13, an amendment to the state constitution (Pilisuk, 1980). The goal of the legislation was to amend the property tax structure, resulting in less money to fund a variety of services, including social services. What actually happened was that fewer professionals were employed, but the number of people in need did not decrease. Human service professionals, serving larger caseloads, felt overworked, ineffective, and devalued. Their jobs seemed to have lost what little status they had; voters had sent a clear message that the services they provided were not supported. Existing programs were cut back, and fewer new programs were funded, but the needs were as great as ever. Self-care, community support systems, and natural helping networks had to assume additional responsibilities. More people in need began to turn to neighborhood groups, churches, friends, and families for assistance.

The passage of Proposition 13 was an early sign of the changing attitude of the American public toward government spending for human services. Ronald Reagan's platform in 1980 illustrated this. His platform called for establishing new priorities in human services, slashing government spending, and reducing the government's involvement in human services. One of Reagan's priorities was to return the administration of human services to the individual states, communities, and private sources. He terminated a number of social programs and drastically cut spending on others. Those affected included "AFDC, childcare, school lunch and other nutrition programs, food stamps, subsidized housing, energy assistance, family planning, public and mental health services, alcohol and drug abuse counseling, legal aid, the Job Corps, and the like" (Trattner, 1999, p. 365). His reelection in 1984 continued to emphasize the economy, defense, and foreign policy. The plight of the poor worsened during this period, and one result was a welfare reform bill designed to help single parents, particularly women, enter the job market. The Family Support Act was signed into law in 1988. Among the programs authorized was the JOBS program, which required single parents on welfare with children older than three years to work or be in training in order to receive assistance. The Act also mandated new procedures for collecting child support payments and one year of support for child care and transportation so that single parents could work or participate in training. For the most part, though, both Reagan administrations largely ignored the plight of the poor and disenfranchised, focusing instead on defense spending and tax cuts.

TABLE 2.6   SUMMARY POINTS: LATE 20TH AND EARLY 21ST CENTURIES

- The election of Richard Nixon in 1968 marked a decline in federal spending that continued throughout the Ford administration.
- Jimmy Carter established the Department of Health and Human Services in 1978 as well as the President's Commission on Mental Health.
- The State of California passed Proposition 13 in 1978, signaling less willingness to support social services with taxes.
- The Americans with Disabilities Act was passed in 1990 during the George Bush Sr. administration.
- Aid to Families with Dependent Children was replaced by the Personal Responsibility and Work Opportunity Reconciliation Act, the legislation that ended "welfare as we know it."
- A major focus of the Obama administration was health care reform, which resulted in the signing of the Patient Protection and Affordable Care Act in March 2010.

As a result of Reagan's policy, there was a shift in service delivery. The number of nonprofit and private agencies in human services expanded, and human service institutions and agencies contracted out for services (Ginsberg, 1987). Reagan also advocated transferring federally owned housing and prisons to the private sector. Just as the labor market tends to respond to economic demands, the human service labor market reflects human service demands. During the 1960s and 1970s, the human service market was growing, and the number of opportunities for employment and for advancement increased. During the 1980s that growth slowed, although some opportunities did develop in the private sector with, for example, the privatization of correctional facilities and the development of **employee assistance programs** in private industry.

George Bush Sr., Reagan's vice president, won the 1988 presidential election and claimed a mandate to continue many of the policies of the Reagan administrations. Generally, Bush's administration is noted for its emphasis on foreign policy and its lack of attention to domestic issues. The most significant human service–related legislation of his four years was the **Americans with Disabilities Act (ADA)**, which was passed in 1990. With little cost to the federal government, ADA was designed to get people into the workforce who otherwise would not be able to enter or who were kept out for other reasons, such as discrimination.

WELFARE REFORM

A declining economy, the growing gap between rich and poor, and the need for **welfare reform** all contributed to the election in 1992 of Democrat Bill Clinton, governor of Arkansas. One of his campaign pledges was to "end welfare as we know it." In 1996, the **Personal Responsibility and Work Opportunity Reconciliation Act (PRWORA)** replaced Aid to Families with Dependent Children, which was the primary welfare law sponsored by the federal government to provide aid to eligible mothers with children. This legislation ended the federal government's six-decade guarantee of aid to the poor. Under the former welfare program, eligibility for support was based on income and was regulated by the federal government.

POLICIES AND PROCEDURES

The key components in the reformed welfare system were state control, work requirements, time limits, and penalties. The states received federal funds in a block grant program called Temporary Assistance for Needy Families (**TANF**), and there was, and still is, flexibility concerning how the states spend their money. Each state receives a fixed amount of money each year, and they must also contribute to the welfare program. Many states have used their funding to provide traditional welfare services, such as cash assistance, employment services, child care, and emergency assistance; however, some states have expanded their services. In addition, the goals of this legislation related to marriage and family formation and included promoting marriage, reducing the birth of children out of wedlock, and supporting two-parent families. The act was extended when Congress passed the Deficit Reduction Act of 2005.

BOX 2.4   EXPLORING THE WEB FOR MORE INFORMATION

Check out the following sources to learn more about health and welfare reform.

Administration for Children and Families (TANF)

Health Care Reform

Health Care Ruling

National Conference of State Legislatures

American Recovery and Reinvestment Act of 2009

Welfare Reform

As a result of the economic downturn during the last half of the decade, the federal government authorized the Emergency Contingency Fund as part of the American Recovery and Reinvestment Act of 2009 that appropriated $5 billion covering 2009–2010 (Administration for Children and Families, 2010). Emergency fund grants were used to provide benefits and services to families that comply with the four statutory purposes of the TANF program: (a) to provide assistance for the care of children at home or in the homes of relatives; (b) to promote job preparation, work, and marriage; (c) to prevent and reduce the incidence of out-of-wedlock pregnancies; and (d) to encourage formation and maintenance of two-parent families. These funds are available until they are expended but they can be carried over for use in a later year.

EVALUATION OF WELFARE REFORM

The debate continues about the effectiveness of welfare reform. Is it really working?

On a practical level, human service professionals working within the framework of the new welfare-to-work programs review the outcomes of the legislation. They applaud the new focus of moving clients off the welfare rolls and into meaningful work that allows them to provide economic stability for their families, but they still see difficulties that their clients have in gaining employment that will support their families. Using a case management approach to provide a multitude of services, they are able to help clients and their families meet basic needs; however, they are concerned about the rules and regulations of the program.

A more formal assessment has been made by the Urban Institute's New Federalism project (Golden, 2005). Their findings include the following:

- More welfare recipients work while on welfare than in the past.
- Although work effort increased after reform, many welfare recipients have multiple barriers to work. These included limited education, little or no work experience, severe mental and physical disabilities, the need to care for a child with disabilities, and language challenges.
- Work activity rose among those likely to use welfare, no matter how stringent the state policy.
- In 2001, only 15% of welfare recipients participated in TANF-funded education and training activities (p. 8).

The findings related to families who left welfare follow:

- Employers are willing to hire welfare recipients.
- Most families that leave welfare have at least one working adult.
- Many former welfare recipients work in low-wage jobs.
- About one-third of these workers have health insurance coverage through their jobs (p. 9).

Significant challenges remain with both the implementation and evaluation of welfare reform. On one level, the various ways that states have chosen to implement welfare legislation is a challenge for any comprehensive evaluation. For example, TANF regulations allow states flexibility with regard to different types of family units and eligibility for benefits. On a national level, the recent downturn in the economy has resulted in high unemployment, layoffs for many who were employed, and tighter state budgets. In turn, funding levels, employment opportunities, and fewer state employees have impacted welfare legislation implementation and consequently, evaluation. These factors make it difficult to predict the future of welfare.

MANAGED CARE

Managed care became increasingly popular during the 1990s and has had a profound effect on the delivery of human services. Its influence is felt by both client and human service professionals as they work together to plan and provide services. Today, managed care organizations administer a large percentage of the group health insurance as well as mental health care, child care, corrections, and other social services.

Managed care is a term used to describe a set of tools or methods designed to manage resources and deliver human services, especially in the areas of health care and mental health. It developed from public demand for accountability of service delivery and from rising costs in health and mental health care. Prior to the use of managed care to allocate resources and services, most care was provided on a **fee-for-service** basis. In other words, a health or human service professional would provide a specific service and charge a standard rate. The payment for these services would come from the client, an insurance provider, or the agency or organization supporting the client care.

THE INFLUENCE OF MANAGED CARE

Managed care influences the delivery of services to clients within the social service network. **External review** of services is one important component of managed care. The external review is used in several ways to monitor and communicate to service providers what they can provide and still receive financial coverage for providing. For example, one type of review authorizes the expense of needed services for a client. For the human service professional, this means that before a service can be provided and before the professional can be reimbursed or paid, the managed care organization reviews the requested service and asks questions such as these:

How do you define the problem?

What treatment do you recommend?

Why do you recommend this treatment?

Do you have any evidence that supports using this treatment?

A guiding principle for managed care review is to approve the lowest level of care that will meet the client's needs. In other words, if hospitalization has been recommended, the managed care reviewer asks, "Could the client also be treated in the home?" If 10 weeks of therapy is recommended, the question is, "Will four weeks be adequate?" If the client needs a vocational assessment, psychological assessment, physical assessment, and a social history, managed care reviewers may recommend conducting the physical and the psychological assessment first before determining whether the others are needed.

Managed care also affects the way we think about and deliver services to specific client populations. Because managed care emphasizes appropriate services for clients and matching services to specific outcomes, both managed care personnel and human service professionals are working to develop standards of best practice for meeting specific client needs. In the past, because of the complexity of problems that client's experience, some human service professionals have had difficulty stating clearly the appropriate services for addressing the needs of their clients—needs that stem from poverty, unemployment, illiteracy, juvenile delinquency, child abuse, and other difficulties. Further complicating the task of developing standards is the complexity and large number of problems that many clients face. When practitioners and managed care personnel work together to define best practices, clients are more likely to receive quality treatment.

MANAGED CARE AND THE HUMAN SERVICE PROFESSIONAL

Managed care has affected the daily work of the human service professional, especially in providing direct service. This interaction has required a shift in the roles and responsibilities of the professional in three ways: an emphasis on case management responsibilities, increasing demands for documentation, and the growing use of gatekeepers.

Today, more human service professionals than ever are using case management in providing services to their clients. The purpose of care coordination or case management by a helping professional, as discussed in Chapter 1, is to oversee the comprehensive care of a client. It can include: (a) assessment; (b) planning, coordinating, and monitoring of treatment; and (c) evaluation. Human service literature describes two ways cases can be managed. One is by a professional in a human service organization who assumes many of the responsibilities just listed; the other is by an employee of a managed care organization. The following examples illustrate their different responsibilities.

Chris Bachman, a rehabilitation counselor, has a caseload of 70 clients. Chris works with each client to develop a plan of services, some delivered by Chris himself but most provided by professionals at other agencies. Chris monitors the delivery of services, authorizes payment on behalf of his agency, and evaluates with the client the services received.

Tasha Jones is a case manager who works for Healthcare Inc., a managed care organization that has clients in five counties. Her major responsibilities include external utilization review and resource allocation. Her contact with human service professionals like Chris Bachman is through applications, forms, or telephone calls. She has never met a client or a human service professional in person.

Another influence of managed care is the increased documentation associated with service delivery. The workload for many human service professionals has doubled as they use the managed care external review process. A request for services can include an initial assessment, a detailed description of the client's problem, a service plan, a periodic assessment of the implementation of the plan and status of outcomes, requests for reimbursement, and termination of clients. Often the documentation required for the managed care process is different from that required by the agency. Thus, unless the managed care organization has established the same information system as the organization, the professional may have two systems of documentation to maintain.

Another change that has emerged is an elaborate gatekeeping function for the initial screening of clients. **Gatekeeping** in the managed care system, especially in the area of mental health, is a method used to control access to services. Often, to receive mental health services, clients must have a referral from a physician. The purpose of this physician referral is to decrease the utilization of mental health services, but the result has been to increase the client load of the physician who must sign the referrals. Gatekeeping also occurs when a special service, not considered part of the standard of good practice, is needed or recommended. The client is not free to take the initiative to seek that service but must have the permission of, and referral from, the primary caretaker—in most cases, the physician. At times, the introduction of the gatekeeper to mental health services places hardships on both the client and the human service professional. Clients see this visit to the physician as a barrier to getting services, and they often encounter physicians who are not sympathetic to their nonmedical problems. Sometimes they must wait to see the physician, and this wait delays their receiving the mental health services they need. For human service professionals, the gatekeeper is another layer of bureaucracy between them and their clients. On a positive note, however, many of these professionals are working with the gatekeeper physicians to help them understand the mental health needs of their clients.

LEGISLATIVE CHANGES IN THE 21ST CENTURY

Several legislative changes mark the federal involvement in human services. These include the passage of a prescription drug act, expanded support of faith-based human services, and health care reform.

The Medicare Prescription Drug, Improvement, and Modernization Act of 2003 (MMA) was passed to provide outpatient prescription drug benefits for individuals on Medicare, Part D. Benefits are available to over 43 million people who enroll in private plans that offer coverage and are approved by Medicare (Henry J. Kaiser Family Foundation, 2010). This plan replaces Medicaid as a source of drug coverage. Implementing this new program has not been easy.

Although pharmacists and physicians believe that MMA has the potential to help their customers and patients, they also say the complicated regulations cause problems for customers and patients (Palosky & Levitt, 2006). Initial problems consumers and patients encountered included: (a) the prescribed drug was not on the chosen plan, (b) customers could not verify that they had enrolled in a plan, (c) customers who were receiving state Medicare could not access their federal plan, and (d) customers experienced serious medical problems because they could not fill prescriptions they needed. As the implementation of MMA matures, the hope is that most beneficiaries will receive adequate prescriptive drug coverage through Part D enrollment or other creditable sources such as drug coverage under employer or union plans.

To help Americans in need, President George W. Bush initiated an effort to bring faith-based agencies and organizations into partnership with the federal government by creating the White House Office of Faith-based and Community Initiatives. He also created **Center for Faith-Based and Community Initiatives (CFBCI)** in 11 federal agencies. The mission of the CFBCI in the Department of Health and Human Services is "to lead the Department efforts to better utilize faith-based and community-based organizations in providing effective human services" (U.S. Department of Health & Human Services [DHHS], n.d.). President Bush stated:

> The paramount goal is compassionate results, and private and charitable groups, including religious ones, should have the fullest opportunity permitted by law to compete on a level playing field, so long as they achieve valid public purposes, like curbing crime, conquering addiction, strengthening families, and overcoming poverty. (DHHS, n.d.)

To reach this goal, CFBCI has developed technical assistance for faith-based organizations in terms of grant writing and service delivery to these organizations, trained departmental and agency staff on ways to develop collaborative efforts, modified governmental policies and regulations so that faith-based organizations can be competitive in securing funding, developed a grant opportunities notebook that outlines possible funding opportunities, and held regional conferences to support partnership efforts. Several of the programs highlighted by the CFBCI are a Compassions Capital Fund, the Mentoring Children of Prisoners, the Access to Recovery program, and a Prisoner Re-entry Initiative. To help faith-based organizations develop programs, the DHHS CFBCI provides a "toolkit" that includes a description of best practices, information about establishing partnerships, supporting documents for grant acquisition and grant management, guidelines for outcomes measurement, information about potential revenue sources, and technical assistance. Bush viewed this effort as an eight-year process that began in 2002 with the Compassion Capital Fund and ended with an assessment of these efforts in 2009 (DHHS, n.d.).

Health care reform, a prominent issue of the 2008 presidential campaign, has been a major focus of the Obama administration. After much debate, Obama signed into law the **Patient Protection and Affordable Care Act** in March 2010. At the center of the debate about health care in the United States was whether a universally accessible health care system should be implemented, that is, is health care a fundamental right of the American people? In 2006, the uninsured in the United States numbered approximately 46 million (DeNavas-Walt, Proctor, & Smith 2007).

This bill attempts to address several issues. Proponents of universal health care argued that the United States was the only wealthy industrialized nation that does not have a universal health care system (Insuring America's Health, 2004). They cited statistics that indicated that the United States ranked last in the quality of health care among developed countries, yet it was the most expensive (America's Uninsured Crisis, 2009; Roehr, 2008). This means that nearly 50 million Americans have no health insurance and receive no care until they are very sick or injured and show up at hospital emergency rooms (The road ahead for health care, 2012)—and someone else pays. In addition, there is great concern that overall health care costs in the United States are on an unsustainable trajectory. Medicare costs, expensive new medical technologies and drugs, and physicians' prescriptions for more tests and treatments contribute to the high costs of health care.

Opponents of the law argued that universal health care is too expensive, taxes would have to increase, and it would have a negative effect on the free enterprise system. The Patient Protection and Affordable Care Act expands health care coverage to millions of Americans previously uninsured. Health insurance exchanges will be created to meet the needs of those meeting criteria using the Federal Poverty Level definitions (Jackson & Nolan, 2010), and beginning in 2014, uninsured people who don't qualify for Medicaid will have to get insurance or pay a tax penalty (See Box 2.5).

BOX 2.5   THE AFFORDABLE CARE ACT

The Affordable Care Act was passed by Congress and then signed into law by the President on March 23, 2010. On June 28, 2012 the Supreme Court rendered a final decision to uphold the health care law.

The Affordable Care Act: An Outline of Title 1.

Title I. Quality, Affordable Health Care for All Americans

This act puts individuals, families and small business owners in control of their health care. It reduces premium costs for millions of working families and small businesses by providing hundreds of billions of dollars in tax relief—the largest middle-class tax cut for health care in history. It also reduces what families will have to pay for health care by capping out-of-pocket expenses and requiring preventive care to be fully covered without any out-of-pocket expense. For Americans with insurance coverage who like what they have, they can keep it. Nothing in this act or anywhere in the bill forces anyone to change the insurance they have, period.

Americans without insurance coverage will be able to choose the insurance coverage that works best for them in a new open, competitive insurance market—the same insurance market that every member of Congress will be required to use for their insurance. The insurance exchange will pool buying power and give Americans new affordable choices of private insurance plans that have to compete for their business based on cost and quality. Small business owners will not only be able to choose insurance coverage through this exchange but will also receive a new tax credit to help offset the cost of covering their employees.

It keeps insurance companies honest by setting clear rules that rein in the worst insurance-industry abuses. And it bans insurance companies from denying insurance coverage because of a person's preexisting medical conditions while giving consumers new power to appeal insurance company decisions that deny doctor-ordered treatments covered by insurance.

The Secretary has the authority to implement many of these new provisions to help families and small business owners have the information they need to make the choices that work best for them. For more information search the Internet using terms such as "healthcare/law" and "Affordable Care Act."

Source: http://www.healthcare.gov/law/full/index.html

Full implementation of the law occurs in 2018 and at that time, many of the questions about it will be clear. Will the law increase the deficit? Will it cut costs? Will more cost-effective treatment result? Under numerous threats of repeal, perhaps the most basic question is about the survival of the legislation as it was passed in 2010.

A FINAL THOUGHT

At this writing, important issues remain unresolved in the United States. Among them are the war on terrorism, the partisan divide between Republicans and Democrats, the Social Security funding crisis, the balance of protection and civil liberties, veterans' services, abortion, and the unrest in the Middle East.

In addition to health care reform and despite prescription drug coverage, the 2006 Voting Rights Act reauthorization, and attempts to improve education and to reform Social Security, a number of Americans have needs that continue to be unmet. In response, human service professionals have renewed their efforts to advocate for their clients and their profession.

KEY TERMS

AFDC

almshouses

Americans with Disabilities Act (ADA)

asylums

Center for Faith-Based and Community Initiatives (CFBCI)

community mental health centers

deinstitutionalization

employee assistance programs

external review

fee-for-service

gatekeeping

health care reform

individualism

laissez-faire

managed care

Medicaid

Medicare

Medicare Prescription Drug, Improvement, and Modernization Act of 2003 (MMA)

National Institute of Mental Health

New Federalism

Patient Protection and Affordable Care Act

Personal Responsibility and Work Opportunity

Reconciliation Act (PRWORA)

poor relief

probation

settlement house

Social Darwinism

Social Security

social workers

TANF

war on poverty

welfare reform

THINGS TO REMEMBER

1. Before the Middle Ages, people believed that mental illness was caused by evil spirits, and early forms of treatment focused on ridding the body of these spirits.
2. Until the 1500s, the Catholic Church was chiefly responsible for providing human services, and it was under the Church's guidance that many institutions were founded for the poor, orphans, the elderly, and the handicapped.
3. The decline of feudalism, the growth of commerce, and the beginning of industrialization made it necessary to find new ways of assisting those in need.
4. Pressures caused by the increasing number of poor in the cities created the need for a large-scale attack on poverty and prompted the passage of the Elizabethan Poor Law of 1601, critical legislation that guided social welfare practices in England

and the United States for the next 350 years.

5. In the early years, the colonists used the English system as a model for their philosophy toward, and services for, the poor and needy. By the early 1800s, however, other philosophies prevailed—ones that discouraged and limited the provision of human services.

6. Major reforms during the late 1800s concentrated on improving the treatment of the institutionalized mentally ill and children.

7. The Charity Organization Society, a forerunner of the Community Chest and the United Way, is an example of society's response to the needs of an expanding urban population.

8. A settlement house was a large house in a slum area that served as a community center, sponsoring such activities as recreation; classes in English, cooking, and citizenship; vocational training; and child care.

9. President Franklin D. Roosevelt introduced the Social Security Act of 1935, which fundamentally changed the federal government's role in providing human services.

10. During the years John F. Kennedy served as president, he set the tone for increased emphasis on the eradication of poverty in the United States, bringing hope to populations that had despaired of changing their situations without assistance.

11. The emergence of human service training programs and the development of a human service philosophy mirror the historical events and presidential leadership from the 1960s to the present.

12. In his 1965 State of the Union address, President Lyndon Johnson declared an "unconditional war on poverty" and developed programs that attacked the roots of poverty in order to create a "Great Society."

13. The National Organization for Human Services and the Council for Standards in Human Service Education have been instrumental in the development of the human service profession.

14. The Nixon and Ford presidential administrations marked a change in the federal government's involvement in social reform with a decline in federal spending.

15. During the presidency of Ronald Reagan, commitment to human services passed from the federal government to state and local governments, the private sector, and needy individuals themselves.

16. The first Bush administration supported the passage of the Americans with Disabilities Act, which provided guidelines to reduce the discrimination of individuals with disabilities.

17. Bill Clinton reformed the welfare system by proposing a new law that emphasized training, education, short-term support, and personal responsibility.

18. Welfare reform has decreased the number of families on the welfare rolls and increased the number of the families who are employed.

19. The Medicare Prescription Drug Bill and the faith-based and community partnership efforts of the second Bush administration are legislative changes to support those in need.

20. Although the Patient Protection and Affordable Care Act was passed in 2010, the debate continues about health care as a fundamental right of the American people.

Self-Assessment

- Describe the major characteristics of helping those in need prior to the Middle Ages, during the Middle Ages, and immediately following the Middle Ages.
- Explain how the Elizabethan Poor Laws influenced colonial America's approach to helping the poor and needy.

- Trace the development of care for the mentally ill and children from the 1850s to the 1930s.
- How was the federal government involved in human services from the 1930s to the present?
- In what ways has major legislation influenced the development of human services?

WANT TO KNOW MORE?

There are several resources you can explore to learn more about the history of human services. Check them out!

Additional Resources: Focus on History

Beers, Clifford W. (1945). *A mind that found itself: An autobiography*. Garden City, NY: Doubleday, Doran.

Clifford Beers writes of his experiences as a three-time patient in mental institutions around the turn of the 20th century.

Herrick, J. (Ed.) (2004). *Encyclopedia of social welfare history in North America*. San Francisco: Sage.

This encyclopedia has 180 entries that provide information about the history of social welfare in the United States, Canada, and Mexico. Included are primary materials, a multinational perspective, suggestions for further reading, appendices, and an index with cross-references.

Jensen, L. (2003). *Patriots, settlers, and the origins of American social policy*. Cambridge, UK: Cambridge University Press.

This book provides an account of the development of America's first entitlement policies during the first 100 years of the United States. It challenges the belief that the United States lagged behind other countries in developing national social programs.

Marshall, Helen E. (1937). *The forgotten Samaritan*. Chapel Hill, NC: University of North Carolina Press.

Marshall has produced a well-written biography of Dorothea Dix, humanitarian and reformer.

Seccombe, K. (2006). *"So you think I drive a Cadillac?": Welfare recipients' perspectives on the system and its reform* (2nd ed.). Needham Heights, MA: Pearson, Allyn & Bacon.

Welfare recipients share their experiences with welfare and their views on its reform. Topics include their plans, hopes, and dreams for the future, as well as their perspectives on work requirements, family caps, and other TANF features.

Sweet, V. (2012). *God's hotel: A doctor, a hospital, and a pilgrimage to the heart of medicine*. New York: Riverhead Hardcover.

Dr. Sweet writes about her 20 years at San Francisco's Laguna Honda Hospital, the last almshouse in the United States.

Trattner, Walter I. (1999). *From poor law to welfare state: A history of social welfare in America*. New York: Free Press.

Trattner gives an overview of social welfare in the United States from the colonial era to the present. He includes highlights of the mental health, child welfare, and public health movements, as well as the beginnings of social welfare as a profession.

Case Study

Jamie is a third-generation welfare recipient who provides a view of welfare before and after welfare reform. You can read her story in Chapter 2 of *Introduction to Human Services: Cases and Applications*, the companion text to this one. Jamie also lives in a rural area which presents other challenges in addition to the new welfare legislation. She lives with other family members and three of her five children in the house where she was born. Her story may also challenge you to think about your own beliefs and values about welfare reform and helping those in need.

REFERENCES

Administration for Children and Families (2010). *American Recovery and Reinvestment Act*. Retrieved from http://www.acf.hhs.gov/programs /ofa/recovery/tanf-faq.htm

Albee, G. W. (1961). Implication of action for mental health. *Perspectives*, 3, 1–5.

America's uninsured crisis: Consequences for health and health care. (2009). *Institute of Medicine report brief*. Retrieved from http://www.iom .edu/Reports/2009/Americas-Uninsured-Crisis -Consequences-for-Health-and-Health-Care .aspx

Beers, C. W. (1945). *A mind that found itself: An autobiography*. Garden City, NY: Doubleday, Doran & Co.

Cranston, A. (1986). Psychology in the Veterans Administration. *American Psychologist, 41*(9), 990–995.

DeNavas-Walt, C., Proctor, B. D., & Smith, J. (2007). *Income, poverty, and health insurance coverage in the United States: 2006*. Washington, DC: U.S. Government Printing Office.

Friedrich, O. (1976). *Going crazy: An inquiry into madness in our time*. New York: Avon Books.

Galbraith, J. K. (1976). *The affluent society*. Boston: Houghton Mifflin.

Ginsberg, L. H. (1987). *Economic, political and social context*. In L. H. Ginsberg (Ed.), *Encyclopedia of social work* (18th ed.) (pp. xxxii–xxxvi). Silver Springs, MD: National Association of Social Workers.

Golden, O. A. (2005). *Assessing the new federalism: Eight years later*. Washington, DC: The Urban Institute.

Harrington, M. (1962). *The other America*. New York: Macmillan.

Henry J. Kaiser Family Foundation. (2010). *Medicare*. Retrieved from http://www.kff.org/medicare/index.cfm

Insuring America's Health: Principles and Recommendations. (2004, January 13). *Institute of Medicine of the National Academies of Science*. Retrieved from http://www.iom.edu/reports/2004/insuring-americas-health-principles-and-recommendations.aspx

Irvine, H. (2002). The legitimizing power of financial statements of the Salvation Army in England, 1885–1892. *Account Historians Journal*. Retrieved from http://ro.uow.edu.au/cgi/viewcontent.cgi?article=1134&context=commpapers

Jackson, J., & Nolan, J. (March 23, 2010). Health care reform bill summary: A look at what's in the bill. *CBS: Political hotsheet*. Retrieved from http://www.cbsnews.com/8301-503544_162-20000846-503544.html

James, V. (1981, April). *Mental health worker news: A forum for the mental health profession. Bulletin: Council for Standards in Human Services Education, 4*.

Kennedy, J. F. (1964). *Remarks on proposed measures to combat mental illness and mental retardation*. Public papers of the Presidents of the United States: John F. Kennedy (January 1–November 22, 1963), 50–51. Washington, DC: U.S. Government Printing Office.

Macht, J. (1990). *A historical perspective*. In S. Fullerton & D. Osher (Eds.), *History of the human service movement, 7*, 90, 9.

Marshall, H. (1937). *The forgotten Samaritan*. Chapel Hill: University of North Carolina Press.

National Institute of Mental Health (NIMH). (1971). *Mental illness and its treatment: Social issues resources issue series, 1*(3), DHEW Publications No [HSM] (72-9030). Washington, DC: Author.

Neugebauer, R. (1979). Medieval and early modern theories of mental illness. *Archives of General Psychiatry, 36*, 477–483.

Palosky, C., & Levitt, L. (2006). *News release: National survey of pharmacists and national survey of physicians*. Retrieved from www.kff.org/kaiserpolls/pomr090706nr.cfm

Pilisuk, M. (1980, April). The future of human services without funding. *American Journal of Orthopsychiatry, 50*(2), 200–204.

Richmond, M. (1917). *Social diagnosis*. New York: Russell Sage Foundation.

The road ahead for health care. *The Week*, July 20, 2012.

Roehr, B. (2008). Healthcare in the U.S. ranks lowest among developed countries. *BMJ, 337*.

Trattner, Walter I. (1999). *From poor law to welfare state: A history of social welfare in America*. New York: Free Press.

U.S. Department of Health and Human Services (DHHS). (n.d.). *The center for faith-based and community initiatives*. Retrieved from http://www.hhs.gov/fbci/index.html

Zimbalist, S. E. (1977). *Historic themes and landmarks in social welfare research*. New York: Harper & Row.

CHAPTER **3**

HUMAN SERVICES TODAY

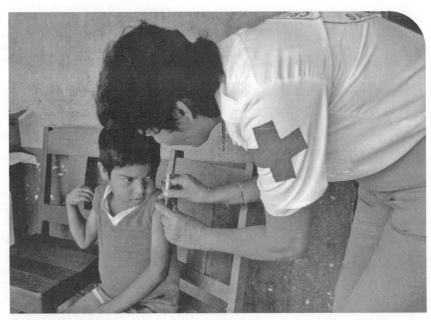

Richard Lord/The Image Works

After reading this chapter, you will be able to:

- Document reasons for the expansion of human service settings.
- Describe nontraditional contexts of human service delivery.
- Identify areas of technology used in human services.
- List the challenges presented by the international dimension of human services.
- Identify the significant trends in human services.

One facet of the definition of human services is how and where services are delivered today. This chapter examines new settings, new skills, and recent trends in human service delivery. As you read this chapter, you will see that human services today has a much broader scope than ever before. It takes place in a variety of settings, addresses global human needs, and reflects recent advances in communication and technology. Human services is also impacted by other changes such as the global recession, the growing number of individuals over 65, and the increasing cultural diversity of the United States. This chapter examines each of these dimensions in more detail to help expand your definition of human services.

SETTINGS FOR HUMAN SERVICE DELIVERY

One way to describe the broadening scope of human services today is to think about where services are delivered and how outreach occurs. In many instances, services continue to be delivered in agencies or institutional settings but with a growing emphasis on making services accessible and comprehensive, service delivery in nontraditional settings has increased. Rural services, military settings, schools, and sites of natural disasters are highlighted in this section.

COMMUNITY-BASED SERVICES: OUTREACH TO THOSE IN NEED

There has been a change in philosophy regarding the delivery of services in institutional settings and in the community. The difference in settings is an obvious factor. Earlier institutions were located in remote places because pastoral settings were believed to be peaceful and calming. These settings may also have been chosen because members of society did not like to be reminded of the existence of people with mental illness. Correctional facilities have been built in rural areas because the criminal population is considered dangerous to others. Again, people did not like to be reminded of this population. Now, however, in mental health, the trend continues toward increasing the number of **community-based services**. The goal of community-based mental health care is to enable clients to interact with their environments in the least restrictive setting in which they can function. It includes reaching out to provide services to clients in homes and on the streets. The commitment to community-based services expands beyond mental health and addresses multiple client needs.

Community-based mental health has changed the nature of service delivery. The focus of treatment has become health and wellness instead of illness. The process involves other social institutions such as schools, recreation facilities, and religious organizations. In addition, the psychological and medical treatment received by clients has been adapted for community-based care. This change requires a helping professional who manages cases and acts as a planner, consultant, and liaison between the mental health agency, the client, and the other supportive institutions. Many of the services are intensive, and the professional may visit the client two or three times a week. Human service professionals also provide help for the families and children.

COMMUNITY-BASED SERVICES: OUTREACH AND WRAPAROUND SERVICES

A concerted effort has been made in community-based services across a broad array of human services to extend the office to the community. Many agencies now include outreach programs that send staff throughout neighborhoods and communities to work with clients where they live, shop, work, or "hang out." Youth in Need is a St. Louis area multiservice agency that reaches homeless and runaway youth on the streets. Box 3.1 profiles this effective program.

Another way of providing community-based services to the multiproblem client, hence serving the whole person, is developing **wraparound services**. These services, especially those associated with children's services, focus on individualized treatment plans within the context of community-based service. In fact, wraparound services refer more to how professionals deliver services rather than the services themselves. One focus of these services is the physical and mental health of

---

BOX 3.1   YOUTH IN NEED

Youth in Need (YIN) is a multiservice agency that serves children, youth, and families throughout Eastern Missouri. The precipitating event in 1974 for the founding of YIN was a teenage girl whose face was bruised from yet another beating. She was brought to the local jail, where at that time all runaway and homeless youth were housed with adult criminals. One of the founders of YIN, Reverend Earl Worley, described the beginning of YIN: "It was late at night and we knew we had talked about opening a youth shelter long enough. Looking at that young girl, we knew that we couldn't let down one more kid." Since that time, YIN has developed a number of programs to make children's healthy development and well-being the community's highest priority.

One of their programs, Street Outreach, is targeted to homeless and runaway youth who are living on the streets of St. Louis and surrounding areas. Staff travel streets and neighborhoods in a specially designed and stocked van to provide blankets, food, and clothing;

most importantly, they are committed to help youth solve their problems and locate needed resources. Their work is illustrated by the following case:

We stopped to talk with a homeless teenager who was downtown near the library. He was upset. He had been in a number of shelters and transitional living programs but just hadn't been successful. He said, "I have a temper. I just want to go home. I've tried to call my dad's phone number." He had gone to the library earlier that day to call but didn't know how to make a collect call. So I gave him a cell phone, something we think is no big deal, and told him to call his dad. They hadn't seen each other in several years. He called: "Dad? It's me." And he started crying. It was a really great moment. It was just a cell phone but he had not known how to make a collect call or to get a phone card that some agencies have. His dad picked him up two or three hours later. It was a pretty rewarding experience—one I won't forget.

children; services also extend to the family. For example, the Brazelton Center for Mental Health Law (2012) describes wraparound services as services that

- are primarily provided in the homes of families and in settings in the community rather than in an office setting;
- are available when families need them, including after school, in the evenings, or on weekends instead of only during office hours;
- emphasize treatment through participation in purposeful activities, giving children the opportunity to practice life skills and make positive choices through involvement in community activities, instead of focusing on treatment through talking about problems; and
- are built around engaging the child and family in activities that interest them and meet their goals instead of just around the goal of stopping negative behaviors.

COMMUNITY-BASED CORRECTIONS   Within the context of youth violence (Office of the Surgeon General, 2001), providing wraparound services, discussed earlier, becomes an important component of both model and promising programs that prevent or address youth violence. Wraparound services help children and families involved in juvenile justice learn and develop problem solving skills, coping skills, and self-efficacy (National Wraparound Initiative, 2012). When services "wrap around" the child and family, professionals provide services in a structured, team-focused, and creative way. In this way, service delivery addresses individual and family needs and helps families integrate into community support systems such as the school, social service agencies, and religious or faith-based organizations. The delivery model, consistent with human service values and principles described in Chapter 1, is strengths-based and focuses on providing clients and families broader life choices and encourages empowerment.

Another focus of community-based care is in adult corrections. These criminal justice programs are designed to take individuals from prisons and local jails and place them in the community within supervised, planned programs. The increasing numbers of individuals in prisons or jails as well as decreasing federal and state budgets recommend community-based care. These programs link educational services, counseling, substance abuse treatment, and employment assistance. Reentry centers, or halfway houses, assist former inmates to integrate themselves back into the community. This includes alcohol and drug treatment for those with abuse issues. In these programs, much of the responsibility falls to the client to take the initiative in using available services (Federal Bureau of Corrections, 2012). Home confinement is one type of community-based care; the individual must stay at home except when working. Electronic monitoring might be one aspect of surveillance and monitor compliance.

COMMUNITY-BASED SCHOOLS   Schools are now a site for human service delivery in many communities. Teachers encounter the problems of children and youth each time they enter the classroom. They ask: "Can learning occur in an environment characterized by gangs, dropouts, teenage pregnancy, substance abuse, AIDS, and violence?" Predictions for the future do not offer much hope. A partnership between human services and education is important to meet the complex needs of children and families, especially in the area of mental health. School-based services or **systems of care** are popular terms that describe the creation of an array of integrated support services in schools where children, youth, and families need to be successful. Substance Abuse and Mental Health Services Administration [SAMHSA] supports school-based violence prevention programs focused on aggressive actions and bullying (SAMHSA, 2012a).

The Substance Abuse and Mental Health Services Administration (SAMHSA, 2012b) developed a Comprehensive Community Mental Health Services program to address the needs of children and youth and their families. This emphasis works in concert with the public and private schools. When schools are part of the system of care, access to assistance is facilitated, crisis situations can be addressed, schools and mental health agencies can share costs, a team approach can meet multiple needs, and children and youth behavior is monitored on a daily basis. There is a relationship between academic improvement and an increase in attendance, with mental health improvement, an increase in positive behaviors, and students remaining in their home schools. Mitchell and Kronick (2011) suggested that the integration of educational, health, and social welfare services may provide support for vulnerable children growing up today. Their full-service school initiatives incorporate universities, corporations, governmental agencies, school systems, individuals, and communities to form a partnership or team. See Box 3.2 for more information about delivering multiple services to those in need. The program described reflects needs related to immigrant families and children as they join schools and communities.

BOX 3.2   MEETING CHILDREN'S NEEDS IN SCHOOL: SERVING BURUNDIAN IMMIGRANTS

Burundi is a small country in the Great Lakes Region of Africa that shares borders with the Congo, Rwanda, and Tanzania. Three main ethnic groups constitute its population: over 80% are Hutus, 15% are Tutsis, and 1% are Twa. Many Burundians farmed or raised cattle before they fled to refugee camps in the Congo or Rwanda in 1972 during the large-scale massacres. Life changed dramatically for them as refugees; they had to abandon a familiar way of life. In 1994, while fleeing from genocide in Rwanda, many Burundians fled to Tanzania. A third move to the southern United States occurred in 2007 after Tanzania restricted national policies on naturalization and property rights.

What was life like for the Burundians who arrived in the United States in 2007? For many of them, refugee camps in Tanzania had been their home since their flight from the genocide in Rwanda. In the refugee camps, families built their own homes and raised small animals, like goats and chickens, and some children attended a primary school. Although the genocide ended, violence in the camps and in the surrounding areas of the camps was prevalent. Coming to the southern United States meant that these Burundians were again outsiders. They faced challenges of language, racial discrimination, and difficulties understanding and negotiating local politics, processes, and procedures in an urban area.

In 2008 through community engagement, I began fieldwork with Burundian children with refugee status and their teachers at a local elementary school and the public housing project where many of the students from the school lived. One teacher identified a small group of children who were disoriented and discouraged by the culture and structure of public school, and she believed that they needed support. My students and I met with these students, read, played, and completed homework with them after school in the public housing project where they lived. On the days when we could not work outside at picnic tables, on front stoops, or in the grass, a ministry center provided shelter for tutoring.

continued

During this time, I began classroom observations and became a classroom volunteer at the local elementary school. Spending time with the children both where they lived and in their school allowed me to understand their experiences and to work with the teachers to develop a tutoring program based on the children's experiences in school and the teachers' recommendations for the tutoring. My students and I tutored the children for the next two years.

Learning English was just one of many challenges for these children. For example, the socialization of American-born children to public school that happens gradually through day care, Head Start programs, and pre-school programs, happened all at once for the Burundian children. In the United States, sitting at a desk for six to seven hours a day in school is common, as is standing in a straight line without touching or speaking to other children, walking silently from room to room in a school, eating quietly at meals and eating only one's own food at meals, responding quickly, politely, and with eye contact when spoken to by an adult; and raising one's hand to seek permission to speak before talking. For these Burundian children, learning without their brothers and sisters was also a surprise. Grades by age artificially separate learning with siblings, and disallowed an older sibling from teaching younger ones, something older Burundian siblings did frequently after school.

Many of the Burundian children climbed trees at recess until the principal and teachers curtailed their scrambling up tree trunks enough times to make them cease. These children needed to be taught that trees at school are not to be climbed but to be admired in full bloom in spring for their aesthetic contribution to the school grounds while playground equipment is to be used for recreation.

Research on children with refugee status indicates that for those who have witnessed violence or survived traumatic experiences, about half of them may be diagnosed with Post-Traumatic Stress Disorder (PTSD). Traumatic experiences can affect young children emotionally, intellectually, and physically. They may need more emotional commitments from teachers, more time to concentrate to learn a task, or a safe space to express and/or process the loss that they feel. Some may experience social isolation while others may become aggressive. Many will experience headaches, stomach aches, and anxiety, particularly about death (Hamilton & Moore, 2004). During the transition for this group of Burundian children, many shed tears and sought isolation daily in the first months of school. When asked to stop crying or coerced to join a group, most cried harder and sat on the edges of a circle of children.

Our work with the Burundian children and their teachers provides a new understanding for us in this particular community regarding the socialization that American-born children and teachers take for granted, and the education that school districts need about children who enter our public schools with symptoms of PTSD and who may need support, time, and guidance to succeed in a new culture. This work also produced a new vision about how universities, public schools, parents, and children can collaborate to make the school and neighborhood environments a welcome place for children to be.

Source: Dr. Allison Anders, University of Tennessee, 2010. Reprinted with permission.

INTERNET EXERCISE

See this text's website at *www.cengagebrain.com* for video exercises. Choose Chapter 3, then Videos.

In this segment Katharine talks about her work with Burundian refugee children in the schools.

After you watch this segment, answer the following questions.

1. *What problems do refugees experience prior to coming to the United States?*
2. *What do they encounter once they arrive?*
3. *What is difficult about school in particular for the children from Burundi?*
4. *What do you think Katharine can do to help?*
5. *What do you think human service students as volunteers have to offer refugees in our country?*

COMMUNITY-BASED HOSPICE CARE   A final example of community-based human service delivery is hospice care, an interdisciplinary approach to providing support to individuals and families during the final stages of life. The goal of hospice is to support the patient and the family in locations such as a patient's home or a nursing home (American Cancer Society, 2012; Hospice Foundation of America, 2012) and to provide quality of care to the patient. The needs of the patient and the family might include, but are not limited to, pain and symptom control, spiritual care, respite care, family support, and bereavement care. The team of individuals providing services could include physicians, nurses, social workers, counselors, clergy, funeral directors, and volunteers. There is a special philosophy of care guiding hospice that is both related to death as a last stage of the life process and with helping patients spend their last days with family in dignity and as pain-free as possible.

Increasingly, graduates are finding that their generalist knowledge and skills transfer to virtually any setting where people may experience problems or need support or assistance. There is every indication that nontraditional settings will increase.

HUMAN SERVICES IN RURAL AREAS

Interest in providing services in rural areas is increasing. Two factors account for this interest. First, historically those living in rural areas, where population is steadily declining, have been disadvantaged and are experiencing a steady erosion in their quality of life. They are more likely to be older, be members of disadvantaged minorities, lack the kinds of opportunities available to their metropolitan counterparts, and need the help of human service agencies and professionals. Evidence also suggests, however, a growing pattern of relocation to rural areas and small towns, which is a reversal of 20th-century migration trends from rural to urban areas.

Small towns and rural areas are attracting those who see advantages in living where there are lower crime rates, opportunities for professional advancement, and larger labor pools with lower wage expectations. Thus, an increasing number of people who are not disadvantaged live in rural areas; indeed, they may have significant wealth. They include property owners, professionals, and business people. Those who are living in rural poverty and those who are not disadvantaged may experience similar problems, such as mental illness, family conflicts, and physical limitations, which require the help of social service agencies and helping professionals.

A second factor for the interest in human services in rural areas is the difficulties or barriers in providing accessible and adequate services. Recruiting and retaining trained health care and helping professionals, the large geographic distances between clients and providers, the cost of services, the maintenance of confidentiality, the isolation, and the coordination of care are all problematic in rural areas. Another significant barrier is the community stigma attached to having problems and receiving services for them. This negative perception may prevent individuals and families from getting the professional help they need. In some cases, individuals seek informal help from the extended family, the church, and social clubs, particularly when formal support systems are lacking.

The provision of mental health services is particularly problematic in rural areas. In addition to the problems mentioned, mental health problems often remain undiagnosed. There exists a "rural stoicism" that relates to working hard, expressing few emotions, and coping without complaint (Waltman, 2011). Rural primary-care providers such as physicians and nurse practitioners are likely to care for those with mental health problems and encounter difficulties in referring them for specialized care. Here again, distance, stigma, and costs are among the barriers that prevent successful referrals.

Recently, new models have emerged for delivering services to rural clients. They represent attempts to meet the unique needs of this population by providing child welfare services, meeting transportation needs, using members of the community for social support, providing home-based care, targeting the identified needs of clients, and asking about clients' needs and preferences. Collaboration among services and providing various services at one location allows service provision at a reduced cost. Using video links and telemedicine provides rural dwellers with access to care providers from other areas. In addition, educators now recognize that service provision in rural areas requires academic preparation that focuses on creative solutions to improve options, improvisation to meet needs, collaboration with a range of other professionals and informal supports, and the building of an infrastructure to provide needed supports to rural residents and communities. Recognizing that professional boundary issues are different from those of urban and suburban practitioners, educators can help rural helpers understand how to help family, acquaintances, and friends and how to maintain professional and nonprofessional relationships.

HUMAN SERVICES AND THE MILITARY

Traditionally, human services has been associated with people in financial need, particularly those who are unemployed or who are labeled as poor. Today, one focus of human service delivery is the military. Meeting basic human needs in the military is different from accomplishing the same in a civilian setting, partly because of the atmosphere of discipline and commitment to the organization. In 1881, the American Red Cross began providing social services to the military out of a concern for the health and welfare of the men and women in uniform. A medical orientation characterized military social service until 1976, when the Service to Armed Forces (SAF) was developed to help the military better serve the families of military personnel. Field offices were established in military hospitals and military installations to assist communication between service personnel and families.

Operation Enduring Freedom (OEF), launched in October 2001, and Operation Iraqi Freedom (OIF), launched in March 2003, reminded us that war can be traumatizing for some military personnel and their families. Often soldiers exposed to combat in OEF and OIF developed mental health problems, such as posttraumatic stress disorder (PTSD), depression, and generalized anxiety. It is hypothesized that one-fifth of troops returning from Afghanistan and Iraq are affected by these issues (Zoroya, 2011). New programs for military personnel and veterans focus on facilitating better access to support services related to medical care, mental health care, family support, and substance abuse issues, to name a few.

In addition, suicide remains a prominent issue for veterans in the field as well as for those returning home (Kristof, 2012; Parrish, 2011). The military built a response to the growing number of suicides that includes education, engagement, and intervention. For example, the program *Total Force Fitness* builds resiliency of families of military personnel. In addition, new training for officers helps identify personnel experiencing difficulties and provides them training for early intervention. Communication to all service personnel emphasizes that help is readily available. In addition, the military is partnering with businesses (current and future employers) to provide workplace stability for returning veterans and their family members. For example, programs and workshops such as "Reconnection Workshops" sponsored by Walmart include support groups focusing on communicating clearly, exploring stress and trauma, identifying depression, relating to children, and working through anger. Finally, the military is addressing the current warrior culture that stigmatizes any mental health issues as a sign of weakness. A suicide hotline and suicide prevention coordinators support the crisis nature of suicide and prevention.

The Veterans Health Initiative provides materials for Veterans Administration (VA) and non-VA service providers (Veterans Health Initiative, 2012). Materials available for human service professionals working with veterans focus on issues related to Agent Orange, the Gulf War, war wounded, traumatic brain injury (TBI), spinal cord injury, PTSD, military sexual trauma, and suicide, to name a few. Each of the areas of focus provides professionals with information related to assessment, epidemiology, care and rehabilitation, and impact on families. In addition, a focus on polytrauma related to TBI, recognizes the complexities of veteran care. "Polytrauma care is for veterans and returning servicemembers with injuries to more than one physical region or organ system, one of which may be life threatening, and which results in physical, cognitive, psychological, or psychosocial impairments and functional disability" (VA Polytrauma System of Care, 2012). This system of care recognizes the complexities of war-related trauma and engages a team of professionals to address the multiple needs of the veteran.

The Wounded Warrior Project (WWP) addresses the needs of wounded service members. Its vision is to "foster the most successful, well-adjusted generation of wounded service members in our nation's history" (Wounded Warrior Project, 2012). WWP's goals are as follows:

- To raise awareness and enlist the public's aid for the needs of injured service members.
- To help injured service members aid and assist each other.
- To provide unique, direct programs and services to meet the needs of injured service members.

The WWP provides holistic services to warriors enlisted in the armed services from September 11, 2001 (9/11), and includes those in Operations Iraqi Freedom, Enduring Freedom, and New Dawn Operation Iraqi Freedom. This includes warriors serving in Afghanistan and the war on terror. Programs address mental health issues, physical health, and work-related issues, to name a few.

In an attempt to make health care more accessible to all veterans, the Veteran's Administration and American Well (2012) announced a new partnership to provide online services. For example, patients can access health care through a web cam by using American Well. Available are assessments, counseling sessions, and

TABLE 3.1   SUMMARY POINTS: SERVICE DELIVERY SETTINGS

- Human service delivery continues in traditional settings such as social service agencies.
- Mental health programs, hospice, corrections, wraparound services, and family services are examples of community-based service delivery.
- Children and youth receive services in school in order to integrate education, mental health, and social welfare services.
- Services for veterans expand to meet the changing needs of this population.
- Rural human service delivery faces many barriers, including distance, cost, confidentiality, and shortages of professionals.

medication management that occur from home, the workplace, or other locations chosen by the client or patient.

A focus on wellness is integrated into the veteran's services (described earlier) for military personnel, their families, and veterans. Using technology to reach this population, newsletters, online communication, and social media help provide information to veterans about how to access services and a focus on ethics and service delivery. Included in the wellness promotion is enhancing exercise, reducing stress, identifying physical symptoms that indicate a need for assessment, complying with physician or counselor instructions, assessing suicide risk or depression, creating a social network, volunteering, and understanding services available.

Another challenge is to provide support for psychiatrists and psychologists who work with military personnel. The difficult problems these professionals encounter and the case loads they carry, at times, result in compassion fatigue (Carey, Cave, & Alvarez, 2009). According to Figley (1995), stress results from working with individuals who have experienced trauma. Helping professionals may begin to exhibit the same symptoms as their clients; in other words, professionals experience secondary trauma accompanied by sadness, depression, anxiety, and other PTSD symptoms. See Table 3.1.

THE IMPACT OF TECHNOLOGY

Technology continues to change the delivery of human services. Human service providers are expanding the ways that they use technology to help their clients both directly and indirectly. Technology is used in the areas of communication, information management, service delivery, and professional development. Development in technology is dynamic, and continued change is the norm. Administrators of services, direct service providers, and clients are all "customers" of the computer systems and software that continue to emerge and we expect growth in the creative use of technology to continue occurring at a rapid pace (Special needs, 2012).

The primary goal for using technology in the human service delivery system is to provide services more effectively and efficiently. Another goal is providing services for clients with limited access. For many human service professionals, use of technology has already helped them provide better quality services in a more cost-effective manner. As these technologies become more interwoven in our lives, they are used simply because they represent the standard way of doing business. One pervading ethical concern about the increased use of technology is the protection of confidentiality. As paper and face-to-face communication have shifted to technology-driven methods, protection of the client and the helping activity must continue to be ensured. In Chapter 9, confidentiality as it relates to technology is explored in more detail. In addition, there is always a question about the nature of help vis-a-vis electronic mediums rather than face to face.

COMMUNICATION

Computer technologies and the advances in satellite communications support the ways many interactions occur in human service settings. **E-mail** continues to be one way human service professionals communicate and share information and files with colleagues, whether they are in the same building or across the state, the nation, or sometimes, the globe. Human service professionals also use distribution lists and listservs to share ideas and concerns regarding ethics, treatment, managed care, and funding. Instant messaging (IM) and SMS (text messaging) continue to help individuals communicate with each other. IM typically represents communication from computer to computer, while SMS is typically between cell phones. Both of these methods of communications allow individuals to communicate synchronously. The advantage of using IM and SMS is the ability to send and receive messages instantaneously.

Another way human service professionals in distant locations can communicate with each other is by **teleconferencing**. Many large organizations find this technology a cost-effective way to conduct meetings and to talk with each other about service delivery, new programming for clients, and ways to learn new information and skills. For example, Nunavut is a Canadian territory created in 1999 that is approximately two million square kilometers and extends from the Hudson Bay to the North Pole. The Inuit comprise 85% of the approximately 29,000 people living in the area. There are 28 settlements, and none are accessible by road (Government of Nunavut, 2012). The Nunavut Department of Health and Social Services is committed to providing a broad range of services to its constituencies by using clinics, clients' homes, outpost camps, and teleconferencing (Department of Health and Social Services, 2012). This is but one example of how teleconferencing is used to stay in touch with other professionals and also to provide services.

Cellular phones and pagers are standard issue for many human service professionals providing direct services to clients. These devices also allow professionals to be available at all times. Professionals working with child abuse cases, community-based mental health, probation and parole, as well as other types of cases, are available 24/7 to meet ongoing client needs. These devices also provide security to many workers when they are in dangerous or isolated situations with clients.

Communications also occur through the **World Wide Web** using individualized Web pages. In this way, many individuals and organizations can provide information to those online. For example, many organizations are using the Web for organizational visibility, direct services, community education, advocacy, and securing resources. Web pages provide Internet users with telephone numbers and e-mail addresses of helplines and relevant offices, as well as information about programs, special conferences and events, and organizational information such as mission and agency structure. Agencies provide online services through chat rooms, e-mail counseling, and online support group meetings. They also use Web logs (blogs) and discussion boards as a way to provide communication and discussion by professionals and those being served. In addition, advocacy efforts involve promoting awareness and support on policy and legislative issues and helping the community find other resources it needs.

Organizations are also using the Web to reach their members and to recruit potential new members, donors, and volunteers. As an example, the web page for the National Organization for Human Services (search the Internet using "National Organization for Human Services") offers information about the organization, with links to its role and mission, the board of directors, the regional organization, and membership.

The World Wide Web is a powerful multicultural tool used to connect people to other people. As you will read later in this chapter, increasing one's understanding of cultures, human diversity, and related ethics is necessary given the rapidly changing demographics of the United States and the world (Chapter 9). The Web allows the sharing of stories, histories, choices, reflections, and interactions that reach beyond what has been traditionally available in books, periodicals, or classrooms.

Web logs (blogs) are sites where individuals can post their diaries, journals, thoughts, and opinions about their experiences or ideas about a particular subject. Blogs provide an opportunity for public information sharing and debate. Numerous blogs focus on human services. **Facebook** is a social networking website where individuals and organizations communicate locally, nationally, and globally. For these organizations, it is a way that users provide updates about services and distribute information about the organization. Many people use **Twitter**, a microblogging service that allows individuals to share minimessages with each other. This social networking tool is also used by human service organizations to foster communication. For example, the Red Cross Heartland Chapter in Nebraska (2012) uses blogs, Facebook, and Twitter to communicate about their organization and the services they deliver.

Just as technology supports better communication, it also offers an improved way of managing information. There are many ways in which computers and their software help manage information within the human service delivery system.

INFORMATION MANAGEMENT

Using computer technology, managers coordinate information from a variety of sources and then organize the data to facilitate planning, decision making, and reporting. Information can also be managed to support evaluation and help tie service delivery to outcomes and cost. The information entered into a human service database can include a client's name and other relevant demographic data (age, gender, race, and marital status), prior use of the human service delivery system, intake information and assessment results, problem identification, treatment plans, treatment records of services provided, and evaluation of those services according to outcomes reached and client satisfaction.

In addition, in this environment of managed care, the information system may also include service costs, payment, the cost of each service delivered, and a record of the interaction with the managed care organization. The interaction record may show the kinds of services authorized by frequency, duration, and definition of the service provider. One advantage of a management information system is its ability to transfer information electronically across organizations and among workers. This feature benefits both human service professionals and clients in several ways. First, the client and the professional save the time and energy required to generate the data for a second or a third time. If the data represent intake or initial assessment information, the professional can review it with the client and request additional information to ensure accuracy. Second, work can begin with the client much earlier because, in some cases, much of the information gathering is complete. Access to broad information gives the human service professional a more comprehensive review of a client's experience within the service delivery system.

Just as technology supports human service work using management information systems, it also helps provide services to clients.

PROVIDING SERVICES TO CLIENTS

The services available through new models of service delivery range from computer programs that assess client knowledge or skill and recommend a plan of action to actual counseling online in real time. A telecommunication system was set up by Rural Assistance Centers for tribal communications in the Midwest (Telehealth Resource Centers, 2012). The services provided include health and legal services to the underserved in rural areas. They have developed one-on-one technical assistance, a Telehealth Inventory, an online technical support tool, and best practice guidelines. This is but one example of the expanded use of telecommunication service delivery.

Many software programs and tools are available to teach clients specific knowledge or skills to enhance their daily living or to increase their vocational potential. Many of the programs are designed for clients who are experiencing difficulties. Several programs focusing on daily living and life skills deal with problem solving and language activities. Other daily living skills such as shopping and buying groceries, sequencing tasks, developing social behaviors, and learning safety behaviors represent a few of the needs of children and adult populations (Special Needs, 2012).

| BOX 3.3 | EXPLORING THE WEB FOR MORE INFORMATION |

Check out the following sources for examples of human service information on the Internet.

Human Services Code of Ethics

American Psychological Association

Counseling

Psychiatry Online

Rural Human Services

Multiple sites that support personal counseling range from information and assessment to the provision of services. For example, consumer mental health sites provide information about psychological disorders, active chat rooms, hosted support groups, journaling opportunities, and psychological tests. Technology-related services for career counseling are widely available. There are software packages that assess functional levels in math and language, aptitudes, and provide opportunities for career exploration (Career Consulting Corner, 2012).

One interesting technological breakthrough relates to assessing signs of depression. Scientists at MIT (Chu, Buckworth, Kirby, & Emery, 2009) are developing software that recognizes indications of depression. Currently speech-recognition software focuses on writing text from the spoken word. This new program will recognize the slow, quiet, and halting monotone used by individuals suffering from depression. As the software becomes more available, professionals will have support as they screen for depression in their clients.

Counseling and other support services are also provided online. This allows human service professionals to be available via e-mail or the Web to work with individuals who are experiencing specific difficulties, thereby increasing access to services. Proponents of online counseling believe that without this venue, many people would not be able to benefit from the knowledge and care of helpers. Others, however, express concerns about confidentiality, informed consent, and competence. Nevertheless, the number of participants receiving services online continues to grow. Certain sites also provide medical consultation and child-care advice. Thus, the phrase "the doctor is always in" reflects the constancy of the Internet and its easy accessibility.

Because of the prevalence of **E-therapy**—online or Internet therapy—and the accompanying concerns of members of the professional community, there are guidelines for those clients who wish to use such therapy. These guidelines address the following types of questions: Are you a good candidate for online therapy? How do you find a credentialed professional? How do you make an appropriate choice among professionals? How do you locate online counseling websites and compare? How do you ensure confidentiality? (ABC's of Internet Therapy, 2012). The American Counseling Association includes guidelines about computer technology in its Code of Ethics (American Counseling Association, 2005). These include understanding the limitations of the client, determining if technology is an appropriate counseling methodology, and explaining to the client the limitations of the computer counseling services.

Online chat forums also help provide support to those in need. They address a range of topics and are accessible on many networks. One example is a chat group for police officers (PoliceOne, 2012). The purpose is for members of the force to get to know one another in an informal environment. Chat services are available for all branches of law enforcement across the globe. There is a restricted login, and the chat room is secure. A second example is the discussion network developed by the Nebraska Network for Children and Families (2012) to focus on elder care. It provides an opportunity for those providing care for Alzheimer's clients, those providing assisted-living services, and those caring for older people. There are both listserv and discussion formats available for those who need social support.

PROFESSIONAL DEVELOPMENT

Professional development is an important aspect of lifelong learning, and technology makes it easier for human service professionals to take advantage of the latest information about populations being served as well as the knowledge and skills of emerging best practice. One way this information is available is by CD-ROM or DVD. Most compact discs of interest to the human service professional can be found in a local university or city library. One advantage of using these CDs or DVDs for research is the easy access to current information.

Another advancement in professional development is the availability of software that facilitates skill development. Programs are available to teach interviewing, problem solving, rehabilitation counseling, decision making, counseling, crisis counseling, organizational assessment, case management, and many other skills. Much of the software is interactive and uses simulation as the primary instructional tool. In teaching problem solving in case management, many programs use simulated cases of individuals with severe problems and difficulties. Students and practitioners are asked to identify and prioritize needs and to choose alternatives and outcomes. Most programs provide the client's current status and other, more detailed information about client history.

Podcasting is another way to deliver audio and video training materials to human service professionals. Podcasting allows users to access information by subscription; in other words, the audio and video transmissions are delivered to the user without the user seeking the transmission. This method of delivery provides up-to-date information to the user quickly and efficiently. For example, the National Institute of Health (2012) and the National Institute of Mental Health (2012) provide live audio reports on human service-related issues such as diabetes, addiction, obesity, and heart disease.

Online educational programs provide access to higher education in human services and other related areas. Programs may be hybrid and include face-to-face and online instruction. Other programs represent only instructional delivery online. The growth of these programs not only reflects the availability of technology but also the need of students to attend college while retaining their employment and remaining in their current location. Best practices for teaching

TABLE 3.2   SUMMARY POINTS: USES OF TECHNOLOGY

- Communication in human services is enhanced by e-mail, listservs, teleconferencing, the World Wide Web, Facebook, blogs, and Twitter.

- Telemedicine, management systems, and care networks are examples of information management systems.

- Direct services to clients by means of technology include assessment, counseling, information, and education.

- Technology allows human service professionals to utilize the latest information about practice, client groups, and skill development.

online articulate effective and efficient ways for instructors to communicate with students (Boettcher, 2009).

In summary, human service professionals are currently using many technologies to improve the ways they communicate with each other, expand the ways information is managed, provide services to clients, and engage in professional development. Human services and technology will continue to develop new ways to address professional and client needs during the 21st century.

THE INTERNATIONAL DIMENSION

Any discussion about human services today without considering its international dimension would be difficult. Everyone on the planet is drawing closer as a result of technological advances in transportation and communication.

Today, people travel the world in a matter of hours rather than days or weeks. Advances in communication keep us instantly informed about developments throughout the world by satellite, e-mail, faxes, and social communication networks. The information superhighway has no borders, with users in most countries around the globe. The world is becoming a smaller place when we consider factors other than physical distance. Thus, we need to know what is happening internationally in terms of human services—the recent changes that have occurred, the challenges that remain, and the lessons from other countries about service delivery. A closer look at the challenges of international human services and their implications for the United States and for you as a human service professional helps us understand their very serious nature and provides insights about future problems.

CHALLENGES IN INTERNATIONAL HUMAN SERVICES

Global population began to increase rapidly in the 20th century, a situation aptly described by the term *population explosion*. This was not a worldwide phenomenon but occurred almost entirely in the developing countries of Africa, Asia, and Latin America. The dramatic contrast in growth between the more-developed and less-developed countries continues to increase. Today, 97% of the world's population growth is in developing countries (World Population Data Sheet, 2012). For instance, developing countries add about 80 million people per year to the world's population compared to the 1 million added in developed countries. By 2050, 86% of the world's population will live in less-developed countries. Middle Africa, followed by western Africa, is expected to be the fastest growing region in the first half of the 21st century, with its population growing 193% by 2050. Limited health care, particularly in rural areas, education, poverty, social unrest, and literacy are challenges in these countries.

Another challenge for the 21st century is international migration. In 2010, there were approximately 214 million migrants worldwide, up from 191 million migrants in 2005. Political upheaval, natural disasters, refugees and asylum seeking, environment and climate change, and economic crisis all account for the increased migration (International Organization for Migration, 2011). Approximately 75% of this number are in 12% of the countries in the world, with most

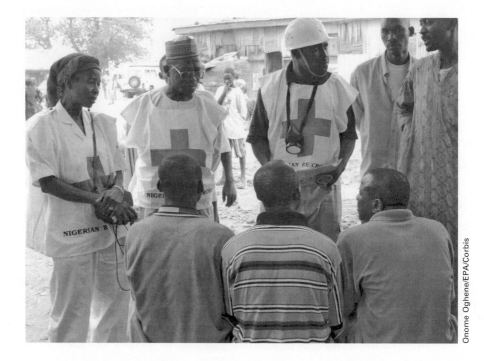

Onome Oghene/EPA/Corbis

moving from one less-developed country to another. For both countries of origin and countries of destination, this movement raises major socioeconomic issues. These numbers are only a small percentage of the estimated global migration that also includes refugees, guest workers, and illegal foreigners.

Another challenge is **urbanization**, a long-term global trend that is most pronounced in poor countries that are least able to cope with its pressures. In developing countries, 90% of the population are living in cities. Today, a third of the world's population do not have the means to meet their basic needs, such as clean water and sewage disposal. For example, Mumbai (formerly Bombay), the largest city in India, has a population of 20.1 million (Indiaonlinepages.com, 2012). By 2025, it will be the second-largest metropolis in the world, with 27.4 million people. In Mumbai, between 200 and 250 families arrive each day, hoping for a better life in the city. Many begin their lives there as pavement dwellers because there is no other place to live. Land is scarce, and rooms and apartments are full. The newcomers may remain on the sidewalks for the rest of their lives, or they may move to a slum dwelling. In either case, clean water, electricity, paved paths or roads, and working community toilets are often nonexistent. Although slum living represents upward mobility in many developing countries, slum dwellers complain about the gangs, high rent, drugs, violence, sewage, and floods.

The challenges in international human services continue to be great. The plights of refugees and migrants, those with AIDS, the homeless, drug users, and the displaced in the aftermath of natural disasters—in addition to the problems discussed here—are some of those challenges.

INTERNATIONAL FOCUS: *A LIBERIAN REFUGEE*

Monique Kolubo-Simpson is an American-Liberian who fled Liberia in 1990 after her life was threatened by rebel forces. She returned there because of her love for her country and to be near family and friends. Her life was threatened again when the rebel soldiers attacked her village. She was frightened for her life and once again fled.

Monique began the day that she left home like any other. She had heard stories of fighting in the area, but she did not realize how dangerous the situation had become until she looked out the window of her home and saw long lines of people leaving the village with only what they could carry. The fighting reached their village as her family decided to leave; already homes were being destroyed and people were being shot in the cross fire. Her father took charge and ordered the entire family to leave. Monique looked back at her home just before she left and grabbed her watch. She thought it might be valuable at some point in her journey.

Instead of fleeing on foot, her family was able to leave by car. As they headed for the American Embassy, they were stopped at a checkpoint. Since it was a peacekeeping checkpoint, they were allowed to go through with little hassle. Further down the road the car was stopped at a rebel checkpoint. They complied with the rebels by answering their questions and letting them search the car and their belongings. Finally they were released, only to be stopped again at a rebel checkpoint headed by a 16-year-old rebel soldier. This last stop was terrifying, but finally they were allowed to proceed.

They reached the embassy where they stayed with little food and bare sleeping quarters. For days no one knew if they would be rescued before the rebel soldiers took the embassy. Finally, a helicopter came to evacuate them. As Monique left the country, she had two primary thoughts. She continued to worry about her friends who had left the country by foot, and she was glad that she would not have to live through the war.

Source: Adapted from U.S. Committee for Refugees and Immigrants. (n.d.). A refugee from Liberia—Monique Kolubo-Simpson. Retrieved from http://www.oakland.k12.mi.us/resources/externships/human/0203/HS%20332.pdf

INFLUENCES ON THE UNITED STATES

How does the international dimension of human services affect the United States? Although most information in this book concerns human services in this country, we must also be aware of its international dimension. Immigrants to the United States increase our awareness of those nationalities that have become or are becoming part of our population. In the early history of the country, immigration was limited primarily to Europeans; 100 years ago, 90% of the immigrants to the United States came from European countries. During the last 30 years, however, the wave of immigration has been primarily non-European, including Chinese, Japanese, Filipino, Korean, Vietnamese, and Indian. Since 9/11, the United States has experienced an increase in immigrants from predominantly Muslim countries in the Middle East, North Africa, and Asia. In 2011, 56,000 refugees were resettled in the United States. Individuals from Burma, Bhutan, and Iraq comprised 75% of these 56,000 (Russell & Batalova, 2012). The states of Texas and California resettle over 75% of these refugees. These are individuals who do not wish to return to their country of origin for fear of persecution.

Another interesting ethnic development is the recognition of **multiracial** individuals. According to the 2010 Census, 9.2% of the population in the United States identified themselves as multiracial. Individuals in this category increased 32% from 2000. There was a 134% increase in the number of individuals identifying as both white and black. The number of individuals identifying as white and Asian increased 87%. There are four multiracial groups that exceed 1 million individuals: white and black; white and "some other race"; white and Asian; white and American Indian/Alaskan Native. The number of those in the population who identify themselves as members of more than one race is expected to increase.

Another important consideration of population in the United States is the 40 million foreign-born people (13% of the population) (U.S. Census Bureau, 2012). The largest population comes from Latin American. Half of this population lives in four states: California, Texas, New York, and Florida. In the state of California one in four individuals are foreign born; in New York one in five are foreign born. Much of the foreign-born population is young (half are between 18 and 44). These foreign born are more likely than natives to be married, less likely to be divorced, less likely to graduate from high school, and more likely to live in poverty.

Today and in the foreseeable future, the United States must grapple with numerous issues related to diversity. Who is a minority? Should changes in immigration laws reduce illegal immigration rates? What efforts should be employed to control immigration? Do immigrants take jobs from unemployed citizens? Are immigrants entitled to public education and other benefits? Should English be the official language of the United States? What impact will these ethnic shifts have on Medicare and Social Security? What about the relationship between terrorism and civil liberties? While these questions are debated throughout the United States, we continue to be part of the global community and play a role in the international human services discussed earlier.

Some human service professionals work as service providers or volunteers in other countries, particularly developing countries. Others are employed by United Nations agencies, the World Bank, or the Peace Corps or volunteer for shorter periods with religious groups, such as the Missionaries of Charity, or for nonprofit organizations, such as Cross-Cultural Solutions or the Red Cross.

Many other human service professionals elect to remain in the United States. Given the population projections, it is increasingly likely that these professionals will work with people of very different backgrounds from them. The Latino population presents an example of the complexity of the situation. In the United States, this group is growing almost five times faster than that of non-Latinos and is now the nation's largest minority. Although ethnic groups from Spanish-speaking countries such as Mexico, Nicaragua, and Argentina are referred to as Latino or Hispanic, those cultures and customs are as diverse as the English-speaking populations. It would be a mistake to assume that they are a uniform, cohesive group that is culturally homogenous. Hispanic or Latino communities are found in Miami, Spanish Harlem, and migrant labor camps, and each is culturally, ethnically, and geographically diverse, making an awareness and appreciation of each group's uniqueness necessary for effective human service delivery.

TRENDS IN HUMAN SERVICES

Human services will be different in this century. We know that change occurs rapidly. In this chapter, you have read about changes already taking place that impact service delivery today. The utilization of technology and the diverse and nontraditional settings for helping activities will continue to impact human services, but other trends will influence what and how services are delivered and to whom. It is appropriate that as part of our discussion of human services today, we devote some thought to the future. It will come quickly. To trigger your thinking about the future, we discuss five major trends to conclude the chapter.

BOX 3.5   INTERNATIONAL FOCUS: *TEACH A MAN TO FISH*

You know the old biblical proverb about "teaching a man to fish?" This phrase captures well the aim of international development, but when I started working in the field it didn't take me long to discover that it just was not that simple. In 2003 I moved to Angola to live with my husband. The Republic of Angola, a country in southern Africa, won a 14-year war for independence from Portugal in 1975. The civil war that followed resulted in the deaths of large numbers of civilians from the fighting and from starvation. One casualty of independence was the departure of skilled European labor. This loss coupled with guerrilla activity took its toll on Angola's economy. The country has been working toward recovery, in part through the development of the lucrative oil and diamond industries, though as is so often the case in countries that are rich in natural resources, but poor in leadership, most Angolans see none of the dividends. I was thrilled to get my first job in international development, hired by a nongovernmental organization that assisted Angolan farmers in communities recovering from the 27-year civil war. It did not take long before I realized that no matter how hard we worked, or how much funding we had, there was only so much we could do to help farmers to help themselves. On paper, everything the organization pursued sounded great. Our training on improved technologies would surely lead farmers to extend the growing season, prevent crop disease, and improve yields. Our assistance on cooperative development would help them become democratically-run advocacy organizations, enabling them to access transport and supplies at better prices and negotiate more effectively with banks, retailers, etc. Further, our facilitation of bank loans should help them acquire the water pumps, seeds, and pesticides they needed to ensure quality and viability of the harvest. We even trained them on postharvest handling, selection, and marketing. With all of this

assistance, and bank credit to boot, how could these farmers go wrong? In fact, the impediments were more complicated than I could ever have imagined. I recall many scenes in which these men and women struggled with the very ideas of change that our organization advocated:

- The day the Boa Esperanca cooperative was electing its leadership, and I saw a few of the women, mostly illiterate, asking (men) whose name they should mark on the ballot.
- One day I sat for hours with a co-op treasurer at a tiny wooden table with a handheld calculator, reviewing the cash flow sheets, explaining basic subtraction.
- When our agronomists introduced a demonstration field to show how "pruned" banana trees (with fewer sprouts allowed to grow from the same root system) will grow faster because they require less fertilizer and water, only two farmers were willing to try it. At least that was the first year, there were probably more the next year.

Of the five cooperatives we helped to strengthen over the course of the project, there were many struggles in leadership. In Bengo, one of the cooperatives discovered their president was stealing fertilizers from the co-op store. Another in Huila province had a president with a claim to ownership of the building the co-op was using as its hub, introducing a conflict of interest. Cooperative elections, almost without exception, resulted in electing individuals who were probably chosen not so much on merit, but because these were people already powerful in the community. Another time we spent an entire day with the Dungo farmer cooperative, teaching farmers how to calculate net profits through estimating production costs against returns. Ultimately, this exercise is useful on an individual basis, where a farmer writes down the inputs

continued

BOX 3.5   INTERNATIONAL FOCUS: *TEACH A MAN TO FISH continued*

and outputs of farming. No one took notes that day. As a practice, they just don't write anything down. Even when the bank agreed to issue loans to farmer groups, our staff's disappointment was tangible with the number of delayed and defaulting loan repayments. During the war, the loans that were accessible to these farmers were generally those issued by the government, and almost never collected on. Though not all of our farmers were identical on this issue, clearly, a culture of credit was lacking. Ultimately, the hopes we have for transformative change through international development are probably not realistic. Most of the successes occur when our intervention happens at the right time and place, and influences individuals or groups that are ready and open to adopt a new way of thinking, or a new approach. For example, there was one fellow in Dungo who was kind of a half-time farmer—Peio split his time between the farm and his family in Luanda. He really

grasped well the concepts we taught about marketing, and internalized deeply the idea that the primary determinant to his moving ahead was himself. Peio had contacts at a military base, and started marketing vegetables from Dungo directly to this and other large-scale buyers. He drove his shoddy passenger car back and forth between the farms and the buyers, learning how to establish client relationships and maintain schedules and quality to clients' expectations, to great benefit to both his clients and his suppliers, the other farmers of Dungo. Eventually, the co-op selected him to run the cooperative store, recognizing his intelligence and initiative, and natural business sense. It may be fair to say that some of our most important work in international development is that which succeeds in catalyzing individuals like Peio with the knowledge and new skills they need to "catch their own fish."

Source: Cathy Hamlin, USAID Staff Member, 2010. Reprinted with permission.

AGING IN AMERICA

Growth and change of the senior population in America rank among the most important demographic developments of the 20th century and will continue their importance in the 21st century. This development has serious implications for the next 50 years. The population in the United States aged 65 and over is expected to double in size within the next 25 years. The number of those 85 and older is also increasing. The Office on Aging (2012) has compiled statistics from the U.S. 2010 Census indicating current status of this population and significant future trends:

- The older population (65 and older) numbered 40.4 million in 2010, an increase of 5.4 million or 15.3% since 2000.
- The number of Americans aged 45–64—who will reach 65 over the next two decades—increased by 31% during this decade.
- Over one in every eight, or 13.1%, of the population is an older American.
- Older women outnumber older men at 23.0 million older women to 17.5 million older men.
- In 2010, 20.0% of persons 65 or older were minorities, of which 8.4% were African Americans.
  Persons of Hispanic origin (who may be of any race) represented 6.9% of the older population. About 3.5% were Asian or Pacific Islander, and less than 1% were American Indian or Native Alaskan. In addition, 0.8% of persons 65 or older identified themselves as being of two or more races.

- Older men were much more likely to be married than older women—72% of men versus 42% of women. Forty percent of older women in 2010 were widows.
- About 29% (11.3 million) of noninstitutionalized older persons live alone (8.1 million women, 3.2 million men).
- Almost half of older women (47%) age 75 or older live alone.
- The population 65 and over has increased from 35 million in 2000 to 40 million in 2010 (a 15% increase) and is projected to increase to 55 million in 2020 (a 36% increase for that decade).
- The 85 and older population is projected to increase from 5.5 million in 2010 to 6.6 million in 2020 (19%) for that decade.
- The median income of older persons in 2010 was $25,704 for males and $15,072 for females.
- The major sources of income as reported by older persons in 2009 were Social Security (reported by 87% of older persons), income from assets (reported by 53%), private pensions (reported by 28%), government employee pensions (reported by 14%), and earnings (reported by 26%). (Office on Aging, 2012).

It is not just the numbers that cause concern, however; some current trends among seniors will be accentuated—and will impact human service delivery.

This group will have increasing education levels and include more minority seniors and more women than men. Many will be reasonably healthy and live independent and active lives, although there will still be a great disparity in terms of income and health status in certain segments of the population. The health of older Americans is improving. Poor health is related primarily to chronic conditions such as arthritis and heart disease (U.S. Census Bureau, 2011). Real median income for older citizens continues to decline. But education is positively correlated with better health, higher income, and a more prosperous retirement. The most vulnerable are older single women with low incomes, baby boomers with less education, and minority groups with low economic status. Those aged 85 and older are also at risk. Life expectancy, medical advances, and improved health and lifestyles make those 85 and, as reported by the Office on Aging (2012), older the fastest-growing age group in the United States. The changes in the American family, particularly divorce, may result in less support for members of the aging population, because the numbers of seniors living alone is increasing (U.S. Census Bureau, 2011).

These changes in the population will present challenges for human services during the next 50 years. There will be a significant number who are troubled by poor health, dependency, and the inability to perform simple tasks. Additionally, those who are in good health will not escape the transition from active and independent living to some form of assisted living. Addressing these needs will present challenges for human services and society at large, particularly in the areas of income assistance, health care, housing alternatives, employment issues, leisure opportunities, and environmental modification. Three such issues—housing, depression, and confronting death and dying—are introduced here.

HOUSING   Living arrangements for those 85 and older are determined by several factors: financial assets, ability to care for self, social support, cultural values, access to social services, and types of housing available. The types of living arrangements vary from renting or owning a home to assisted living.

First, many individuals own or rent their own homes, and their first choice is to "age in place." Services such as mobile meal delivery or home health care make this possible. Often in the United States, older Americans do not choose the second alternative, living with their children; they want to remain independent and fear they will be a burden. When parents do live with their adult children, as an alternative to independent living, mutual consent contributes to a successful coexistence. A third choice, **assisted living,** is a relatively new choice for those 85 and older. The number of individuals choosing this option is increasing, because level of care can be matched to individual need. Assisted-living environments offer a combination of personal space and social services to meet the needs of their clients. An increasing number of older adults live in institutions (Office on Aging, 2012). Although a stigma about nursing home care exists, trained professional staff, broad programming, hygienic and safe conditions, and support from governmental services contribute to quality care.

DEPRESSION   Just as important as the living arrangements for the aging population are the mental health issues that many of them face. One important issue is depression. Many individuals have experienced episodes or times of depression throughout their lives, but for others, this first occurs in the 80s or even 90s. There are several difficulties in diagnosing depression in those over 65, mostly related to stereotypes about aging, culture, values, and lack of knowledge about the disease. Many individuals believe that depression is just a natural part of the aging process and goes hand in hand with decline in later years. An assumption is made that the difficulties associated with getting older are just part of the aging experience and that it is natural to feel stressed and "down." Others, aware of the stigma related to mental health, hide their depression or refuse to seek treatment. Many older people or their families simply know little about the disease and do not recognize when it is present. Fear of the treatment itself or the cost of treatment also keeps many people from seeking help.

There can be serious consequences for not seeking help from depression, such as suicide or a higher mortality rate. While depression is linked with an inability to sleep, physical deterioration, overwhelming sadness, being a woman, and mourning the loss of a loved one, the highest rate of suicide is for older white males (Papalia, Olds, & Feldman, 2011). In addition, many individuals experience depression after a stroke or heart attack or related surgery.

CONFRONTING DEATH AND DYING   Although many members of the aging population do not experience depression, sadness and grief over loss are inevitable. These emotions are natural and predictable reactions to leaving home, deterioration of health, developing a disability, and losing independence and the ability to care for one's *self.* Death of a spouse and the process of dying present special challenges. According to Erikson (1963), in the final stage of life—ego integrity versus despair—one comes to terms with both the meaning of life and the place of death within the experience of living. For most individuals over 65, several issues around dying and death, such as care for a loved one, require social support and social services.

Bereavement is the "loss of someone to whom a person feels close and the process of adjusting to it" (Papalia, Olds, & Feldman, 2011). One of the most difficult losses for those over 65 is the death of a spouse. The survivor is likely to experience a wide range of emotions, such as denial, disbelief, confusion, shock, sadness, and despair. In addition to emotional turmoil, adjustments to daily living require new skills in order to perform roles previously assumed by the former spouse (paying bills, washing clothes, cooking, home and auto repairs) and require revising social connections as a widow or a widower. During this time, the survivor works through stages of grief that include shock and disbelief, preoccupation with the memory of the dead person, and resolution (Hiller & Barrow, 2007). Older widows are more likely to seek out social support during this time, while widowers tend to isolate themselves. However, both older female and male survivors have more coping skills than younger survivors and often deal with death and loss more effectively.

In recent years, attempts have been made to make the dying process more humane both for the dying spouse and for the survivor. Attention to the psychosocial needs as well as the medical needs has expanded services beyond physicians and hospitals to social support networks and home and family. Hospice care provides patient-centered care to patients and their families, with the focus on providing palliative care by keeping the patient comfortable, pain free, and within a familiar setting. Although hospice services are typically provided in the patient's home or the home of a family member, hospitals or hospice centers also offer these services. In each of these settings, medical professionals, social service professionals, and the family form a team to serve the patient's needs. Support is also available for the family members.

Human service professionals play a major role in assisting those 65 and over as they grapple with the issues of the aging process. Because of this, the need for a variety of social services and human service professionals will expand in the coming decades.

A NEW FOCUS Even though the aging process is often fraught with difficulties, there is an increasing recognition that those 65 and beyond may retain much of their vitality and interest in maintaining productive lifestyles. This reflects the emergence of a new life stage in which individuals envision retirement as a time to continue working or engage in public service (Adler & Goggin, 2005). Motivations include staying cognitively sound, maintaining good physical health, wanting to be useful,

---

BOX 3.6	EXPLORING THE WEB FOR MORE INFORMATION

Check out the following sources on the Web to learn more about older adults or children of older adults.

AARP

Aging with dignity

Elder Web

Elder law

Estate planning

Living wills

Depression in the elderly

finding enjoyment, hoping to help others, and needing additional income, to name a few. In fact, these individuals could have an exciting place in the field of human services (Miller, 2009) as volunteers, part-time employees, or full-time engagement in a second career.

AN EMPHASIS ON DIVERSITY

Typically, when we think about **diversity**, it is the ethnic makeup of our country that comes to mind. In fact, earlier in this chapter you read about the changing demographics of both the United States and the world and how those changes will impact human services. It is accepted today that as you enter the human service profession you will encounter clients who are different from you. You will also be working with other helping professionals who are different from you. For example, at an agency in Miami, a team of human service professionals represents a variety of countries: Spain, Cuba, El Salvador, Romania, and the Dominican Republic. Not only do the members of the team differ in the countries where they were raised, but they also speak different languages, come from different economic backgrounds, are of different ages and genders, and entered the United States under various circumstances.

You can prepare for working relationships such as these by learning about multicultural counseling, reading the plethora of books that address ethnic diversity, and increasing your awareness of other cultures through travel, interaction with other students, and television, books, and movies. Diversity, however, has a much broader connotation than ethnic diversity, and it is an understanding of this more sweeping concept that will help us address the challenges of 21st-century problems.

Diversity is inherent to the American way of life. The term *diversity*, broadly conceived, is used to refer to many demographic variables, including age, color, disabilities, gender, national origin, race, religion, and sexual orientation (U.S. Department of the Interior, 2012). America draws strength from its diversity; for example, contributions from racial and ethnic minorities have enriched all our lives. During the 21st century, emphasis will be placed on the broader definition of diversity. Since 9/11, there is a growing awareness of differing spiritual beliefs, and issues surrounding homosexuality such as equal rights and the right to marry have sparked debate in Congress and in state legislatures.

The Ethical Standards for Human Service Professionals (National Organization for Human Services, 2000) recognize "an appreciation of human beings in all of their diversity" as a basic tenet of human service delivery. Specific standards further address "the respect, acceptance, and dignity" due each client (#2), the need to be advocates "for the rights of all members of society, particularly those who are members of minorities and groups at which discriminatory practices have historically been directed" (#16), and the provision of services "without discrimination or preference based on age, ethnicity, culture, race, disability, gender, religion, sexual orientation, or socioeconomic status" (#17). Human service professionals are also "knowledgeable about the cultures and communities within which they practice" (#18), and they are "aware of their own cultural backgrounds, beliefs, and values" (#19). Although there is concern about service delivery within the limit and scope of one's professional knowledge and skills (#26), human service professionals engage in continuing education, professional development, and supervision in order to work effectively with culturally diverse groups (#21). This, then, is the challenge of the 21st century: to develop the knowledge, skills, and self-awareness to be effective in delivering human services.

Both the changing demographics and the ethical standards that address diversity give additional importance to understanding the concept of "worldview." Each person has a worldview that affects our thoughts, decision making, lifestyle, and behavior; it also encompasses our attitudes, values, and opinions. Most importantly, it affects how we see each other and the world. It is a critical concept for human service professionals. Individuals who are different from you racially, ethnically, or in other ways will probably have a different worldview than you do. This may result in the helper attributing negative traits to the client (Sue & Sue, 2012). Another consequence is the influence worldview has on the helping relationship, for example, the client's view of the helping process and the helper, and the helper's approach to problem assessment and the choice of interventions. The challenge for human service professionals is to become aware of and understand their own worldview, to expand their worldview to become effective cross-culturally, and to be sensitive to the worldview of their clients. We will explore three areas of diversity. As you read, think about your worldview and its impact on service delivery with these potential clients.

RACIAL AND ETHNIC DIVERSITY   Racial and ethnic diversity often come to mind first when the word *diversity* is mentioned. According to federal classifications, African Americans (blacks), American Indians and Alaska Natives, Asian American and Pacific Islanders, and white Americans (whites) are races. Hispanic American (Latino) is an ethnicity and may apply to a person of any race (Office of Management and Budget, n.d.). This example reflects the reference of the term **ethnicity** to a common culture, heritage, and shared meaning. It may include religious groups (e.g., Jews), country of origin (e.g., China), or any other facet passed from generation to generation. These terms are important in the United States where the ethnic and racial structure is changing as discussed earlier in the section on influences in the United States. For example, the percentage of nonwhites in the United States continues to increase. In 2012, for the first time, nonwhite births outnumbered white births. The 2012 U.S. Census reports increasing number of nonwhite populations living in metro areas; the most prominent is the increase in Hispanic population. It is both the changing statistics and our ethical standards that require us to learn as much as possible about minority worldviews. There will not be enough minority helpers for each racial or ethnic group to have its own.

We must also be sensitive to the fact that equal opportunity underlies the American belief system, yet racial and ethnic minorities bear a greater burden from unmet mental health needs. As a result, they suffer a greater loss to their overall health and productivity (Mental Health: A Report of the Surgeon General, 2012). There are many reasons for this: the cost of care or services, societal stigma, fragmented services, and the client's fear and mistrust of treatment. Other barriers may come from the helper's lack of awareness of cultural issues, bias, or inability to speak the language. Whatever the barriers, the fact remains that equal access to services has not been achieved. The Office of Minority Health outlined Cultural and Linguistically Appropriate Standards (CLAS) (For more information, search the Internet using terms "Office of Minority Health" or "Cultural and Linguistically Appropriate Standards") to make services more accessible and effective. Areas of focus for the standards include culturally competent care, language access services, and organizational support for cultural competence. These standards reinforce the need for increased sensitivity to the special needs of minority populations.

RELIGION   Diversity in the United States also embraces religious differences. In fact, the United States has been called the most religiously diverse nation in the world, primarily because it is a nation of immigrants. America was already home to Native American traditional spiritualities when the colonies were settled by those who established different Protestant churches. During the 19th and 20th centuries, the immigration of Roman Catholics, Jews, and people who practiced Chinese religions, Islam, and Sikhism further diversified religion in the United States. Most recently, a 1965 change in immigration law was the most significant development in bringing about cultural change, particularly in increasing religious diversity (Buck, n.d.). The Hart-Celler Bill ended a closed-door policy in place since the 1920s, replacing national and ethnic quotas with quotas based on occupation and family reunification. As a result, the settlement of significant communities of Muslims, Hindus, Buddhists, Sikhs, and Jains occurred. Today, of those 18 years of age or older in the United States, 78.4% are Christian (Catholic, Baptist, Methodist, Lutheran, etc.). Other religions (Jewish, Islamic, Buddhist, etc.) total 4.7%. Those specifying no religion comprise 16.1% (U.S. Demographics for Religion, 2009).

Religious diversity brings both challenges and opportunities to a community. As a challenge, religious difference is a main factor in social conflict on local, national, and global levels as shown by the political impact of religious fundamentalism and ethnoreligious groups. Some object to the presence of other religious groups in their communities, citing the vandalism and violence against certain groups, negative stereotypes, discrimination, and ignorance.

Religion is an area of strongly held beliefs and emotions. Those who see diversity as an opportunity or strength are also intense about their beliefs. They cite the richness of significant religious holidays and observances and the increasing number of ecumenical and interfaith organizations as positive forces in religious diversity. They also believe that religious diversity facilitates a dialogue that enables the exploration of new and old questions. How has America dealt with religious difference historically? What are today's challenges for communities, schools, and public institutions?

SEXUAL ORIENTATION   Another emotional diversity issue is sexual orientation. This is now a regular topic on radio and television talk shows, and increasingly in casual conversations. Because these interchanges frequently involve public policy, legal issues, and religious beliefs, they become intense and often polarizing. Misconceptions and fear contribute to heightened emotions.

Perhaps the most prevalent misconception is that homosexuality is a disease. Neither the American Psychological Association nor the American Psychiatric Association considers homosexuality to be an emotional or mental disorder. There are serious issues that confront people in a sexual minority such as lesbian, gay, bisexual, and transgender (LGBT), particularly the social stigma they experience. This segment of the population often does not have the same basic rights as other citizens. In many states and cities, a person within the LGBT community can legally be denied housing, employment, and public accommodation on the basis of sexual orientation. These inequalities, coupled with the desire for equal rights and equal protection of those rights and the inability to offer financial and legal security to their families, have led many to be involved in civil rights issues.

How do we work with those who are different from us? All people are shaped by the culture in which they were raised, including those who consider themselves the dominant culture in the United States (Sue & Sue, 2012). What do you know about your own culture and how it is perceived by others? Are you open to learning about others whose worlds are different?

The ability to work effectively with diverse groups means establishing relationships based on the trust and respect for others, increasing our awareness and knowledge of other ways, listening without judgment, and appreciating the worldview of others. The challenge to human service professionals in the 21st century is to take the lead to work effectively with others, whether that is a client, a neighborhood, a regional population, or other professionals.

THE CHANGING WORKPLACE

Prior to the 2008 Great Recession, the U.S. workplace had begun to change. Trends included a "distribution" of the workplace, signaling an end to an actual building or common site for all workers to conduct their work. Many workers commuted to the office from time to time but primarily worked from home (Ouye, 2011). Taking advantage of developing communication technologies, workers collaborated with colleagues and clients using cell phone, e-mail, social media, and synchronous technology allowing real-time communication. In addition, the types of jobs available shifted from manufacturing to the service sector, and many jobs reflected this change in education and skills. In response to these changes, human service professionals helped their clients understand the changing workplace, adapt a flexible attitude about the dynamic nature of the world of work, and begin to understand they would, in all probability, have multiple work experiences throughout their work life.

The Great Recession and its economic aftermath present human service professionals with additional challenges well beyond the increased need for education and flexibility. Resulting from the cascading effects of the drop in real estate values, followed by the decrease in wealth and consumer spending, the financial market spiraled downward. Business and industry, unable to sustain the reduction in spending, suffered closures or downsizing, and approximately 8.4 million jobs were lost (The Great Recession, 2012). The very nature of individuals and their relationship to work has shifted dramatically (Reeves & Leonard, 2009).

Four types of workers emerge from the Great Recession:

- Employed—those individuals who work full time at a job commensurate with their education and skill level.

- Unemployed—those individuals who are ready to work but cannot find paid employment.
- Underemployed—this is an individual who has part time work but wishes to work full time or is overqualified for the job he or she holds.
- Marginally attached worker—this individual wants a job but has stopped looking for work. (The Great Recession, 2012).

It is important to note trends that predict the future of work and project what the new work opportunities will be. In fact, as the economy recovers, individuals will return to a different workplace. The changes in the workplace reflect many of the current work-related demographics and the nature of the compensation for work. Several trends are well known to professionals working in the human service arena. Those in young adulthood are not finding full-time jobs; college graduates are less able to find work commensurate with their education. More senior individuals are delaying retirement; fewer individuals are moving from job to job. Women are more likely to find employment than men.

Experts predict that as the economy recovers the types of jobs available will also change (Career Consulting Corner, 2012). For instance, workers will be asked to work more for less compensation, and there will be fewer benefits (e.g., health insurance, retirement benefits) (Reeves & Leonard, 2009). Many jobs will require fewer skills and less education. Business will retain the adjustments they made during the Great Recession such as furloughs, fewer and longer work shifts, and maintaining layoffs.

As the Bureau of Labor Statistics reports in "The 30 fastest growing jobs in America," (2012), jobs in America are changing. Nineteen of the jobs do not require a college education; several of the jobs do not require a high school education. Jobs preparation at the undergraduate or graduate level includes those required to be a veterinarian, mental health counselor, medical scientist, cost estimator, health educator, audiologist, physical therapist, marriage and family therapist, marketing research analyst, interpreter and translator, meeting convener and planner, or biomedical engineer. An associate degree prepares students to meet the increasing demands for veterinarian technologists, physical therapist assistants, diagnostic medical sonographers, and occupational therapists, to name a few. A high school diploma or below helps individuals assume positions as personal-care aides; home-health aides; brick, block, or stone masons or tile or marble cutters' helpers; carpenters' helpers; reinforcing iron and rebar workers; pipe layers, plumbers, and pipefitter helpers; and glaziers. This list, although projective in nature, describes the types of jobs available for many of the clients we serve.

NEW ROLES AND SKILLS FOR CLIENTS AND HELPERS

As the 21st century begins, one well-accepted change is the role of the client in the helping process. For many years, the client was a passive recipient of services—accepting the decisions, following the direction of a helper, and generally assuming little responsibility for what occurred in the process. With the recognition of clients' rights, the emphasis on consumer satisfaction, and the advent of welfare reform, the participation of the client in human service delivery has increased greatly; in many instances, the client becomes actively involved in the helping process.

This change has necessitated efforts on the part of human service professionals to engage the client as a partner in the helping process. Establishing a collaborative relationship calls for skills that promote a climate of trust and a sense of partnership. Taking time to get to know the client, considering the client's point of view, and exploring client expectations are part of this process. Once a relationship exists, the client becomes an active participant in assessing the problem and the situation, collecting information, determining a course of action, and evaluating the process. As a result of these actions, the client shares responsibility for the success or failure of the endeavor.

For human service professionals, this shift in the client's role has some benefits. First, the client shares the responsibility with the helper for the effectiveness of the helping process. A client's active engagement in the process increases the likelihood that he or she will follow through on whatever tasks are necessary and will be more satisfied with the results. Second, the establishment of a relationship with the client also impacts the client's satisfaction. Having a good relationship with the helper means that clients believe that the helper listened, spent time with them, and provided follow-up services. Finally, clients have much to teach the human service professional about themselves, their problems, and the services they need. Ignoring these aspects of service delivery leads to ineffective and inefficient services. These are important lessons for helpers that will carry over to their work with other clients.

Just as the client assumes a new role in the helping process, 21st-century human service professionals need different helping skills. Advocacy—recognized, accepted, and taught as a human service skill—will continue to be emphasized in the future and will be critical for successful service delivery.

As human services changes, there may be both positive and negative reactions. It is possible that services will become more streamlined yet less available, and cost containment will save money but become an overriding factor in limiting treatment and other services. It is even possible that legislation unfair to some groups or individuals will become law. These possibilities make vigilance on the part of human service providers particularly important as they look out for the interests of their clients.

Advocacy means speaking out on behalf of clients or those who cannot speak for themselves. It frequently involves clients, their families, the community, and other professionals. Direct advocacy efforts may take many forms: empowering clients to act; improving environments; acting on behalf of a client by writing letters, filing forms, and so forth; informing clients about programs, services, and policies; and guiding a client through choices and changes. There are also situations that require advocacy on a larger scale. Are needed services provided? Are they available and accessible? Is the public policy fair and equitable? In these instances, a human service professional may act as a spokesperson to inform the public and legislators about what exists or what is needed. It may also be necessary to act as part of a collaborative effort for common agreement or support about an issue. The advocacy role of the human service professional is discussed more completely in Chapter 6. As you think about the future and the skills you will need to be an effective service provider, you will also want to think about how to prepare for this role.

Returning to a consideration of the **whole person** is more important than ever before within the context of the current economic downturn. Loss of employment or change in employment status not only influences self-esteem and has a negative influence of internal locus of control, it also affects one's ability to afford housing, pay bills, access health care, and provide basic care for other family members. Another issue that influences the status of individuals and families is the problem of mortgages and foreclosures. What begins as a single issue, either loss or change of job status or threat of foreclosure, leads to multiple challenges. The responsibilities of human service professionals broaden to an assessment of financial issues, making knowledge of available services, especially those related to the economic downturn, critical to support clients and meet needs.

The number of individuals and families with mental health issues is increasing. As discussed earlier, individuals who suffer job loss or a change in the status of their jobs such as reduction in hours or a reduction in pay are currently increasing. Depression and risk of suicide appear to be increasing; in addition, those unemployed are less likely to report any increase of alcohol or substance abuse or mental health-related matters. The Substance Abuse and Mental Health Services Administration (2011) provides advice for those in need for getting through tough economic times. They recommend ways the individuals can assess their difficulties and provide areas within the human service delivery system where they can receive help, including helping professionals, health-related professionals, and community resources.

A CLIMATE OF PARTISANSHIP

Politics in the United States reflects a two-party system; each party represents a range of ideas about the role of government in general and the role of government regarding specific issues such as rights of individuals, states' rights, taxation, and the responsibility of government to help those in need. Within the context of the two-party system, the elected representatives of the legislative and executive

TABLE 3.3   SUMMARY POINTS: TRENDS

- The effect of urbanization in poor countries will continue to create difficulties in meeting the basic needs of people.

- Demographic shifts in the United States raise questions about immigration policies, language, employment, and entitlement programs.

- One important shift is the growth and change of the older population, which indicates an increase in the number of seniors as well as changes in their characteristics.

- Economic downturns create human service challenges for individuals and families, including changes in the workplace.

- Clients will remain active participants in human service delivery.

- Advocacy as a helping skill continues to be increasingly important.

branches of federal and state governments usually belong to one of the two. **Partisanship** is a term that indicates strong support of the party platform and a rejection of the other party's platform or proposed policies. The term *bipartisanship* describes a time when politicians from all parties come together to support common goals.

At the time of this writing, bipartisanship does not reflect the reality of the Congress, especially as it relates to issues of health care, immigration policy, and climate change, among others. A rise in the number of citizens who consider themselves as Independents in the political process reflects, to some degree, the lack of cooperation between the two parties. Thinking about partisanship in terms of two parties does not reflect the complexities of the political system. For example, several moderate Republicans support Democratic efforts to policy issues while some conservative Democrats have positioned themselves against them.

How does this climate of partisanship affect human service professionals and the clients they serve? Human service agencies and organizations may be affected in different ways, depending on their relationship to federal and state governments, their funding sources, and their missions. Governmental policies determine who are clients and ways that clients may be served; funding influences the resources we have to help the increasing number of those in need. Advocacy efforts mentioned earlier continue to be critical and reach beyond the politics of Republicans and Democrats alike to bring voice to client needs and increase the likelihood that helping others can be a bipartisan effort.

In summary, human service educators recognize that their field continues to change rapidly and that innovative approaches to traditional helping may be needed to meet the demands of service delivery in the 21st century. It is also important to retain those traditional skills that are effective. As human service professionals, our challenge is to stay abreast of both societal trends and new developments in order to provide quality services to those who need assistance.

KEY TERMS

advocacy	E-therapy	systems of care	Web logs
assisted living	ethnicity	teleconferencing	whole person
community-based services	Facebook	Twitter	World Wide Web
diversity	multiracial	urbanization	wraparound services
e-mail	partisanship		

THINGS TO REMEMBER

1. Human services are delivered to populations in a variety of settings, including rural areas, the military, schools, and other community-based settings, all of which increase the number of clients who can be reached.

2. Schools have become a site for service delivery, especially mental health services, where teachers and human service professionals share the same clients.

3. The trend toward providing more services in community-based settings and less in institutional ones is helping to serve clients in the least restrictive environment. Wraparound services help provide quality services to the multiproblem client.

4. Community-based services were first used with clients with mental illness who were deinstitutionalized; now, populations receiving community-based services include those in the criminal justice system, the developmentally disabled, and seniors.

5. The barriers to service delivery in rural areas include shortages of workers, the large geographic distances between clients and providers, the cost of services, confidentiality issues, and coordination of care.

6. Technology has begun to change the way human service professionals meet their responsibilities, particularly in the areas of communication, information management, service provision, and professional development.

7. Communication avenues used by human service professionals include e-mail, listservs, the World Wide Web, cellular phones, and teleconferencing.

8. Computer technology is available to help human service professionals manage information and use data to make decisions about planning programs, establishing costs, and reporting.

9. Technology is being effectively used to provide services to clients, including diagnosing and assessing, teaching new skills, and assisting those with disabilities or impairments.

10. As technological advances draw the world closer, we become more aware of the human service challenges in an international context, such as increases in the global population, international migration, and urbanization.

11. In the international context, many individuals live in large cities in poor countries, where they struggle to meet basic needs and have little access to housing, sanitation, and nutritious food.

12. Among the trends in the United States that will influence future human service delivery are the growth and change of its aging population, the increasing diversity of clients and professionals, the increasingly active participation of clients, the dynamic nature of the workplace, and the development of new and, in some cases, nontraditional skills.

SELF-ASSESSMENT

- Explain why human service delivery has expanded beyond the traditional settings.
- How has technology changed the delivery of human services?
- Why is it important to understand the international dimension of human services?

- How will the trends occurring in the next few decades affect human service delivery?
- Describe how religious diversity challenges and brings opportunities to a community.

WANT TO KNOW MORE?

There are several resources you can access to learn more about human services and many of the concepts discussed in this chapter. Check them out!

Additional Resources: New Trends

Finley, E. P. (2011). *Field of combat: Understanding PTSD among veterans of Iraq and Afghanistan.* Cornell, NY: Cornell University.

The author explores the nature of the military experience and how veterans and families negotiate the return to the United States.

Gamble, R. (2012). *The distance between us*. New York: Simon and Schuster.

The author presents a personal memoir of migrating to the United States from Mexico.

Hall, L. K. (2008). *Counseling military families: What mental health professionals need to know*. New York: Taylor and Francis.

The author describes the need for expertise in counseling military families, the unique culture of the military and the needs that emerge, and strategies that work for family, marriage, and individual counseling.

Howard, C. (2008). *The welfare state nobody knows: Debunking myths about U.S. social policy*. Princeton, NJ: Princeton.

The author describes the United States welfare system and helps readers understand the comprehensiveness of this public program.

Kelly, U. A. (2009). *Migration and education in a multicultural work: Culture, loss, and identity*. Boston: Palgrave/Macmillan.

The author explores the global migration occurring in the 21st century and describes the struggles and barriers the migrants encounter. She advocates recognizing migrant needs and helping individuals honor their lost home and culture and transition into new spaces.

Moorehead, C. (2006). *Human cargo: A journey among refugees*. New York: Holt.

As an experienced writer about human rights for 25 years, the author presents an overview of the fate of refugees who are either searching for a better life or seeking asylum after persecution, rape, torture, and genocidal massacres.

Moody, H. R. (2009). *Aging: Concepts and controversies*. Thousand Oaks, CA: Sage.

The author explores aging from the historical, developmental, and theoretical perspectives. He describes the psychological, biological, and social aspects of aging. He explores the myths that exist about aging and challenges a more comprehensive understanding of the process.

Case Study

If you'd like to know more about the work of human service professionals, read the discussion among five human service professionals in *Introduction to Human Services: Cases and Applications*, the companion text to *Introduction to Human Services*. These professionals work in five different settings with five different client groups.

They represent the fields of community mental health, case management, educational interpreting, employee-assistance programs, and a nonprofit agency. Their discussion touches on a number of issues and challenges that will improve your understanding of the "real world" of human services.

REFERENCES

ABC's of Internet Therapy. (2012). *Talk to a therapist online*. Retrieved from http://www.metanoia.org/imhs/

Adler, R. P., & Goggins, J. (2005). What do we mean by "Civic Engagement"? *Journal of Transformative Education*, 3(3), 236–253. doi: 10.1177/1541344605276792.

American Cancer Society. (2012). *What is hospice care?* Retrieved from http://www.cancer.org/Treatment/FindingandPayingforTreatment/ChoosingYourTreatmentTeam/HospiceCare/hospice-care-what-is-hospice-care

American Counseling Association. (2005). *2005 Code of ethics*. Retrieved from http:// www.counseling.org/Resources/CodeOfEthics/TP/ Home/CT2.aspx

American Well. (2012). *Online care to serve America's veterans*. Retrieved from www.americanwell.com/veteransaffairs.htm

Boettcher, J. (2009). *Designing for learning: Teaching online for the first time*. Retrieved from http://www.designingforlearning.info/services/writing/ecoach/tenbest.html

Brazelton Center for Mental Health Law. (2012). *Wrap around services*. Retrieved from https://www.bazelon.org/Where-We-Stand/Success-for-All-Children/Mental-Health-Services-for-Children/Wraparound-Services-.aspx

Buck, F. (n.d.). *Religious diversity works to define 21st century America*. FACSNET. Retrieved from http://www.facsnet.org/issues/faith/williams.php

Career Consulting Corner. (2012). *Links*. Retrieved from http://www.careercc.com/

Carey, B., Cave, D., & Alvarez, L. (2009). Painful stories take a toll on military therapists. *New York Times*. Retrieved from http://www.nytimes.com/2009/11/08/us/08stress.html

Chu, I. H., Buckworth, J., Kirby, T. E., & Emery, C. F. (2009). Effect of exercise intensity on depressive symptoms in women. *Mental Health and Physical Activity*, 2(1), 37–43.

Department of Health and Social Services. (2012). *Government of Nunavut*. Retrieved from http://www.gov.nu.ca/files/Building%20Our%20Infrastructure.pdf

Erikson, E. (1963). *Childhood and society*. New York: Norton.

Federal Bureau of Corrections. (2012). *Community corrections*. Retrieved from http://www.bop.gov/locations/cc/index.jsp

Figley, C. R. (1995). *Compassion fatigue: Coping with secondary traumatic stress disorder*. London: Brunner, Routledge.

Government of Nunavut. (2012). *Government of Nunavut*. Retrieved from http://www.gov.nu.ca/english/

Hamilton, R. J., & Moore, D. (2004). *Education interventions for refugee children: Theoretical perspectives and implementing best practices*. London: Routledge/Falmer.

Hiller, S. M., & Barrow, G. M. (2007). *Aging, the individual, and society*. Belmont, CA: Wadsworth/Thomson Learning.

Hospice Foundation of America. (2012). *Choosing hospice*. Retrieved from http://www.hospicefoundation.org/

Indiaonlinepages.com. (2012). Mumbai population 2012. Retrieved from http://www.indiaonlinepages.com/population/mumbai-population.html

International Organization for Migration. (2011). *World migration report 2011*. Retrieved from http://publications.iom.int/bookstore/free/WMR2011_English.pdf

Kristof, N. D. (2012). A veteran's death, the nation's shame. *New York Times*. Retrieved from http://www.nytimes.com/2012/04/15/opinion/sunday/kristof-a-veterans-death-the-nations-shame.html?pagewanted=all

Mental Health: A Report of the Surgeon General. (2012). *Mental health: Culture, race, and ethinicity: A supplement to mental health: A Report of the Surgeon General*. Retrieved from http://www.migrantclinician.org/files/20120113153854406.pdf.

Mitchell, L., & Kronick, R. (2011). Service-learning in a community school: AmeriCorps VISTA and the university, *Community Works Journal*. Retrieved from http://www.communityworksinstitute.org/cwjonline/articles/aarticles-text/kronickvista.html

Millier, N. (2009). *Aging and activism: New trends in the new millennium*. Presentation for the 2009 National Organization for Human Services Conference, Portland, Oregon.

National Institute of Health. (2012). *NIH audio reports*. Retrieved from http://www.nih.gov/news/radio/radio.htm

National Institute of Mental Health. (2012). *NIMH audio*. Retrieved from http://www.nimh.nih.gov/media/audio/index.shtml

National Organization for Human Services. (2000). *Code of ethics*. Retrieved from http://www.nationalhumanservices.org/

National Wraparound Initiative. (2012). *Wraparound basics*. Retrieved from http://www.nwi.pdx.edu/wraparoundbasics.shtml

Nebraska Network for Children and Families. (2012). *Answers 4 Families*. Retrieved from http://www.answers4families.org/

Office of the Surgeon General. (2001). *Youth violence*. Retrieved from http://www.ncbi.nlm.nih.gov/books/NBK44294/

Office of Management and Budget. (n.d.) *Revisions to standards for the classification of federal data on race and ethnicity*. Retrieved from http://www.whitehouse.gov/omb/fedreg_1997standards

Office on Aging. (2012). *A profile of older Americans: 2011*. Retrieved from http://www.aoa.gov/aoaroot/aging_statistics/Profile/2011/docs/2011profile.pdf

Ouye, J. A. (2011). *Five trends that are dramatically changing work and the workplace*. Retrieved from http://www.knoll.com/media/18/144/WP_FiveTrends.pdf

Papalia, D. E., Olds, S. W., & Feldman, R. D. (2011). *Experience human development* (12th ed.). Boston: McGraw Hill.

Parrish, K. (2011). *Battaligia calls reducing suicides a top priority. U.S. Department of Defense*. Retrieved from http://www.defense.gov/news/newsarticle.aspx?id=66431

PoliceOne. (2009). *Police community*. Retrieved from http://www.policeone.com/police-forums/

Red Cross Heartland Chapter. (2012). Home. Retrieved from http://www.redcrossomaha.org/index.asp?IDCapitulo=V4N8M8Z9T9

Reeves, J., & Leonard, C. (2012). How the Great Recession is changing the American workplace. *Insurance Journal*. Retrieved from http://www.insurancejournal.com/news/national/2009/10/05/104296.htm

Russell, J., & Batalova, J. (2012). Refugees and asylees in the United States. Retrieved from http://www.migrationinformation.org/USfocus/display.cfm?id=907

Special needs. (2012). *Daily living & life skills*. Retrieved from http://www.especialneeds.com/computer-software-daily-living-life-skills.html

Substance Abuse and Mental Health Services Administration. (2012a). School-based violence prevention programs to reduce bullying and aggressive behaviors. Retrieved from http://www.nrepp.samhsa.gov/pdfs/bullying_review5.pdf

Substance Abuse and Mental Health Services Administration. (2012b). Implementation cooperative agreements for the expansion of the comprehensive community mental health services for children and their families program. Retrieved from http://www.samhsa.gov/grants/2012/sm_12_003.aspx

Substance Abuse and Mental Health Services Administration. (2011). *Getting through tough economic times*. Retrieved from http://www.samhsa.gov/economy/

Sue, D. W., & Sue, D. (2012). *Counseling the culturally diverse*. (6th ed.) New York: Wiley.

Telehealth Resource Centers. (2012). Home. Retrieved from http://www.telehealthresourcecenter.org/

The Great Recession: Unemployment and under employment. (2012). The State of Working America. Retrieved from http://stateofworkingamerica.org/great-recession/unemployment-and-underemployment/

The 30 fastest growing jobs in America. (2012). *Business Insider*. Retrieved from http://www.businessinsider.com/the-30-fastest-growing-jobs-in-america-2012-2?op=1

U.S. Census Bureau. (2012). Foreign born population in the United States. Retrieved from http://www.census.gov/prod/2012pubs/acs-19.pdf

U.S. Census Bureau. (2008). Mapping Census 2000: The geography of diversity. Retrieved from http://www.census.gov/population/www/cen2000/atlas/index.html

U.S. Census Bureau. (2010). Aging boomers will increase dependency ration. Retrieved from http://www.census.gov/newsroom/releases/archives/aging_population/cb10-72.html

U.A. Census Bureau. (2011). 2010 census shows nation's population is aging. Retrieved from http://2010.census.gov/news/releases/operations/cb11-cn147.html

U.S. demographics for religion. (2009). *U.S. Demographics*. Retrieved from http://www.teachingaboutreligion.org/Demographics/map_demographics.htm

U.S. Office of the Interior. (2012). *Policy, management and budget offices: What is diversity?* Retrieved from http://www.doi.gov/pmb/eeo/what-is-diversity.cfm

VA Polytrauma Systems of Care. (2012). What it is and how it works. Retrieved from http://www.polytrauma.va.gov/system-of-care/

Veterans Health Initiative. (2012). Public health. Retrieved from http://www.publichealth.va.gov/vethealthinitiative

Waltman, G. (2011). Reflections on rural social work. *Families in Society*, 92(2), 236–239. Retrieved from http://www.familiesinsociety.org/ArticleArchive/2011/92-2_Waltman.pdf

World Population Data Sheet. (2012). *World population data sheet 2012*. Retrieved from http://www.prb.org/Publications/Datasheets/2012/world-population-data-sheet/data-sheet.aspx

Wounded Warrior Project. (2012). Mission and vision. Retrieved from http://www.woundedwarriorproject.org/mission.aspx

Zoroya, G. (2011). Rise in PTSD cases from two wars strain resources. *USA Today*. Retrieved from http://www.usatoday.com/news/military/story/2011-11-29/PTSD-cases-rise/51476604/1

CHAPTER **4**   MODELS OF SERVICE DELIVERY

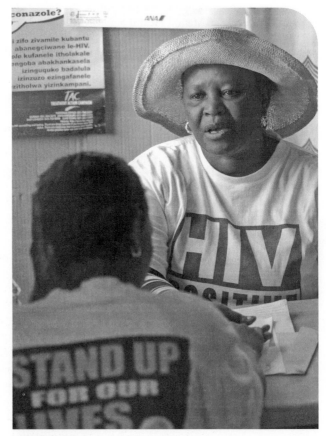

Louise Gubb/Corbis

After reading this chapter, you will be able to:

- Define three models of service delivery.
- Trace their development.
- Illustrate the use of these models in human service delivery today.
- Apply the three models to a human service problem.

In developing a definition of human services, we have discussed its various characterizations, briefly traced the history of service provision, and explored recent developments, emphasizing human services today. Another approach to defining human services is to examine the way it benefits service recipients. This chapter describes three models that represent different orientations in service delivery: the medical model, the public health model, and the human service model. The chapter concludes with a case that illustrates the interaction of these models.

In this chapter, you will meet clients who have received services delivered in the context of these three models. The cases of Robert Smith and Ralph Jones illustrate services provided by the medical model. Sean O'Reilly was a recipient of services provided by the public health model. Susan, her husband, Ted, and children, Matthew and Justin, illustrate the complexities of client needs that may require multifaceted, long-term intervention.

All three models are used to deliver services today, and depending on the problem, an integration of all three models may be most effective. In practice, some agencies may prefer one over the others, and one model may be more effective than the other two in some situations. Helpers may be skilled in following one particular model, but they are likely to be working closely with practitioners who follow the other models. Therefore, you should know the characteristics of each model, its historical development, and how it is used. To help translate this information into human service practice, we examine a relevant social problem from the perspective of each model.

Each of the three models of service delivery has certain philosophical assumptions that guide its practice. These assumptions reflect beliefs about the causes of problems, their treatment, and the role of the professional in the model. To illustrate, we consider the nature of mental disorders from the perspectives of each of the three models.

The medical model is based on an orientation developed by the medical profession; it assumes that mental disorders are diseases or illnesses that impair an individual's ability to function. The disease or illness, in this case the mental disorder, has an organic basis and responds to medical interventions such as medication, laboratory studies, and physical therapies. Often the individual, or **patient**, receives treatment from a physician in a hospital or medical clinic.

The public health model resembles the medical model in its diagnosis and treatment process, but the models differ in recipients of services and methodologies of treatment. Whereas the medical model emphasizes *individuals*, the public health model focuses on *groups* in the population who may be identified by geography (community, country, region, or state), types of problems (abuse, poverty, specific illnesses), or specific characteristics such as age (children, the elderly). This model views mental disorders as the result of malfunctions or pressures created by the environment or by society. The mental disorder is evaluated for its impact not only on the individual but also on society at large. In addition to treating the individual, this model emphasizes preventing the problem through supporting activities such as use of films, speakers, school programs, pamphlets, and internet resources, all aimed at educating the population about the problem.

The **human service model** is concerned with the interaction between the individual and the environment, stressing the need for balance between the two. Although recognizing both the medical and the public health perspectives, this model focuses on the interpersonal and environmental conflicts that may result from the problem (in this case, a mental disorder). Perhaps the individual (or **client** or **consumer**) has problems resulting from genetic predispositions, biochemical imbalances, faulty learning, lack of insight into behavior that may be inappropriate, a physical or mental disability, or influences from the social environment. Whatever the situation, the client is experiencing interpersonal and emotional difficulties that affect behavior. Treatment in this model encompasses services to both the individual and the environment through work with the client as well as the people and the institutions with which the client is involved. An important consideration in the model is the focus on client strengths rather than on inadequacies. Each model provides a different perspective on the same problem. We now look at the development of each one.

THE MEDICAL MODEL

DEFINITION

The **medical model** sees the person coming for help as an individual whose problem is a disease or a sickness. The individual is "sick" or "ill." Often called *patients,* these individuals depend on the physician or service provider to prescribe a treatment or cure for the "disease." Historically, this model can be summarized as a system that involves the following elements: symptom–diagnosis–treatment–cure (Reinhard, 1986).

The medical model, with a history that includes shamans, medicine men and women, and witch doctors, is perhaps the oldest of all treatment models. In fact, other models used it as they were developing. For example, in Chapter 2 we discussed the beginning of the new profession of social work at the turn of the 20th century. Mary Richmond, author of *Social Diagnosis* (1917), used the medical model to describe social casework. Believing that the presenting problem was rooted in the individual, she suggested that pauperism was a disease. The friendly visitor, therefore, became a social physician whose duty was to heal the complex conditions of poverty (Trattner, 1999; Zimbalist, 1977).

The corrections field also adopted the medical model during the 1930s, when its emphasis shifted from punishment to treatment. The change was based on the assumption that criminal behavior was the result of physical or environmental aspects of an individual's life, requiring treatment (Clear, Resig, & Cole, 2012). Theoretically, prisons were to become therapeutic communities, where inmates would be rehabilitated to reenter society. Unfortunately, budget constraints limited this change to one of name only; departments of prisons became "departments of

| BOX 4.1 | INTERNATIONAL FOCUS: *MODELS OF SERVICE DESIGN* |

Thinking about models of service design in developing countries, Howard N. Higginbotham (1979) suggested three basic models of service design: traditional psychiatry, the public health approach, and the village system. He believed that the "the first model, traditional **psychiatry**, is similar to North American or European psychiatry, which has not been modified for use in non-Western settings." The focus of this model includes using residential facilities that means that recipients must travel to find help. Residential services range from long-term confinement or therapy like farming or doing daily chores. New admits and long-term clients may receive psychotropic medication and electroconvulsive shock therapy (ECT); few patients receive traditional **psychotherapy**.

The second model is a public health approach to services where prevention and training volunteers or paraprofessionals is emphasized. Patients are helped outside a residential setting using consultation with family and education of the patient and the family and other community resources.

Because the Western models have not worked well in developing countries, the village system has emerged as a viable option to treatment for those with mental illness. It uses native healers, therapeutic relationships, psychotropic drugs, and the natural therapeutic elements of the village, which include confession, dancing, and rituals.

Source: Adapted from "Culture and Mental Services," by Howard N. Higginbotham. In Anthony J. Marsella, Roland G. Tharp, and Thomas Ciborowski (Eds.), *Perspectives on Cross-Cultural Psychology*, pp. 205–236. Copyright 1979 by Academic Press.

corrections," but punishment continued to be the reality. Structurally, the system already included parole, probation, and the indeterminate sentence. All that remained to complete the incorporation of the medical model was the addition of a classification system to aid in diagnosis and treatment (Clear et al., 2012).

HISTORY

As mentioned in Chapter 2, institutions developed as a way to meet the needs of some segments of society. Asylums were established primarily to care for people with mental illness, shifting care from the local community to rural institutions and replacing local financing with state funding. Responsibility for the care of people with mental illness rested with the medical profession.

Psychiatry emerged as a discipline at the end of the 18th century when Philippe Pinel became head of the Hospice de Bicêtre and later of Salpêtrière (mental institutions in France). Some mental disorders had been recognized as such early on, but Pinel's removal of chains from patients and other humane acts emphasized the belief that pathological behavioral disorders had organic origins and that their treatment belonged to medicine. Accordingly, those diagnosed as mentally ill were to be treated as patients by physicians in hospital settings, just like other patients with medical problems. Pinel, hoping to create a science of mental disease, is credited with introducing the medical model into psychiatry by stressing clinical diagnosis and appropriate medical treatment. (See Box 4.2.)

Until the end of the 19th century, insanity was socially defined: "An insane was a person whose behavior for pathological reasons was so disturbed that he

---

BOX 4.2 PHILIPPE PINEL

Philippe Pinel (1745–1826) is famous in the history of medicine and mental health. In revolutionary France, Pinel courageously campaigned to secure a new status for persons with mental illness as people suffering from disease rather than being possessed by demons or manifesting the consequences of sin. Pinel argued, practiced, and taught that such persons require medical care rather than persecution or punishment, and that they are entitled to be treated with respect as persons and citizens. This was a revolutionary idea.

In 1792, apparently because of his connections with the Ideologues, Pinel was appointed Physician of the Infirmaries to the Hospice de Bicêtre, a Parisian custodial institution for ailing indigent men.

During this time, Pinel published three significant works: *Philosophical Nosography* (1798), *Treatise on Insanity* (1801), and *Clinical Medicine* (1802). The first book would serve for years as a text for the classification of diseases; the second would lay the foundation for modern psychiatry; and the third, published in three successively enlarged editions, would spread his methodology and fame among the next generation.

In 1794, Pinel transferred to the Hospice de la Salpêtrière, an institution that housed nearly 7,000 destitute women. He administered, practiced, and taught in this hospital for 30 years, applying the principles that gave him the reputation as a founder of modern psychiatry.

With regard to mental health, Pinel is often given credit for what he learned from the uneducated but experienced and successful keeper of the insane at Bicêtre, J. P. Pussin (1746–1811): namely, that the mental patients could be managed without cages, chains, or cruelty. Pinel brought Pussin to Salpêtrière in 1802 to aid him in caring for the many unruly patients. Pinel combined Pussin's practical management principles with his own medical knowledge to develop his famous "moral method" for treating mental illness. This method assumes that mental illness is due to some imbalance in the patient, which the physician can treat and rectify. The crux of this method is extensive observation and knowledge about the patient. This knowledge makes possible detailed therapy, which the physician must carefully supervise. Pinel's approach is radically different from bleeding, beating, purging, and imprisonment, which had been the usual methods of treating the insane.

Pinel's concern for humane treatment of persons with mental illness was realized in France and made that country a world leader in the enlightened treatment of mental illness. When Dorothea Dix traveled in Europe in the late 1850s, extending her great American crusade to reform in the treatment of the insane, she had only small changes to recommend to the French and to the Turks in Constantinople, who had been trained by the French.

Source: Used by permission of H. Phillips Hamlin (2010).

---

had to be segregated in special institutions" (Pichot, 1985, p. 10). With the emergence of psychiatry as a medical specialty, a body of knowledge was established to explain the nature and causes of insanity. The discovery and application of the most effective treatments became a priority. Insanity became medically defined, meaning that the institution of treatment had to be a hospital instead of a prison, and the care of the patient would be handled by a physician, not a warden.

After the middle of the 19th century, use of the medical model to treat mental illness predominated. By the end of the century, however, the medical model was changing. A new school of thought rejected medical treatment and advocated psychotherapy for treatment of people with mental illness. The new philosophy was based on the assumption that diseases of the soul were completely separate from diseases of the body. Psychiatry concerned itself with the medicine of the soul; psychosis was the disease of the soul, and **neurosis** was the disease of the nerves (Pichot, 1985). Sigmund Freud's work reflected this orientation.

Early in his career, Freud was a researcher and clinician in biology and neurology; he made outstanding contributions to both fields. He used the scientific method, insisting that medical problems of mental illness be studied in the rigorous laboratory setting. Later, Freud rejected his earlier training and revolutionized the study and treatment of mental illness. He developed a method of therapy commonly known today as the **psychoanalytic method**. In this method, the clients or patients share all thoughts with the therapist. The therapist interprets this material to explain to patients the nature of their repressions and the influence of these repressions on their present problems. Freud also developed a theory of neurosis and one of the normal mind based on the assumption that mental disorders were psychologically rooted.

Although Freud's impact was profound, psychoanalytic theory did not completely change the medical model or become the preferred method of treatment, for several reasons. First, its success was difficult to evaluate and to document. Second, it required too much time and expense to be a viable treatment for large numbers of people.

The treatment of people with mental illness continued to develop in the 1940s; however, more psychiatrists and improved treatment were needed. A common treatment during this decade was electroconvulsive or **electroshock therapy**. This treatment involved administering an electric shock of 70–130 volts to the brain, leaving the patient unconsciousness or in convulsions. On regaining consciousness, the patient sometimes experienced confusion and memory loss, but problem behaviors diminished after several weeks of treatments. Electroshock therapy was effective with depressed individuals, but it was used less successfully to treat other mental disorders. Its abuse during the 1960s resulted in negative perceptions of this treatment method, and these perceptions contributed to the growing popularity of psychotropic medications.

Psychiatric drugs, which act on the brain, are now among the most widely used treatments for mental disorders. Many human service professionals work with clients taking these medications and need to be knowledgeable about the drugs their clients are taking. The science of the preparation, uses, and effects of drugs is pharmacology. The branch of pharmacology of most interest to human service professionals is **psychopharmacology**, which focuses on "the psychological effects of drugs and the use of drugs to treat symptoms of mental and emotional disorders" (Ingersoll & Rak, 2006, p. 3).

One example of the necessity for knowledge about psychiatric drugs is on-label and off-label prescriptions. On-label means that the drug has been approved by the Food and Drug Administration (FDA) to treat a specific disorder; however, many psychiatric drugs are prescribed off-label. This means that they are not specifically approved by the FDA for a certain disorder. Rather, the medical professional believes, based on case studies and other evidence, that the drug will help the condition or disorder of the client. Neither label guarantees a drug is totally safe or effective for everyone.

Psychiatric medications can be divided into four major categories: antipsychotic drugs, antidepressant drugs, antianxiety drugs, and narcotic pain medications. **Antipsychotic drugs** are effective in managing psychotic disorders such as manic and depressive psychosis, schizophrenia, and schizoaffective disorder. Although these drugs do not cure psychosis, they help to control certain psychotic behaviors such as suspiciousness, hallucinations, and impulsiveness. Terms used to describe the general category of antipsychotic drugs include neuroleptics and psychotropics (Buelow, Hebert, & Buelow, 2000). Stelazine (trifluoperazine), Thorazine (chlorpromazine), Clozaril (clozapine), Zyprexa (olanzapine), and Mellaril (thioridazine) are well-known examples of antipsychotic medication.

Antidepressant drugs, the second category, relieve depression. There are several classes of antidepressant drugs: the tricyclic antidepressants, the monoamine oxidase inhibitors (MAOIs), selective serotonin reuptake inhibitors (SSRIs), and serotonin norepinephrine reuptake inhibitors (SNRIs). Human service professionals will likely come in contact with tricyclic antidepressants such as Elavil (amitriptyline), Sinequan (doxepin), or Tofranil (imipramine). Less frequently, a second class of antidepressant drugs, MAOIs, are generally used only with those who are nonresponsive to other antidepressants. Marplan (isocarboxazid) and Nardil (phenelzine) are in this class. Drugs such as these are often prescribed for patients with decreased appetite, weight loss, lack of interest in people or objects, and a family history of depression. SSRIs such as Prozac (fluoxetine), Paxil (paroxetine), Luvox (fluvoxamine), and Zoloft (sertraline) and SNRIs such as venlafaxine (Effexor) and desvenlafaxine (Pristiq) have become increasingly popular in recent years because of fewer side effects. An example of a miscellaneous antidepressant is Wellbutrin (bupropion).

The most widely used psychiatric medications are the **antianxiety drugs**: *sedatives* and *hypnotics*. Prescribed to relieve anxiety, fear, or tension, these medications may be classed as barbiturates, benzodiazepines, or antihistamines. Benzodiazepines such as Valium (diazepam), Klonopin (clonazepam), Xanax (alprazolam), Tranxene (clorazepate), and Librium (chlordiazepoxide) are especially popular because they reduce anxiety without significantly reducing overall performance.

The final category of psychiatric medications is those used for pain. Chronic back pain, headaches, and chronic pain in the elderly due to cancer or arthritis are examples of diseases that are responsive to traditional pain medications such as acetaminophen (Tylenol) or ibuprofen (Advil). Narcotic analgesics such as codeine, Demerol (meperidine), Oxycontin (oxycodone), and MS Contin (morphine) are in this category. Psychiatric medications have revolutionized mental health by facilitating deinstitutionalization, but the effects have not always been positive. For example, critics say that antianxiety drugs mask symptoms so that individuals avoid dealing with the real problem. Clients who take psychotropic agents over a long period of time may suffer dangerous side effects, such as tardive dyskinesia, a neurological disorder characterized by abnormal, involuntary mouth or tongue movements. Table 4.1 lists other common side effects of the four major categories.

Today, those who deliver services in the medical model face several challenges. One is that the symptom–diagnosis–treatment–cure process more realistically leads to cure *or* control. Particularly with psychiatric illnesses, controlling the symptoms and making the patient functional are the guides for treatment. Complicating this

TABLE 4.1   POSSIBLE SIDE EFFECTS OF PSYCHIATRIC MEDICATIONS

Antipsychotic Drugs	Convulsions
Feeling of heaviness	**Antianxiety Drugs**
Sluggishness	Drug tolerance
Weakness	Stumbling gait
Faintness	Slurred speech
Drowsiness	Drowsiness
Dizziness	Conjunctivitis
Tremors	Dry mouth
Seizures	Constipation
Tardive dyskinesia	Urinary problems
Loss of muscle tone	**Narcotic Pain Medications**
Tricyclic Antidepressants	Euphoria
Dry mouth	Drowsiness
Blurred vision	Mental confusion
Constipation	Nausea
Urinary retention	Vomiting
Lowered or raised blood pressure	Constipation
Agitation	Sedation
Raised temperature	Lowered blood pressure
Hallucinations	

issue are the numerous new drugs that appear with increasing frequency. There are now many drugs that do not fit neatly into the four categories of psychotropic drugs just described.

Human service professionals need not be experts in psychiatric medications, but there are reasons they should be familiar with them. It is often the case that a human service professional may have more regular contact with a client than the prescribing physician and therefore be more aware of any problems, side effects, or break-through symptoms. In some cases, the human service professional may even act as the liaison between clients and physicians. The role of educator may also fall to the human service professional. Since physicians often have a limited amount of time with a patient, explanations of how medications work, the importance of complying with the regimen, and increasing awareness of side effects may be information the human service professional can offer to the client (Shawcross, 2012).

As you can see, the subject of psychiatric medications is a complex one, and helping professionals may often feel like they are reading or speaking a foreign language. It is the responsibility of the human service professional to know about psychiatric medications, their use, and their side effects. Consulting the *Physicians Desk Reference* (PDR), the *DSM-5*, and other medical guides is always good practice.

INTERNET EXERCISE

See this text's website at *www.cengagebrain.com* for video exercises. Choose Chapter 4, then Videos.

Dr. Glenn Farr, a professor and a pharmacist, discusses the role of psychotropic medications in human service delivery. Watch Dr. Farr, then answer the following questions.

1. *According to Dr. Farr, why does the human service professional need to know about pharmacology?*
2. *What is the role of drugs in our culture and in the human service profession?*
3. *Relate Dr. Farr's presentation to the three models of service delivery.*

A second challenge is determining who controls medical services. Is it the physician, the patient, insurers or managed-care organizations, employers, or the government? To varying degrees, all seem to have a role. For example, the intrusions of government become greater each year. Although it is sometimes difficult medically to separate the organic and psychiatric states, it has happened at some state government levels; that is, diagnosis and reimbursement guidelines have differentiated physical and mental conditions. A second example is the impact of managed care discussed in Chapter 2. Typically, in a managed system, physicians receive a fixed amount per patient to take care of medical problems. A small part of the capitation fee is for behavioral health care. Once again, physicians are faced with an arbitrary separation between physical and psychiatric conditions. They also grapple daily with wanting to do the right thing but at the same time contain costs. Achieving this balance is difficult when physicians attend to the "whole" patient, which includes a consideration of the patient's environment and social circumstances. In some instances, physicians have lost their right to choose which drugs to prescribe because managed-care staff overrule their recommendations in favor of less expensive medicines.

The past 30 years have demystified psychiatric illness and made its acceptance widespread. The future may include new perspectives. One perspective may be an awareness that we treat mild disease too aggressively. A second perspective is that in some cases it is society that is malfunctional, not the individual—that is, society places people in situations that are not normal but expects them not to behave abnormally. For example, think about the "malfunctional" mother who has a full-time job as well as responsibility for the home and the children. The problem may not be that she is malfunctional but that society's expectations are unrealistic. See Table 4.2.

BOX 4.3	EXPLORING THE WEB FOR MORE INFORMATION

Learn more about psychiatric medications using search terms such as "psychiatric medications," "mental health medications," and "NIMH mental health medications."

Descriptions, diagnoses, and treatment and research findings are provided for the most common mental disorders. These sites provide an extensive list of psychotropic medications, their descriptions, indications, contraindications, warnings, adverse effects, dosage, and research findings.

TABLE 4.2   SUMMARY POINTS: HISTORY OF THE MEDICAL MODEL

- Individual is "sick."
- Recipient is called patient.
- In the 18th century, Philippe Pinel removes chains of mentally ill.
- Pinel stresses clinical diagnosis and treatment.
- Psychiatry emerges as a medical specialty.
- Mid-19th-century psychotherapy emerges as treatment.
- Freud develops psychoanalytic method.
- Electric shock is introduced in the 1940s.
- Psychotropic drugs become the most widely used treatments.

CASE STUDIES

One obvious example of the medical model's application to human service problems is its use in treating mental illness. Two illustrative case studies follow. The case of Robert Smith describes the mental illness and treatment of a man in the late 1870s. This narrative not only illustrates the orientation of the medical model but also the attitudes of that time toward mental illness. The case of Ralph Jones represents the use of the medical model over 100 years later. The medical model in the second case reflects the use of prescription medication and other physical treatments for Ralph's illness. In both cases, note that the clients are considered ill and their treatment is based on this diagnosis.

ROBERT SMITH

Robert Smith was the fourth of six children and the third son. His family, third-generation immigrants from England, lived in Philadelphia. Robert was quiet and withdrawn as a child, and while he did the work the family found for him, he was never very energetic in seeking it out.

The Smith family was relatively poor. Their fortunes improved somewhat during the Civil War, when they were able to find employment in the war-related metal industry, but after the war they descended again into poverty.

In his late 20s, Robert began to have episodes of "mania," as a doctor later called it. While still usually quiet and withdrawn, Robert would become violent and aggressive if crossed by members of his family or neighbors or if frustrated by events. These episodes of mania cost him his job, and soon the family was having to watch him all the time. During an episode, he would sometimes attack anyone who tried to communicate with him; when the episode passed, he would again become withdrawn and listless.

When Robert's aggressiveness began to be expressed toward the neighbors as well as toward family members, the family began to seek help for him. They took Robert to physicians, who examined him but did not know what to do for him. By the time he was 32, Robert Smith's behavior had become so distressing that his family was desperate. He had been arrested more than once for destroying property in the neighborhood and threatening neighbors. His family had only barely kept him out of prison. His father took him to the county commission, which, after hearing the testimony of the family and the local sheriff, agreed to send him to the Blockley Almshouse in the fall of 1875. Blockley Almshouse was a huge collection of buildings maintained by the city of Philadelphia for its insane poor. When it was time for Robert to go there, the combined efforts of several family members and neighbors were necessary to overcome his resistance and subdue him.

At first, Robert was kept in the general hospital to recover from the injuries he had received in resisting the move to Blockley. Then he was transferred to a crowded asylum building, where he was nominally under the care of Dr. Isaac Ray, whom he actually never saw except from a distance. Robert had to sleep on a night bed put on the floor in a corridor. When his violent episodes occurred, he was put in a straightjacket, which reduced his ability to attack other patients or attendants. The ward was generally noisy and turbulent. There was little chance for a good night's sleep, nor was there anything much for the patients to do during the day except to excite each other, creating almost continual disturbances.

After a year in Blockley, and weeks in a straightjacket, Robert became less violent and more depressed. Cold-water treatments seemed to reduce his violent episodes while he was in Blockley. His family noticed that he had lost weight and they became worried about his physical health. They found the hospital dreary and depressing, but they were reluctant to have Robert discharged because they were afraid of what he would do outside. They were torn by their desire to get help for him and their concern that conditions at Blockley were unhealthy.

In the fall of 1876, the Smiths decided to move to Albany, New York. Because Robert seemed more manageable, if not better, they decided to take him with them. He made the journey all right, but the new environment seemed to bring on upsetting manic episodes such as those he had had in Philadelphia. Within months, the family was again trying to decide what to do with him.

The business they had joined, begun by Mr. Smith's oldest brother, was modestly successful, so the family's financial resources were improved. When Robert's condition worsened, his family took him to a well-known local physician. After futile attempts to treat Robert, the doctor suggested that they take him to the Lunatic Asylum for the State of New York at Utica. The physician assured them that this asylum was a reputable one, much better than Blockley, and he signed a Certificate of Insanity, which helped them get Robert's admission to the asylum approved by a justice of the court.

In the early summer of 1877, Robert was taken to Utica by his father, uncle, and two older brothers. They traveled by boat, a short distance up the Hudson River, and then west on the Mohawk, a journey of some 150 miles.

The Smiths were impressed and encouraged by the asylum at Utica. They were shown the ward where Robert would stay; it was large, cheerful, and well furnished with large windows. None of the other patients were in straightjacket, and the Smiths were told that Dr. Gray, the superintendent, did not believe in mechanical restraints. Rather, he believed in an organized regimen of treatment that involved engaging the patients' minds and bodies in healthy activities, such as walking, bowling, gardening, and the mechanical arts.

Robert improved somewhat at Utica. The frequency and intensity of his manic episodes decreased, and within a year he was able to go home on a parole of about six months. However, he was never able to remain outside the asylum longer than that because his mania would return and intensify. He spent most of his remaining life in the asylum at Utica and died in 1890 from pneumonia, which he caught after a bout with influenza (Hamlin, 2010).

RALPH JONES

Ralph Jones has had a hard life. The third youngest of seven children, he apparently witnessed the suicide of his natural mother when he was 6. His natural father was either unable or unwilling to keep the family together, and all the children were sent to foster homes and orphanages.

Ralph was adopted at age 10 by a minister and a psychiatric social worker. He had a hard time getting along with them. He began dealing and using drugs when he was about 13 years old, abusing pot, phencyclidine (PCP), acid, and alcohol. He may have become an alcoholic by the age of 16. Ralph says that his adoptive parents were kind to him, but he just could not seem to do what they wanted, and after a while relations between them became very strained. At 16, Ralph was brought to the local youth program at the mental hospital because of his drug problems and violent acting out.

He did not complete high school but managed to get a GED while studying mechanics at a local vocational school and living in a group home. Ralph served 18 months in the army. He was discharged with partial disability, caused by an injury to his left leg which he incurred playing football.

Ralph tends to be violent and lacks self-control when he has been drinking. Because of this behavior, he has lost many different jobs. Once, while drunk, he robbed and assaulted an elderly man in Florida—a crime for which he spent one year in jail. Also, he has been in several accidents, suffering injuries to his head and his back. He complains frequently of back pains.

Within the last five months, Ralph has been in jail twice and also in the state mental hospital. He was jailed on charges of driving while intoxicated. While there, he committed acts that were taken to be suicidal gestures. The first time, he cut his wrists superficially, and the second time, he slashed his throat with a razor blade. Both times, Ralph was brought straight from the jail to the mental hospital. The second incident occurred only three days before his jail term was to be completed.

A case review was undertaken after three weeks at the mental hospital. Admission notes were reviewed: Ralph was unclean, nonverbal, depressed, and lacking in judgment. He claimed to be suffering from alcohol withdrawal at the time of admission. The doctor who admitted him said that Ralph looked "psychotic" at the time.

A number of features of Ralph's situation came out during the case review. During his previous stay at the mental hospital, he had received shock treatments and was heavily sedated most of the time. He was given Thorazine, a tranquilizer used to control psychotic behaviors and calm patients, and another drug to counter the side effects of Thorazine. The two psychiatrists he saw noted that he was uncooperative and lacked understanding of his suicidal, violent, alcoholic, and abusive behavior.

Today his situation remains complex. First, Ralph admits to several suicide attempts or gestures, dating back to when he was 18, but he is not willing to talk about them other than to say that he is depressed all the time. Second, his left leg remains impaired, and he limps as a result. In addition, when the weather is damp, he must use a walker.

Third, Robert has a fiancée, whom he plans to marry within a year. She visits him regularly, dominates communication between him and the staff when she is around, and believes that he would be better off discharged. Also, she reports that he is well behaved, even gregarious, around her family. Ralph has virtually no other social contacts. She has been encouraging him to go to AA meetings and accompanies him when he does attend. In a conversation with a social worker, Ralph said he was afraid that she would press charges for a beating he gave her eight months ago.

Fourth, Ralph's contacts with his siblings and adoptive family have been minimal. He says he would like to live with his adoptive family, but they absolutely refuse to have anything to do with him. He has had no contact with any of his siblings in over two years.

Fifth, Ralph apparently does well at skilled manual work and is only about one term short of completing training as a mechanic at a vocational school. When asked about his plans for the future, he says that he wishes to complete his schooling, get a job, and then get married.

Sixth, he was married in his late teens and fathered two children (ages 7 and 8 now) before getting divorced at age 22. However, it is unknown where this family is and what connection, if any, he has with them.

Finally, it seems clear that Ralph is a depressed, angry person who can be dangerous to himself and others. His antisocial tendencies seem to have been established early in his life, and they are exacerbated by his alcohol problem. It is not at all clear that he has even begun to work through what was perhaps the central trauma of his childhood, his mother's suicide.

Two weeks ago Ralph was discharged and placed in a community halfway house. Ten days later he was readmitted to the mental hospital (three days ago) after he beat his roommate and then slashed his own wrists. The treatment team, composed of a case manager, a nurse, a physician, a social worker, a psychologist, and a teacher, is not sure whether Ralph should be discharged again so that he can pursue the goals he articulates. The team is not convinced that he can handle life outside the hospital. The alcohol problem remains and seems to precipitate actions dangerous to Ralph and others; yet he still has goals, and apparently his fiancée remains supportive. If he were to establish a relationship with someone at a mental health center to secure help for him at his lowest points and if he were to attend AA meetings and stop abusing alcohol, some members of the treatment team believe that he might be able to get his life together and be placed in the community again (Hamlin, 2010).

These case studies describe two treatments of mental illness. As you answer the following questions, you will come to understand better the characteristics of the medical model.

- What problems did Robert Smith face? Ralph Jones?
- What treatments did Robert receive? Ralph?
- Why are these treatments classified as part of the medical model?

THE PUBLIC HEALTH MODEL

DEFINITION

Public health is a concept that is sometimes difficult to define. One challenge is its multidisciplinary nature, which leads to difficulty in understanding it as a whole and defining its operations. We can approach the definition of public health in three ways. The first approach is to define it by examining its historical development, achievements, and health successes. The next section will provide a brief review of this perspective. A second approach is to examine its mission, which is to promote physical and mental health and prevent disease, injury, and disability (National Center for Life Health Statistics, 2008; Public Health in America, 2008). This mission determines its goals. For example, preventing epidemics, protecting against environmental hazards, preventing injuries, and promoting healthy behaviors are among its goals. Because the concept of health changed during the 1800s and 1900s, a third approach to defining public health reflects its dynamism and adaptability. For example, until the past few decades, health has meant the absence of disease and disability. Today, health has a more positive meaning—the capacity to live fully, which entails maintaining the physical, mental, and social reserves for coping with life's circumstances in a way that brings satisfaction.

In recent years, a series of natural disasters have presented new challenges for public health. Throughout the world, typhoons, hurricanes, tornadoes, forest fires, and erupting volcanoes have created havoc for people, governments, transportation, communication, and basic health and safety. In the United States, hurricanes Katrina and Isaac, western wildfires, and midwestern and southern drought areas have required responses on a much larger scale. You can read more about a natural disaster and public health responses in Chapter 4 of *Introduction to Human Services: Cases and Applications*. Another public health challenge facing the United States is obesity. Some even call it a severe public health crisis (Griffin, 2012), particularly its incidence among children. There was a dramatic increase in obesity nationwide from 1990 through 2010. In fact, no state met the goal of *Healthy People 2010* to lower obesity prevalence to 15% (Obesity and Overweight for Professionals, 2012). This is a public health problem because it increases the risk of a number of health conditions, including heart disease, stroke, some cancers, hypertension, and type 2 diabetes. Very simply, eating too much and exercising too little cause obesity so a major response has been educating the public about food choices and physical exercise. Public awareness campaigns offer both information and resources to attack the problem.

The **public health model** bridges the medical and human service models but is more obviously linked with the medical model. Diagnosis and treatment of individuals through the use of medicine and surgery are the core of clinical medicine. Those physicians who are cognizant of social, environmental, and biological factors and see disease as it affects populations have moved toward the public health model.

Public health is sometimes not separable from human welfare. Improving public health means improving education, nutrition, safe food and water supplies, immunization, and maternal and child health. It is particularly difficult to dissociate ill health from poverty.

In conclusion, a number of characteristics of the public health model distinguish it from the other two service delivery models. The public health model, like the medical model, is concerned with individuals who have problems, but it extends the concept of health care beyond the traditional medical model. In the belief that individuals' problems may be linked to other social problems, the public health model serves larger populations rather than just individuals. Societal control is a prime concern of the public health model, as it attempts to solve many of society's social problems. This model approaches social conditions by collecting data from the public and from examining individuals with problems. The public health model applies a multicausal approach to studying the causes or origins of problems and emphasizes **prevention**. The preventive component also distinguishes this model from the medical model. The general aims of the American public health service system include not only a more equal distribution of health care services (as elsewhere) to all segments of the population (including the elderly, people with disabilities, and the impoverished), but also identification of social, nondisease problems and methods of attacking their causes and contributing factors. This is also the case in southern Africa, where HIV continues to spread. Public health efforts focused on prevention combine education about abstinence, condoms, and fidelity. The objective of the public health model is to improve the present and future quality of life and to alleviate health problems that have consequences for society in general.

HISTORY

Communicable diseases, poor sanitation, and lack of medical knowledge have been community health problems since ancient times. During the colonial period in North America, smallpox, yellow fever, and cholera were major health problems. Laws such as the Massachusetts Poor Law of 1692 gave local authorities the power to remove and isolate the afflicted. By the end of the 18th century, establishment of the first dispensaries and the first local boards of health had laid the foundations for voluntary organizations and public health agencies.

In the early 1800s, people migrated from the country to urban areas around burgeoning industrial plants. Severe disease outbreaks resulted from the poor nutrition, overcrowding, filth, and excessive work requirements of the inhabitants living in these slums. Lemuel Shattuck, a Boston city councilman, prepared a report financed by the Massachusetts legislature that presented the first plan for an integrated health program in the United States. The 1850 Shattuck Report in the United States precipitated both a sanitary awakening and social reform that constituted public health at that time (Afifi & Breslow, 1994).

The report declared the need for improved sanitation and disease control in Massachusetts and recommended establishment of state and local boards of health, collection of vital statistics, institution of sanitation programs, and prevention of disease (Shirreffs, 1982). Although widely ignored at the time, Shattuck's report has come to be considered the most farsighted and influential document in the history of the public health system (Committee Study of the Future of Public Health, 1988). By 1868, Massachusetts had established the first state public health department in the country.

The social philosophies of the early 19th century also impacted public health as they reflected two beliefs about disease. The first belief was that disease was providential. Like poverty and natural disasters such as floods, disease occurred as a result of God's wrath toward an individual. Therefore, the obvious solution to the problem was improved behavior. The second belief linked disease to the disorderly and filthy cities with their unpaved streets, poor drainage, untethered animals, and outside privies. Intuitively, people realized the impact of environmental factors on disease. Many believed that the solution was to eliminate dirt and filth to create a healthier environment.

A second important event was the organization in 1861 of the U.S. Sanitary Commission, the first major public health group in America. It is significant to the public health movement because its efforts were primarily preventive; it alerted the public to the benefits of preventive sanitary measures. Appalled by the poor conditions in army camps and hospitals, a group led by Dr. Henry Bellows, Louisa Schuyler, and Dr. Elisha Harris organized this voluntary citizen effort. A central focus of the commission was to unite all voluntary groups to aid governmental agencies in meeting the physical and spiritual needs of men in uniform. Initially, their efforts were directed toward teaching proper personal hygiene and inspecting and supervising living arrangements in camps and field hospitals. Their later efforts included recruiting nurses, distributing supplies, and assisting in communication between soldiers and their families.

Prevention emerged as a major component of the public health movement when Dr. Louis Pasteur and Robert Koch demonstrated that germs—not God or dirt—cause disease. The "golden age of public health" (1890–1910) included the discovery of causes for typhoid, tuberculosis, and cholera. Personal cleanliness, inoculations, serums, and hygienic laws became the basis of reform, and preventive medicine developed beyond research and lab diagnosis. Preventive medicine included a social focus, with well-organized public health education programs. Today, the Public Health Service is part of the Department of Health and Human Services. It focuses on interventions aimed at disease prevention and health promotion that shape a community's overall profile.

Industrialization and its spread around the world during the 19th and 20th centuries stimulated the problems of communicable disease; these were followed by the difficulties that accompanied epidemics of chronic disease—coronary heart disease, cancer, diabetes, and chronic obstructive lung disease. Public health responded to the first set of problems and has made strides toward controlling the second set of problems. A third set of problems that has emerged in the past two decades consists of HIV/AIDS; domestic, school, and street violence; and substance abuse.

Many changes have occurred in public health over the years. In 1789, the Reverend Edward Wigglesworth assessed the health of Americans and produced the first American mortality tables. By 1900, influenza, pneumonia, tuberculosis, and gastrointestinal infections were the main causes of death in the United States. Average life expectancy at birth was 47 years. This last statistic has seen a phenomenal rise, with life expectancy at birth extending to 68 years by 1950, a change attributable to improvements in diet and sanitation and the development of antibiotics and vaccines. By 2009, life expectancy at birth was 78.2 years. Today, leading causes of death are heart disease, cancer, and stroke. Leading causes of death differ by age group: infants, congenital malformations; people 1 to 44 years, unintentional injuries; cancer for adults 45–64; and heart disease for adults 65 and older (Kochanek, Xu, Murphy, et al., 2011).

The Healthy People Initiative, begun in 1979 and reformulated each decade, is the prevention agenda for the United States. It is a national effort to provide a vision for improving the health of all Americans and to guide decisions and actions. Led by the Public Health Service, the initial objectives for 1990 were

---

BOX 4.4   WHAT'S NEW IN *HEALTHY PEOPLE 2020?*

Healthy People 2020 is committed to the vision of a society in which all people live long, healthy lives. This decade, several new features will help make this vision a reality:

- Emphasizing ideas of health equity that address social determinants of health and promote health across all stages of life.
- Replacing the traditional print publication with an interactive website as the main vehicle for dissemination.

- Maintaining a website that allows users to tailor information to their needs and explore evidence-based resources for implementation.

Healthy People 2020. (November 2010). Washington, DC: U.S. Department of Health and Human Services, Office of Disease Prevention and Health Promotion, ODPHP Publication No. BO132.

TABLE 4.3   SUMMARY POINTS: HISTORY OF THE PUBLIC HEALTH MODEL

- The model fulfills society's interest in assuring healthy conditions.
- Massachusetts Poor Law of 1692 empowered governments to act to promote healthy conditions.
- Local boards of health were established by the end of the 18th century.
- English Public Health Act of 1848 was passed.
- Shattuck (1842) and Chadwick (1850) reports apprised citizens of public health problems.
- The U.S. Sanitary Commission was established in 1861.
- Massachusetts established the first state public health department in 1868.
- By the 1900s, public health adopted a social focus.
- In 1979, the Healthy People Initiative was established.
- The objectives of *Healthy People 2020* were released in 2010.

established in 1980 and expanded for 2000 to include topics such as HIV infection and cancer. The focus areas for *Healthy People 2010* included chronic kidney disease, disability and secondary conditions, health communication, medical product safety, respiratory diseases, and vision and hearing. *Healthy People 2020* was released in 2010. Features of the new set of goals and objectives are summarized in Box 4.4. You can follow its progress at HealthyPeople.gov on the Internet. To access this information use the search term "Healthy People 2020."

The major challenge has been to shift the national emphasis to prevention, with some of the following successes. Since the 1970s, stroke death rates have declined by 58% and coronary heart disease death rates have declined by 49%; a 32% decline in the death rate from car crashes is attributed to the increased use of safety restraints. Unfortunately, cases of AIDS, tuberculosis, asthma, and birth defects have increased.

The Internet has also greatly influenced health care. Health information has proliferated so rapidly that no one knows for certain how many health websites exist. This type of information can be a powerful tool in coping with diseases or maintaining one's health, but oftentimes fast and easy access does not equal accuracy of information. Knowing who disseminates the information, checking for frequent updates, and looking for conformity to the Health on the New Foundation's Code of Conduct (HON Code) are clues to the accuracy of information. See Table 4.3.

CASE STUDIES

The following case study illustrates historical problems that are the primary focus of the public health model. It tells of Sean O'Reilly, who lived in the 1850s in New York City. The study illustrates the living conditions that called attention to public health concerns in America. Especially in larger cities, the problems of immigrants living in poverty greatly challenged public health professionals. The second case study illustrates a major public health effort today.

SEAN O'REILLY

Sean O'Reilly, age 25, was the first member of his family to emigrate from Ireland to America. He joined the great numbers of Irish who came to America in the wake of the potato blight that devastated Ireland in the middle of the 1840s. His journey, in a wooden sailing vessel from Liverpool, took 40 days. The voyage was very difficult. Like most poor immigrants, he traveled in steerage, a lower deck below the water line, reserved for third-class passengers. The space was 4–6 feet high and lined with two berths of wooden bunks. The floor was crowded with baggage, water, and cord wood. The only fresh air for the steerage area came from the hole in the deck for the hatchway.

After the six-week crossing, Sean emerged from steerage looking pale, weak, and 20 pounds lighter than when he started. He had not succumbed to cholera or dysentery, as had several other passengers. The starvation, filth, and crowded conditions he had encountered during the passage to America were just a continuation of the hardships he had experienced in Ireland, which had driven him to emigrate.

The ship docked in New York. Even though Sean did not feel well, he was not eligible for medical treatment from the Marine hospital on Staten Island, as he did not have a communicable disease. Nor did he have enough money to enter Bellevue, the city hospital. He ignored the "runners" who accosted him on board, trying to get him to travel to other cities for a "small" fee. He left the ship and joined hundreds of other new arrivals, mostly Irish like himself, in search of a place to live and a job.

Although Sean had been a farmer in Ireland, he felt that the land had somehow rejected him. He wanted to stay with other Irishmen, near the sea, so he decided to remain in New York City. Sean found work before he found lodging. The first night, he slept in an alley, and the next day he joined a construction gang, moving earth to build roads in the city. The men he met at work suggested that he live with them in a tenement building that housed other newly arrived Irish immigrants. His first Saturday night in America, he was invited to and attended a "kitchen racquet" (get-acquainted party) organized by the family who lived downstairs.

Shannon Stapleton/Reuters/Corbis

Housing was the most difficult problem Sean faced; laborers' jobs, the sort of work he could do, were plentiful but irregular. Slum lords, who took advantage of immigrants in dire need of housing, crowded families into small, filthy, dimly lit, poorly ventilated tenements situated on narrow, unpaved streets with inadequate drainage. Partly because there was no integrated health program or municipal board of health, the city was disorderly, dirty, and disease ridden.

From the time he landed, Sean became part of the considerable Irish community in New York. He shared two rooms with a family of six. His living conditions never significantly improved. He held several jobs constructing roads, buildings, and sewage ditches. The jobs involved long hours, hazardous working conditions, low wages, and frequent short periods of unemployment.

Any money he made beyond bare living expenses went to the church and to his small account in the Emigrant Industrial Savings Bank of New York. This account enabled him to bring his family to America through the system known as "one bringing another," in which each immigrant worked and saved for a prepaid ticket for the next member of his family to come to America. By the late 1850s, most of Sean's family had joined him in New York.

REMOTE AREA MEDICAL VOLUNTEER CORPS

The Remote Area Medical (RAM) Volunteer Corps is a charitable organization with no paid employees, which uses an airborne force of volunteers dedicated to serving humankind and providing free health care, veterinary services, and technical and educational assistance in remote and rural areas in the United States and around the world. Its history is deeply rooted in the adventuresome nature of its dreamer, designer, and founder, Stan Brock. He lived for many years in the Amazon region of Guyana, South America, where he managed the world's largest tropical ranch. The only medical care was many days' walk away in Georgetown, the nearest city. After ranch owners acquired a small aircraft, he would transport sick or injured people and fly in basic medical necessities. He became a sort of "jungle quack," doing his best to get aid to the rain forest dwellers. When he left there to co-host the "Wild Kingdom" television series, he traveled extensively, still discovering people who were medically helpless all over the world. He vowed that some day he would find a way to take medical care to people who had none.

The vow became reality when RAM was incorporated in March 1985 and subsequently received tax-exempt charity status by the Internal Revenue Service. Since then, there have been as many as 34 yearly expeditions, serving thousands of people and animals on a conservative budget amounting to over $7.5 million. There is a medical record on every person and animal treated.

RAM has used the services of over 3,500 volunteers from throughout the United States, Canada, Europe, and South America. RAM volunteer health care delivery teams consist of physicians and surgeons of all specialties, nurses, dentists, dental assistants, optometrists, opticians, technicians, veterinarians, and administrative and logistical-support personnel who travel to destinations as far away as India or who work here in the United States. Team members pay their own expenses and are asked to procure medicines and other supplies. A team might have as few as 10 members or as many as 40.

RAM teams go only where they are invited. Word of mouth, an expedition nearby, a news article, and often unknown sources familiarize a group or community with its services and frequently generate invitations. The team carefully assesses the area's needs, visits the site, and when appropriate, arranges an expedition. In addition to activity in this country, RAM has programs underway in Guatemala, Haiti, the Dominican Republic, India, and South America. Foreign expeditions can be 10 days to 3 weeks in length, during which team members might treat as many as 4,000 patients.

RAM medical services run the gamut from a basic blood pressure check to full-scale surgery. Operating teams repair cleft lips and palates, remove cataracts, correct eye muscle problems, and perform trauma surgical procedures. Internal medicine, family practice, or emergency specialists provide treatment for skin disorders, intestinal parasites, tropical diseases, and routine ailments and injuries. Dental teams offer emergency extractions and restorative work. Eye care professionals check visual acuity, examine for ocular disease, and dispense free eyeglasses. Thousands of pairs of eyeglasses a year are secured from the Lions Club Eyeglass Recycling program and carried overseas. In this country, RAM's portable optical lab enables skilled technicians to make new glasses to prescription on site. All providers strive to educate patients, their family members, and the community about the basics of oral and physical health, first aid, hygiene, food handling, clean water, animal management, and self-care.

RAM is unique in the scope of services it offers, the frequency with which teams are dispatched, its local and international focus, the variety of destinations selected yearly, and the success of its multifaceted mission. It is truly a relief organization by people of the world for people of the world.

The following questions will help you clarify the role of public health today.

- How do the public health problems in RAM compare with those Sean O'Reilly encountered?
- How do these two case studies illustrate what you have read about the history of the public health model?
- How do the solutions in public health in the 1850s differ from those today?

THE HUMAN SERVICE MODEL

DEFINITION

A primary focus of the human service model is to provide services that help individuals solve their problems. As Table 4.4 shows, this model differs considerably from the medical model and the public health model. According to the human service model, problems are an expected and even necessary part of everyday life. They occur because human existence is a complex process, involving interaction with other individuals, groups, institutions, and the environment. The human service model considers the problem of the individual within the context of the environment. If an individual must be temporarily removed from the environment to provide effective treatment, then treatment within the context of the environment will continue once the individual reenters that environment. In addition, human service professionals work with clients in a culturally sensitive manner, fostering empowerment and self-sufficiency.

Individuals are one of the "clients" or "consumers" of the human service system. Clients can include smaller groups such as families, larger geographic populations such as neighborhoods or communities, and populations having problems in common such as the homeless and substance abusers.

The primary method of treatment or service is **problem solving**, a process focused on the here and now that maximizes the identification and use of client strengths. The first phase, problem identification, is critical to the entire process. Correctly identifying the problem, be it uncontrollable anger, unemployment,

TABLE 4.4 AN OVERVIEW OF THREE MODELS OF SERVICE DELIVERY

	View of the problem	Who is the client?	Who is the worker?	Where does the treatment occur?	Method of treatment	Goal of treatment
Medical	Individual has a physiologically based illness or disease	Individual who receives services is called a patient	Trained professional in health sciences (physician, nurse, dentist, psychiatrist)	Office Institution	Diagnosis Treatment Behavioral prescription Medication Psychoanalysis	Return individual to prior state
Public Health	Individual, groups, and society have disease or illness Environmental and social pressures also contribute to problem	Individuals and special populations or geographic areas (community, neighborhood, state, nation) can be clients	Public health training combines medical knowledge with community action skills	Office Community	Medical diagnosis Prescription Education Mobilization of resources Advocacy for special populations	Prevention Social action
Human Services	"Problems in living" may be internal, environmental, or intrapersonal	Individuals, families, special populations, and environment can be clients	Volunteer Paraprofessional Entry-level human service worker who works with abuse, rehabilitation, education, etc. Professionals (rehabilitation or mental health counselor, social worker, psychologist)	Offices/agencies/institutions serving individuals, families, and children Community	Problem-solving process Strengths identification	Enhance client's well-being and quality of life Teach client problem-solving skills Prevention

chronic tardiness, housing, or substance abuse, for example, focuses the process on resolution. Incorrectly identifying the problem may result in client frustration, the perception of the helper as ineffective, and a continuing problem. For these reasons, human service professionals take time to build a relationship with their clients, fully explore the problem or situation that the client is experiencing, and identify any strengths or resources that the client may have, the context in which they live, and the culture aspects that influences their lives.

Once the problem is accurately identified, client strengths determined, the context described, and the culture understood, some type of intervention may occur. The goal of the intervention varies depending on the problem. Generally, problems occur in one or more of three areas: emotions, thoughts or beliefs, and behaviors. Problems that deal with feelings or emotions such as feeling inferior or lacking self-awareness may respond best to strategies that encourage the verbal and non-verbal expressions of feelings or sensory imaging (Okun & Kantrowitz, 2008). If problems relate to how one thinks, for example solving problems or interpreting situations, then learning coping skills, reframing, or restructuring may be helpful. Violence, a habit like smoking, and self-defeating actions are examples of behavioral problems that may respond to strategies such as reinforcement, contracts, and homework assignments. More complex problems like eating disorders, phobias, and depression may be a combination of all three areas and consequently require an intervention that addresses all areas.

Identifying strengths follows the same process of enumerating emotions, thoughts, or beliefs and behaviors that have helped clients succeed in the past. The client is encouraged to match personal strengths to identified problems as a way of planning interventions. This may be a difficult task for a client whose previous experiences with human services have focused on problems or deficits. In a **strengths-based approach,** the helper encourages the client to think about past problems or situations that were resolved effectively. This approach emphasizes strengths, resources, coping, possibilities, and resilience. In addition, many problems require help with basic needs such as food, housing, and safe living conditions. See Table 4.5.

The problem-solving approach is used in this model for several reasons. First, the process provides a systematic way of thinking about complex situations. Problem identification suggests ways to describe situations in clear, understandable

TABLE 4.5 SUMMARY POINTS: THE PROBLEM-SOLVING PROCESS

- Process focuses on here and now.
- Process begins with problem identification and identifying client strengths.
- Process then moves to decision-making stage.
- Process terminates in implementation.
- Evaluation is important throughout the process.
- Meeting people's needs comprehensively and effectively requires an understanding of the relationship of the "whole person" and (the) environment.
- Meeting the whole person's needs means that the resources of many disciplines should be cooperatively mobilized to meet the needs of the whole person.

terms, encouraging the client and the worker to prioritize the problems that need to be addressed and discouraging impulsive, reactive behaviors. As a part of this approach, **client strengths** focus on the positive rather than deficits, an encouraging approach for clients. Second, the effectiveness of the process can be assessed at each stage. If the worker or the client discovers new information or if the problem or the environment changes, then the process can be revised. Third, clients can learn this problem-solving process and use it themselves when they no longer require services. Clients have the opportunity to improve their own problem-solving skills by working with a human service worker to solve problems and by rehearsing the behaviors under the worker's direction. Fourth, the outcomes of the process support the philosophy of human services by fostering client self-esteem and sense of personal responsibility as clients work successfully through the process. In addition, the results of the process improve the quality of life for the client. Fifth, the approach is a tool for identifying other problems that may occur and determining strategies to prevent future problems.

PHILOSOPHY

In its broadest sense, the philosophy of human services was solidified during the 1940s. It included the following beliefs:

- People had the right to expect their society, through its technology and other resources, to prevent their deprivation and provide for their basic human needs.
- The society, through its government, had the irrevocable responsibility for providing people with adequate human services.

The community health movement, directly related to deinstitutionalization, contributed to the development of a human service model. Community mental health centers often were modeled after other public health efforts. Bringing services to those in need within the framework of community health helped broaden the definitions of care, services, recipients, and goals of intervention. At about the same time the medical field began to recognize the goals of the human service field. The medical profession began stressing patient responsibility for diet, exercise, recreation, and rest. A third factor contributing to the growth of the human service model was the support of President Jimmy Carter who publicized the fact that Americans did not have access to adequate mental health care. This was attributed to residence, gender, race, and age. Carter's understanding of the mental health dilemma reflects the human service philosophy of the 1940s, with its emphasis on both the responsibilities of society and the importance of working with the whole person.

Most authors agree that a model of human service delivery should include the following characteristics or themes (Burger, 2011; Eriksen, 1981; Harris, Maloney, & Rother, 2004; Mehr & Kanwischer, 2010):

1. The **generic focus** is critical in both human service training and delivery.
2. Services should be accessible, comprehensive, and coordinated.
3. The "problem-solving approach" emphasizes the here and now. Included in this approach are the acts of helping the client solve the problem and teaching the client problem-solving skills while building on client strengths.

4. The model works with the person and the environment, taking into consideration the impact of social institutions, social systems, and social problems.

5. Treating the whole person is best accomplished when the worker recognizes client needs in relation to others and to the environment. Interaction and treatment is culturally sensitive.

6. Advocacy is a major focus of this model.

7. Human services is accountable to the consumer. Clients are active participants in the human service model, making decisions, taking action, and accepting responsibility for themselves.

CASE STUDY

The following case study illustrates several concepts you have read about in this chapter. It presents four possible clients who are experiencing problems and who have different perspectives on their problems. This situation also illustrates both the individual and the family as clients. Let us focus first on the human service model of service delivery.

Consider yourself the human service professional who has received the following case. As you read it, think about these questions:

- How have Susan, Ted, Justin, and Matthew solved problems in the past?
- How do you think each person in the case study will define the problems?
- As you consider problem solving as a systematic way of thinking, how would you as a human service professional approach the problems Susan faces?
- Identify any strengths of any of the four individuals that might be helpful in addressing problems.
- Describe the cultural considerations that are important when working with the individuals in the family and with the family unit.
- How will the themes and characteristics of human services guide your work with this case?

SUSAN AND TED

Susan and Ted met in college, where she was studying to be a teacher and he was studying to be an engineer. Ted was from an upper-middle-class family; Susan, from a religious, working-class family. Even while they were dating, Ted was a heavy "social drinker," but Susan ignored his drinking. She wanted to marry a man with a college education and have a large family. She came from a small, close-knit family and had only one sister. She remembered her family as having few luxuries while she was growing up, but much love and nurturance. Ted's family was also small, but not close. Ted had little contact with his family, even though they lived in the same town as the university.

Ted and Susan decided to marry during Ted's senior and Susan's sophomore year. They were living together and talked about a life together. When Susan became pregnant, they talked with both of their families about the pregnancy. Both families saw marriage as the "right thing to do." Susan's family promised to help care for the baby. Ted's family agreed to pay tuition and basic living expenses until Ted graduated. Ted continued in school; Susan dropped out to concentrate on building their home. Her religious tradition placed value on her responsibilities as a wife and mother.

Ted felt he was leaving behind a happy, carefree life without responsibility. He was now beholden to his parents for financial support. He was determined to graduate so he could take his place in the world and earn a decent salary. His dreams did not include children; he saw college and career as a way to enhance his social status and pay for an exciting lifestyle that included fast cars and an active social life. He now faced an uncertain future.

Susan tried to be the "perfect wife" her mother had been. She was determined to work before the baby was born. After the baby was born, she would assume the role of homemaker and mother. Susan and Ted did not discuss their finances together. Susan felt that Ted should assume the role of the financial planner. She was happy to have an allowance for food and other expenses. She deposited her check from work into their account. Ted felt that Susan had no business in the financial affairs. That was a husband's role. In addition, Ted's parents were paying many of their expenses. Susan's small financial contribution did not merit her involvement.

Ted began drinking heavily after they married. His grades were slipping. He did not spend much time at home. When Ted came home he seemed angry. He did not resemble the man Susan married. He threatened to hit her several times. Susan was sure that she must be doing something wrong. She thought her mother was a good wife and she followed her mother's example, so she was lost about what else she could do. She was scared that she might lose Ted if she complained. Ted turned to drugs, and the relationship deteriorated further. Susan was alone and depressed but did not confide in her family, because she did not want to upset them.

Susan knew that Ted was intent on completing school. He was often away for days. As Susan's pregnancy progressed, Ted would come home after class frustrated and angry. He began to hit her. Once, he beat her so badly that he cracked two of her ribs and broke her nose. He also attempted to strangle her. She told no one and lied to her doctor, coworker, and friends about the injuries. Ted "came to his senses" and tried to make amends, but he began drinking heavily once again and in a fit of rage kicked her in the stomach, bringing on labor. Susan delivered a son in the sixth month of her pregnancy. Justin weighed 3 pounds, 2 ounces, and had difficulty breathing. He was placed in an intensive-care nursery for six weeks before his parents could take him home. During this time, Susan worked and Justin continued to be sickly, suffering from chronic ear infections and colic. Ted had trouble adjusting to his new son and refused to help, so Susan quit her job and took care of Justin alone.

Susan worried about the medical bills related to Justin's premature birth and subsequent medical treatments. Anytime she brought up questions about finances, Ted yelled at her, saying she did not trust him to manage that part of their lives. He forbad her to open the mail. She complied; she still could see the stack of letters or bills stacking up on the living room desk. Justin was so sick that she could not go back to work. After Ted graduated Susan hoped that their relationship would improve. Ted took a job at a local company; Susan believed that the job would be less stressful than school and Ted would have fewer pressures.

Justin continued to have many health problems and was constantly under the care of physicians. He was often hospitalized with pneumonia and severe dehydration. When Justin was 14 months old, Ted deserted them. Susan had no money, no job, and no car. She turned to her parents for a small loan and took a job in a department store making minimum wage. She had to work, but it distressed her to leave Justin with her mom. She felt that she should be able to care for her own son. Being a single parent was difficult. By the time she paid the rent, the bills, and the babysitter, there was no money left. She was desperately unhappy but determined to make the best of things.

Several months later, Ted returned. He had a new job making good money and was ready to "work things out." He continued to drink and he still beat her, but she now wanted him at any cost. He soon learned this fact. One year later, Susan had another son, Matthew. At this point, Ted and Susan bought a house and proceeded to raise their family. For Ted, this consisted of nightly bouts with the bottle in front of a television set, long sessions on the computer, and forcing himself sexually on Susan. Whenever Susan thought about leaving, she concluded that her life included two very important aspects: she was financially secure and she was not raising her children alone.

Since Justin and Mathew both needed special services, financial stability was critical. Justin was diagnosed with Asperger's syndrome when he was three. He attended a special day care for two years and now attends elementary school. Justin continues to be in ill health. Just last year he was diagnosed with severe allergies. He has had pneumonia twice in the past year; he was hospitalized three times for various illnesses. Mathew is visually and hearing impaired. Each was diagnosed at his two-year-old pediatric exam. Mathew responded poorly to developmental and physical tests; after subsequent visits to specialists, doctors recommended therapeutic intervention. Every day Susan was grateful for Ted's insurance coverage. Even with the coverage, their medical expenses were about $1,500 a month.

Susan's stability ended the day that Ted announced he had lost his job. He was to pack up his office by the end of the week. He received one month's severance pay. Susan had feared this would be the result of the recent downsizing in many of the local industries. The entire community was feeling the effects of the economic downturn; all she had to do was drive to the neighborhood grocery store to see the devastating effects. Along this route, five houses were for sale on their street; several restaurants, the hardware store, one dress store, and two beauty shops had closed their doors in the last six months. Susan hoped that Ted would be spared. Susan was afraid that Ted would not be able to handle the layoff. She tried to talk with him about next steps in looking for alternate employment and applying for unemployment benefits. Ted's answer was escalating violence and drink. He left a week later.

Susan knows that she needs help. In fact, she is overwhelmed by her problems. She tries to make a list of what issues she faces, but despairs 10 minutes into the activity. She applied for a part-time job and has asked her mom and dad if they could take care of the boys when she is working. She worries about Ted's whereabouts and health. Her connection with him survived such hard times, and, for her, it is difficult to imagine a world without him. And then there are the day-to-day financial pressures that confound her. How will she pay the rent, utility bills, and medical bills? What about food and transportation expenses? Susan wonders who she can turn to for help. What can she do? Where can she go?

As you think about these clients' needs from the human service perspective, you quickly realize that a part-time job and child-care support from Susan's parents solve only immediate problems. The larger problems that Susan, Ted, Justin, and Matthew face are much more complex and will require comprehensive, coordinated service delivery.

You have learned in this chapter that human service professionals use three primary models of service delivery. In taking charge of this case, you will function within the context of the human service model. To promote the well-being of the whole person and to provide the comprehensive services necessary to that end, you may rely on professionals whose service delivery is guided by the public health model or by the medical model. To minimize duplication of services and to promote coordinated service delivery, you need to maintain active links with other professionals who may work with the same clients as you do.

Now that you are familiar with the history of Susan, Ted, Matthew, and Justin, review the problem-solving process. Select one of the individuals in the case study as your client and ask yourself the following questions:

- What is the mindset of this client now?
- What problems and subproblems does the client face?
- How does culture influence the issues?
- What alternatives are possible to solve these problems?
- How would you as the helping professional use the human service model in this case? How would you blend the three models?
- What services might be provided by professionals who practice the medical model, the public health model, or both?
- How can a human service professional facilitate the interaction of all three models in resolving client problems?

Using models is a helpful way of identifying the different approaches to clients' problems. The distinctions among the models are not arbitrary, for each has a separate history and has developed in response to different social needs. From the human service perspective, however, each model has a part in the problem-solving process. The worker is responsible for blending the models, and the treatments or services they represent, in response to client needs. Indeed, one strength of human services is the focus on clients' needs and the flexibility to use approaches from various models to meet those needs.

KEY TERMS

antianxiety drugs	electroshock therapy	prevention	psychopharmacology
antidepressant drugs	generic focus	problem solving	psychotherapy
antipsychotic drugs	human service model	psychiatric drugs	public health model
client	medical model	psychiatry	strengths-based approach
client strengths	neurosis	psychoanalytic method	
consumer	patient		

THINGS TO REMEMBER

1. Three different models represent orientations in service delivery: the medical model, the public health model, and the human service model.

2. Underlying each of the three models is a set of philosophical assumptions that guide the delivery of services and shape beliefs about the causes of problems, their treatment, and the role of the professional in service delivery.

3. The medical model views the person coming for help as a "patient" whose problem is diagnosed as a disease or sickness and treated by a physician or service provider who prescribes a treatment or cure for the "disease."

4. At the turn of the 20th century, Mary Richmond, author of *Social Diagnosis*, used the medical model to describe social casework.

5. Until the end of the 19th century, insanity was socially defined, but when psychiatry emerged as a medical specialty, insanity became a medical label.

6. Psychiatric drugs are now among the most widely used treatments for mental disorders. Psychopharmacology, the study of the effects of drugs on mental health, is an area of interest to human service professionals.
7. The public health model, like the medical model, focuses on individuals and larger populations; it attempts to solve many of society's social problems.
8. Communicable diseases, poor sanitation, and lack of medical knowledge have been primary community health problems since ancient times. Laws such as the Massachusetts Poor Law of 1692 and the Public Health Act of 1848 in Great Britain initiated efforts to improve public health conditions.
9. The U.S. Sanitary Commission was the first major public health group in the United States. Its efforts were primarily preventive, alerting the public to the benefits of preventive sanitary measures.
10. A primary focus of the human service model is to provide services that help individuals solve their problems, including a consideration of client problems and strenghts within the context of their environments.

11. Individuals are among the clients of the human service system, as are small groups, larger geographic populations, populations defined by lifestyle, and populations that have problems in common.
12. The primary method of treatment is problem solving, a process focused on the here and now that encompasses three phases: problem identification, decision making, and problem resolution.
13. Integral to the human service model is a strengths-based approach to client knowledge, skills, and behaviors and includes approaching clients with cultural sensitivity.
14. The human service philosophy emphasizes both the responsibilities of society and the importance of working with the whole person.
15. Advocacy is an important role for the human service professional.
16. Themes characteristic of human service delivery are its generic focus; accessible, integrated services; problem-solving approach; treatment of the whole person; and accountability to the consumer.
17. Using models is a helpful way to identify the different approaches to clients' problems.

Self-Assessment

- Outline the differences among the medical model, the public health model, and the human service model.
- What principles of the medical model and the public health model are present in the human service model?
- Compare the treatment of mental illness in the three service-delivery models.

- List the key factors that contributed to the development of the human service model.
- Describe how the three models might suggest services to address a human service problem such as teen pregnancy.

Want to Know More?

There are several resources you can tap to learn more about mental illness and some of the other concepts introduced in this chapter. Check them out!

Additional Resources: Focus on Mental Illness

Amador, X. (2007) *I am not sick I don't need help.* Peconic, NY: Vida Press.

This highly readable and practical book is written for the families of individuals with mental illness, specifically those who are schizophrenic or bipolar.

Beam, A. (2009). *Gracefully insane: The rise and fall of America's premier mental hospital*. New York: Public Affairs.

"Alumni" of McLean Hospital, one of the most famous, elite, and luxurious mental hospitals in America, include Frederick Law Olmsted, Robert Lowell, Sylvia Plath, James Taylor, and Ray Charles. This biography traces the hospital's history from its founding in 1817 through today as a downsized, downscale institution trying to stay afloat.

Hine, R. V. (2006). *Broken glass: A family's journey through mental illness*. Albuquerque: NM: University of New Mexico Press.

A father shares the story of his family's struggle to keep a daughter with a serious personality disorder on track and functional. Challenges included delusions, medication, and eventually helping her raise her own children.

Kotuiski T. (2006). *Saving Millie: A daughter's story of surviving her mother's schizophrenia*. Madelia, MN: Extraordinary Voices Press.

The author recounts her experiences with her mother to serve as a resource for families dealing with schizophrenia and a broken health care system.

Morey, B., & Mueser, K. T. (2007). *The family intervention guide to mental illness: Recognizing symptoms and getting treatment*. Oakland, CA: New Harbinger Publications.

This reference covers a broad spectrum of concerns and discussions of good steps, bad steps, wish lists, pitfalls, and recipes for success.

Torrey, E. F. (2005). *Surviving manic depression: A manual on bipolar disorder for patients, families, and providers*. New York: Basic Books.

This book provides a guide to living with bipolar disorder—symptoms, treatments, and advocacy.

Whitaker, R. (2011). *Anatomy of an epidemic: Magic bullets, psychiatric drugs, and the astonishing rise of mental illness in America*. New York: Broadway.

The author documents the alarming rise of disability and increasing number of people on Social Security Supplemental Income (SSI) and Social Security Disability Insurance (SSDI) due to mental illness over the last 50 years. He reveals the damage that can, and often does, result from the long-term use of psychotropic drugs.

Case Study

If you would like to learn more about the application of the concepts discussed in Chapter 4, read about the McNeary family in Chapter 4 of *Introduction to Human Services: Cases and Applications*, the companion text to *Introduction to Human Services*. The McNeary family lives in a coastal area that is hit by a hurricane. The case study illustrates what happens to a family and a community when there is a disaster and illustrates the application of the three models of service delivery in a crisis.

REFERENCES

Afifi, A., & Breslow, L. (1994). The maturing paradigm of public health. *Annual Review of Public Health, 15*, 223–235.

Buelow, G., Hebert, S., & Buelow, S. (2000). *Psychotherapist's psychiatric medications: Issues of treatment and referral*. Belmont, CA: Brooks/Cole Thomson.

Burger, W. R. (2011). *Human services in contemporary America* (8th ed.). Pacific Grove, CA: Brooks/Cole.

Clear, T. R., Resig, M. D., & Cole, G. F. (2012). *American corrections*. Belmont, CA: Wadsworth/Thomson.

Committee Study of the Future of Public Health–Institute of Medicine. (1988). *The future of public health*. Washington, DC: National Academy Press.

Eriksen, K. (1981). *Human services today*. Reston, VA: Reston Publishing.

Griffin, R. M. (2012). Obesity epidemic "astronomical." WebMD. Retrieved from http:/www.webmd.com/diet/features/obesity-edpemic-astronomical

Hamlin, P. (2010). *Experiences in mental institutions: Case studies*. Unpublished manuscript.

Harris, H. S., Maloney, D. C., & Rother, F. M. (2004). *Human services: Contemporary issues and trends* (3rd ed.). Boston: Pearson.

Ingersoll, R. E., & Rak, C. F. (2006). *Psycho-pharmacology for helping professionals: An integral exploration*. Belmont, CA: Thomson Brooks/Cole.

Kochanek, K. D., Xu, J. Q., Murphy, S. L. et al. (2011). Deaths: Preliminary data for 2009. *National Vital Statistics Reports 59*(4). Hyattsville, MD: National Center for Health Statistics.

Mehr, J., & Kanwischer, R. (2010). *Human services: Concepts and intervention strategies* (10th ed.). Boston: Allyn & Bacon.

National Center for Life Health Statistics. (2008). *Health, United States, 2008*. Hyattsville, MD: U.S. Government Printing Office.

Obesity and Overweight for Professionals. (2012). Centers for Disease Control. Retrieved from http://www.cdc.gov/obesity/data/adult.html

Okun, B. F., & Kantrowitz, R.E. (2008). *Effective helping: Interviewing and counseling techniques* (7th ed.). Pacific Grove, CA: Brooks/Cole.

Pichot, P. (1985). Remedicalisation of psychiatry. *Psychiatrial Fennica, 16*, 9–17.

Public health in America. (2008). Retrieved from http://www.health.gov/phfunctions/public.htm

Reinhard, S. (1986). Financing long-term health care of the elderly: Dismantling the medical model. *Public Health Nursing, 3*(1), 3–22.

Richmond, M. (1917). *Social diagnosis*. New York: Sage.

Shawcross, L. (July 2012). Client, counselor, pre-scriber. *Counseling Today*, 38–42.

Shirreffs, J. H. (1982). *Community health: Contemporary perspectives*. Englewood Cliffs, NJ: Prentice Hall.

Trattner, W. I. (1999). *From poor law to welfare state: A history of social welfare in America*. New York: Free Press.

Zimbalist, S. E. (1977). *Historic themes and landmarks in social welfare research*. New York: Harper & Row.

CLIENTS AND HELPERS IN HUMAN SERVICES

John Birdsall/The Image Works

Questions to Consider

- What types of problems lead people to human services?
- How do people find help?
- What are helpers like? What are the different ways of categorizing professionals who deliver human services?
- How do human service professionals provide services to those who want or need them?

Part II focuses on the people who are involved in the practice of human services, either as recipients or as service providers. Chapter 5 introduces the client or consumer—who may be an individual, a group, or a population—and gives examples of these different types. The chapter examines how they get help, barriers they encounter, and their perspectives on help.

Chapter 6 shifts to the human service professional, the provider of human services, with an examination of helpers' motivations, values, and characteristics. It also provides an overview of the categories of human service professionals and insights about them. The chapter concludes with a description of the roles and responsibilities of human service professionals.

The primary purpose of Part II is to further refine the definition of human services by considering the individuals who are involved in service delivery. As you read the two chapters in Part II, think about the Questions to Consider.

THE CLIENT

CHAPTER 5

AP Photo/Steve Gates

After reading this chapter, you will be able to:

- Define "the whole person."
- Differentiate among six perspectives of client problems.
- Define "client(s)."
- List the ways people get help.
- Identify the barriers to getting help.
- Summarize the influence of client expectations on the helping process.

The purpose of this chapter is to explore the recipient of human services. This individual may be called a *client*, a *consumer*, or a *customer*. Some consumer groups are concerned with the "client" label because of the stereotype it generates. The term *consumer* is used to emphasize the business nature of the delivery of services. The term *customer* connotes an individual who is actually purchasing the services and the need to be accountable to that individual. The term **client** describes the engagement of a professional in order to get advice and services. For this text, we have elected to use the term *client* since it is most often used in agency settings. Understanding the client is critical to any study of human services. Indeed, the client is the reason there are helpers and a helping process. Part I has already established that some people, in some circumstances, need assistance from others to survive and to develop the ability to help themselves.

In an effort to define the term *client* comprehensively, this chapter introduces several ways of thinking about the user of human services. One way of viewing the client is to study the meaning of the phrase "working with the whole person." This guiding principle in human services focuses on the many components that define an individual and the areas of support a helper must consider when providing assistance.

Describing the problems that clients experience is also an important consideration in defining the client. Problems can be considered in various ways. Several possible theories can be used to define the problems and difficulties that confront individuals. The developmental theory approaches problems from the life-span perspective and defines them in terms of life crises or tasks that occur during a lifetime. The situational perspective describes problems that occur from accidents and other traumatic points in time. Meeting human needs, both physical and psychological, is another approach to explaining the problems that individuals encounter. A wellness model describes a strengths-based approach to understanding experiences. The feminist perspective provides insights into the role of power in the social context. Finally, culture may also be a critical factor in understanding the problems an individual or group experiences and may present challenges to the human service professional to consider its influence. Each of these perspectives is defined and its impact on the delivery of human services is described in this chapter.

The term *client* has many meanings. In some cases, clients are individuals; in others, the client may be a small group such as a family, or even a larger population such as the residents of a geographic area. In this chapter, you will meet several individuals who are clients: Mary, who was hit by a car; two individuals who share first-person accounts as victims of random violence and nonphysical assault; Kisha, a homeless teenager; and a pregnant teenager who is involved in a gang. In the international arena, you will also read about countries in crisis. These accounts will illustrate the concepts introduced in this chapter.

Finally, in defining the client, we explore the experience of getting help from the client's perspective. Sometimes it is difficult for human service professionals who themselves have never been clients to understand thoroughly what it is like to ask for and receive services. We discuss the many ways of getting help, the barriers to be surmounted, clients' expectations, and their evaluation of services.

THE WHOLE PERSON

Clients enter the human service delivery system as individuals with multifaceted perspectives that include psychological, biological, cultural, social, financial, educational, vocational, and spiritual components. These components encompass life experiences such as family, friends, health, school, work, legal status, residence, safety and security, finances, play, well-being, and accomplishments. These perspectives are integrated within the individual to form the **whole person** that the human service professional encounters. During the helping process, the professional is continually aware that the client does not simply represent "a housing issue," "a food-stamp dilemma," or "a child-care consideration." Problems for clients are rarely single issues, and the human service professional should approach each client with the expectation of more than one problem. In fact, one problem can cause, influence, or at the very least be related to other difficulties.

The case of Mary is a good example of how problems in one area influence problems in other areas. The following is from the official record.

> The client, a 38-year-old white female, was involved in an accident while standing on the corner of a busy street in her hometown. She was hit by an automobile driven by a drunk driver. She sustained a severe head injury, a neck injury, and multiple orthopedic injuries at the scene of the accident. She was rushed to the hospital by ambulance and suffered cardiac arrest in route. Her recovery was slow and she was in the hospital for over three months. She was moved to a rehabilitation facility in a town 60 miles away. After three months in rehabilitation, the professionals involved in Mary's staffing indicated that she would need at least six additional months of rehabilitation. She was unable to speak, had limited daily living skills and limited ambulation, and could communicate slowly. The case manager, the team leader of the human service professionals working with Mary, spent time on funding issues. At present, and projected for the future, Mary needed 24-hour support to sustain her activity and her safety. Her husband, Seth, worked in their hometown and visited each day.

The initial concerns for Mary were physical. She sustained multiple injuries and experienced cardiac arrest, so attention to her physical well-being was of primary importance. Once her physical condition stabilized, human service professionals involved with planning and providing her care—using the whole-person perspective—established the following treatment plan that addressed other issues.

> *The Intervention.* Client receives 0.5 hour of occupational therapy 2 days a week. Client receives physical therapy for 1.5 hours per day, 5 days per week or as tolerated. Client has been tested by speech therapist; the test indicated that she does not respond to interaction or treatment.

Mobility. Client is not mobile. This immobility places the client at risk.

Nutrition. Client's usual weight is approximately 130 lbs. Client eats poorly and currently weighs 115 lbs.

Communication. Professionals report the client will not interact with others. The client does not make eye contact. The client does watch television.

Elimination and urination. Client is unable to eliminate and urinate without assistance.

Daily living. Client is able to help with bathing and dressing, but does not appear interested in expanding or improving skills. Client is uninterested in these activities.

Mental health assessment. Client is seen by a psychiatrist once a week. Medications have been used consistently for clinical depression.

Safety. Client needs to be supervised 24 hours, seven days a week.

Social history. Client is married and having difficulty with home visits. The client rejects help from spouse but cannot manage daily living skills. It is difficult for the spouse to visit during the day since he works in a neighboring town. The spouse indicates that there were marital problems before the accident.

Spiritual assessment. The client received visits daily from the hospital chaplain. She talked with Mary each day and visited with her husband a couple of times each week. Mary is a member of a local church that will provide support for her and her family once she returns home. Her husband attends the church on special occasions.

This treatment plan illustrates a multiproblem client who is receiving help in the human service delivery system. Note that, in this case, severe physical problems affect other areas, such as psychological functioning, relationships with family, vocational limitations, spiritual needs, and financial difficulties. Although the financial and vocational are not addressed specifically in the treatment plan, advocates for the client are currently trying to find financial resources for her as she does not have long-term care benefits or home-care benefits. Vocational needs are addressed by recognizing that the client will not be able to work and will need 24-hour supervision or care.

As a human service professional, the critical point to remember is that the client is an individual comprised of psychological, social, economic, educational, vocational, and spiritual dimensions and possibly will have needs in many of those areas. Even if a client appears only to be looking for housing, the helper realizes that the client may possibly have other difficulties such as unemployment, lack of literacy, or a lack of child care. If single problems are solved with little attention to the other difficulties the client is experiencing, then that person may not be able to become self-sufficient.

A majority of clients enter the human service delivery system because they are experiencing problems. Those problems can be defined in many ways.

PERCEPTIONS OF CLIENT PROBLEMS

Problems are a normal part of life. This concept is central to understanding who a client is and what problems the client encounters. As you recall from Chapter 1, the "problems in living" approach, which is basic to our definition of human services, has been a major factor in shaping the human service model (as described in Chapter 4).

DEFINING PROBLEMS

Thinking about problems is one way to understand the concept of "problems in living." Problems usually indicate something exists that is causing the client to experience trouble or discomfort. Usually the act of problem solving is an associated action, indicating that the problems, whether short- or long-term, have solutions or that there are possible ways of addressing them. Problems in living, from the human service perspective, can have two components: a description of the problem and a course of action leading to its resolution. First, the problem is described as a situation, event, or condition that is troublesome for the client. It can be as simple as a married, pregnant 20-year-old's request for information about prenatal care programs or as complex as an unmarried, pregnant 15-year-old's need for counseling. The second component occurs in several stages: The problem is identified and discussed, solutions are formulated and implemented, and the results are evaluated.

One complicating factor in identifying and resolving problems is the difficulty of predicting what an individual will experience as a problem. Factors such as the cultural values of the society and the developmental needs of the individual influence how problems are defined. For example, an increasingly common problem in this society is adult children caring for aging parents and relatives. The extended family that once cared for elderly relatives has been replaced by the smaller nuclear family, a unit whose living space and lifestyle are sometimes not suitable for the care of others. This new generation of caregivers is known as the "sandwich generation." Many of them are caring for children at home while assisting aging relatives with their needs.

Some problems can be addressed and solved while other problems are long-term. For persistent problems, work with clients includes understanding the reality of the situation and assessing how problems might be addressed. For many clients, learning how to live with a difficult situation or management of the challenge becomes the focus of the helping process. Addiction, disability, and grief represent problems clients face that have no easy solution.

How clients view their own situations and what they perceive to be problems are important factors in problem identification. It is possible that individuals lack either the resources or the skills, or both, to solve the problem. It is also possible that the client and the helper may disagree about the client's situation. For example, the helper may believe the client lacks resources or skills, while the client may perceive no problem at all. In the client's **environment**, unemployment, poor school attendance, and lack of literacy may be normal conditions among neighbors and family members. The client experiences these conditions as a way of life, not as situations that must be corrected or problems that need to be solved. The helper, on the other hand, may view these conditions as problems that should be faced and resolved.

Even if clients recognize the existence of problems, there is no guarantee that they will seek assistance. If they do ask themselves whether help will alleviate the problems they have, they may conclude that it will not. They may see the condition as something to be endured, or they may feel that having the difficulty is preferable to seeking assistance.

TABLE 5.1 SUMMARY POINTS: CLIENT PROBLEMS

- It is difficult to predict what an individual will experience as a problem.

- The individual perspective is part of the problem definition.

- A person often lacks resources or skills, or both, to solve problems.

- Some problems may be managed by the client but not solved.

- No guarantee exists that an individual will seek help.

UNDERSTANDING CLIENT PROBLEMS

Despite the difficulties of identification, **problems** are still a useful way to address the identity and needs of the client. It is because individuals have unmet needs that they come in contact with the human service delivery system. The system uses a variety of conceptual frameworks to aid in identifying problems. Various models and strategies exist. This section introduces six ways to think about client situations: (a) developmental and (b) situational problems, (c) hierarchical needs, (d) wellness and strengths-based perspectives, (e) power-related (feminist) perspectives, and (f) environmental influences.

A DEVELOPMENTAL PERSPECTIVE According to developmental theorists, individuals engage in certain tasks or activities at different points in their lives. Describing the **developmental process**, experts in developmental psychology suggest that human development is a continuous process and that there are certain phases and stages that individuals experience during the life span. The development begins at the point of conception and ends at the time of death. During the time between these two points, the individual experiences systemic changes. The change of dependent children into independent adults was studied by Erik H. Erikson, a psychoanalyst and expert in adult development, whose major contribution to the understanding of human development was his description of the "eight stages of man" (Erikson, 1963). Erikson's stage model is one of many perspectives on development. His stages, summarized in the list that follows, reflect the tasks through which individuals work during the different stages.

Basic trust versus basic mistrust. Infants learn to trust in an environment that consistently provides for their needs—that is, one in which the caretaker is sensitive to the needs of the infant. A person who does not experience this warmth and caring in infancy will have difficulty trusting others in later years.

Autonomy versus shame and doubt. In this stage, the toddler wishes to "let go" and try new things but does not know the alternatives and consequences of such actions. The child at this stage needs both urging to try new things and gentle protection from the consequences of his or her lack of experience. A toddler who does not experience such support may later be reluctant to try new things and may doubt his or her abilities.

Initiative versus guilt. The child who moves beyond the stage of autonomy is able to define a task and work to complete it. Initiative means cooperative effort, enthusiasm for new things, and acceptance of responsibility. When a person experiences success at this stage, he or she will generally become an adult who is willing to accept moral responsibility and takes pleasure in developing his or her abilities. A child who does not develop the ability to take initiative becomes an adult who is unable to take risks and meet new challenges.

Industry versus inferiority. In this period of growth, the child begins to experience life as a worker and provider. Receiving instruction and evaluation (in the culture, in school), the child learns to enjoy work and develops good work skills, such as the ability to concentrate and to manipulate the tools of the society. If the child does not develop a sense of being capable, he or she may later have a fear of inadequacy, resulting in poor performance, low expectations, or both.

Identity versus role confusion. In this stage, the adolescent begins to combine the identity formed in the previous stages with the work he or she must accomplish in the future. The stage is complicated by physical growth and sexual maturation. The adolescent rebels against those who previously provided support and relies on peers and heroes and heroines for guidance and care. During this stage, the individual struggles to make sense of an adult world in terms of childhood experiences.

Intimacy versus isolation. The young adult, having formed an identity during the previous stage, desires to establish intimate relationships that may include the components of mutual love, sexual intimacy, and parenting. An inability to establish intimacy with others may result in isolation.

Generativity versus stagnation. The adult assumes the responsibility for "parenting" the next generation, guided by the children's needs, as described for the previous stages. This parenting responsibility is required of all adults, not just those who are biological parents. During this stage, acceptance of this role helps the adult avoid stagnation and loss of purpose.

Ego integrity versus despair. The ego integrity that is possible at this stage represents the culmination of the successful development of identity through the previous seven stages. The older adult understands and accepts life as it has been experienced, assumes responsibility for that life, and accepts death as the final part of the life cycle.

Erikson's stages provide the foundation for thinking about human development, but other theorists have expanded what we know about the life-span perspective for adults. For instance, midlife development is often a complex time as adults face issues such as balancing work and family. During this time, adults perform at their peak in terms of work and relationships, while at the same time they experience crises of identity. Research on midlife confirms that development is varied and difficult to categorize. One aspect of development that influences the helping process is the midlife search for a sense of wholeness and meaning rather than perfection; individuals begin to see their lives within a cultural context and feel they belong to a community. This often leads midlife adults to ask for help. Research on the aging "baby boomers" indicate that the most recent seniors will reflect a new way of aging since they expect to live longer than other generations (Pew Research, 2012). Productivity and health become a focus for the later adult years, and a very positive orientation becomes the focus for many in the later years.

Developmental theorists view life as a process from birth until death, from the beginning to the end. Although everyone goes through the same developmental stages, individuals experience these stages in different ways. Development may be affected by the social context in which the individual lives—the home, family, community, culture, country, and sociopolitical climate. A person's characteristics, including traits, wishes, values, and childhood experiences, may also influence the way that person experiences each stage. Sometimes an individual is deeply focused

---

---

on the tasks of a certain developmental stage, but there are also times of transition between stages, when the tasks are being completed and the individual is only beginning to formulate the questions that will signal the next stage (Upton, 2011).

Using a developmental model to view problems may be helpful to the human service professional because it provides the helper with a basic understanding of the process of growth and change that individuals normally experience. Helpers can use Erikson's stages to help describe problems in terms of current tasks that require the client's focus, as well as to determine whether the previous developmental tasks have been adequately completed.

Human service professionals can also use developmental models to provide a framework for identifying problems not regarded as normal. For example, certain problems associated with mental illness (such as hallucinations and delusions) and with criminal behavior (such as aggressive, violent behavior) are labeled deviant. In any attempt to account for this deviance, Erikson's developmental model is a starting point for identifying whether a problem can be categorized as a problem in living or as a departure from the expected. With clients who have very serious problems not classified as problems in living, it may be necessary to use several problem identification perspectives.

A Situational Perspective Another way of viewing problems in living is from the situational perspective. Problems resulting from accidents, violent crimes, natural disasters, and major changes in life—such as loss of housing, a move, job change, unemployment, or divorce—are all defined as **situational problems**. The characteristics of these problems are very different from those of the developmental problems discussed in the preceding section. First, these problems usually occur because the individual is in a particular place at a particular time. It is difficult for

TABLE 5.2 Summary Points: Erikson's Developmental Perspective

- Individuals engage in certain tasks or activities at different times during their life.
- Stages are experienced differently by each person.
- The social context affects movement through developmental stages.
- Traditional stages are changing as society changes.

individuals to "be in the world" without experiencing some situational problems. Such problems can occur even if the individual has not done anything to contribute to or cause them. In such cases, individual responsibility begins once the situation has occurred and is identified as a problem situation. Linking situational problems with a specific event may be difficult because the event might be only a marker of a more complex situation. For example, with divorce or a geographic move, there are obviously contributing factors that precede the event. However, the problem may still be characterized as situational because of the existence of the marker—a clear problem on which the client and the human service professional can focus.

Another characteristic of situational problems is that they can lead to short-term or long-term difficulties, or both. Most such problems require, at a minimum, immediate action. The complexity and quantity of assistance required depend on the severity of the problem and the state of the client when the situation occurs. Situational problems may require additional help after the short-term assistance has been provided. Yet another characteristic is that individuals experiencing situational problems are often viewed as victims—people who suffer injury from their own fault or that of others. One of the first responsibilities of the helper is to move the client from the role of victim to the status of taking responsibility for personal actions and thoughts.

> I first became involved with human services in January. As a victim of aggravated assault, attempted murder, and mayhem in a case of random violence, my situation was severe. As the result of the assault, I was blinded in my right eye and impaired in my left eye. The first person I saw was my physician, who gave me the prognosis and told me what medical treatment I would need, including surgery. The second person was a hospital administrator, who told me I had no major insurance that would cover my needs and the costs of surgery. The third person I talked to gave me hope. He was a case manager who worked with victims of violent crime. He talked with me for two hours about what legal processes were involved, how to apply for assistance, and who to see in the different agencies. He told me to have faith in the system. And he told me that his job was to help link me to services that I need and then monitor progress.

Violent crime, such as the assault just described, is a situational problem experienced by Americans every day. Problems also include the unreported violence that occurs behind the doors of homes, workplaces, and institutions and the nonphysical assaults that go unreported. The emotional sufferings of these victims can be the most serious result. One explanation for this finding is the damage that occurs after the crime to previously psychologically healthy individuals. After the crime, even healthy individuals are likely to experience depression, anger, shame, and anxiety. They begin to question their previous sense of social order and to redefine their ideas of fairness and justice. Women in particular experience a sharp increase in physical and psychological stress after such victimization, feeling both powerless and helpless. The following account describes the fear and terror that accompanied a nonphysical assault.

> It was an ordinary day like any other, exceptionally cold and dreary. The walk to class was an ordinary walk, exceptionally quick in order to keep warm from the cold. Few people were walking so the pace and the tempo were the only interests keeping me alert. A hand, his hand, dipped to below his belt whereupon he unzipped his pants.

Odd, I thought. In order to keep warm, I kept walking. Not only was he unzipping his pants but he was showing me the most private part of his body. The only tempo I felt now was that of pounding beating inside my chest in sheer and utter panic. I was moved to another place, another time, another element. I panicked. I was terrified. What would he do from here? The ordinary day became a tangled net of confused thoughts, options. Where do I go? Where was he? Where did he go? Was he behind me? Watching me? Would he try to get me, touch me, hurt me? The numbers were all mixed up in my head. They were simple numbers. I know them. The police dispatch woman talked me through the incident quicker than it happened. Sirens, lights flashed, and uniformed men pounced. Safety. Was it safe? Am I safe? Can I move? Breathe? Walk? Think? Was it a dream? Did this just happen to me? The litany of questions confirmed my story as truth. The story was told again. And again. And yet again. The story will be told a fourth time on Tuesday to a judge and then again to an administrative hearing board for the university. My story. Will he be convicted? Will he go to jail? Will he be expelled from this university? He never touched me, yet he scarred me irreparably. The terror and the fear will never escape me. (Willis, 1999)

Differences in behavior, customs, or traditions that are cultural often cause situational problems for people. The behavior or custom in question may be considered normal in one culture but unacceptable in another.

For example, in the United States, it is common for babies to sleep in their own beds when they come home from the hospital. In other parts of the world, especially in Asian, mothers sleep with their babies until they are two or three years of age. East African mothers co-sleep with their babies, feed babies on demand, and attend to the child's needs throughout the day. Immigrant women with different child raising practices negotiate between American culture and their own continually (Mangione, 2011; Natural child column, 2012).

Another situation that creates problems is unemployment. During the economic recession, corporate downsizing, the closing of mills and factories, and the high rate of small-business failures are factors that have made unemployment a situational crisis for many individuals. These new unemployed are finding it difficult to secure jobs comparable to the ones they lost. Their jobs are part-time or temporary; the pay is less than at their previous jobs with fewer benefits and often less job satisfaction. Overall, the affected individuals feel ashamed and unappreciated. In today's context, short- and long-term unemployment remain a problem. The situation also creates economic difficulty that the whole family faces as the chief breadwinner's ability to provide the basics such as food, clothing, and shelter is threatened.

MEETING HUMAN NEEDS Another way of defining human problems is to identify basic human needs and ask, "Which of these are being met and which are not being met?" Abraham Maslow developed a **hierarchy of needs** that is helpful in the problem identification process. Maslow's hierarchy begins with the most basic of physical human needs and ends with the need of individuals to become self-actualized, to strive to develop their understanding of themselves and their environment (see Figure 5.1).

According to Maslow, these needs exist in a hierarchy, which means that individuals cannot address higher-order needs until their most basic needs have been

Copyright © Cengage Learning®

FIGURE 5.1   HIERARCHY OF NEEDS PROPOSED BY MASLOW

TABLE 5.3   SUMMARY POINTS: SITUATIONAL PROBLEMS

- Such situations occur because an individual is in a particular place at a particular time.
- Problems can lead to short- or long-term difficulties or both.
- Experience results in a variety of feelings for the person.
- A person experiencing situational problems is often viewed as a victim.

Copyright © Cengage Learning®

met. If an individual is hungry, cold, scared, or in a life-threatening situation, this person will have difficulty concentrating on love and belonging needs. Likewise, people who get little acceptance or respect from others will have difficulty involving themselves in activities that will lead to self-actualization.

The importance of meeting basic needs is a primary consideration in the case of child abuse and neglect. When children are abused and neglected, many of their basic needs are threatened, including their physical, safety, social, and self-esteem needs. Even though experts agree on the needs that are not being met, they have not always agreed on the way to restore children to a supportive environment (U.S. Department of Health and Human Services, 2009).

During the 1960s and 1970s, the emphasis was on removing the abused or neglected child from the home and placing the child in foster care. During the 1980s, the approach was to leave the child in the home and provide services to parents that helped them better meet their child's needs. Today, the debate continues about whether foster care or family reunification is the best approach to meet the abused or neglected child's basic needs.

On a larger scale, natural disasters such as hurricanes, tornadoes, floods, and earthquakes may result in human needs by many people at the same time. Immediate needs may be physiological, safety, or both (e.g., food, clothing, shelter, and water). When these needs are met, concern shifts to higher-order needs. Moving from a shelter to more permanent housing, returning to school and jobs, and dealing with the longer-term emotional effects of a large-scale disaster will be the focus of many victims.

WELLNESS OR STRENGTHS-BASED PERSPECTIVE   The Greek philosopher Aristotle wrote about wellness in the 5th century BC. Aristotle presented well-being as *eudemonia* or happiness (Garfield, 2012). The Golden Mean or living moderately provided a key guideline for achieving this well-being or wellness. Today, helping approaches such as positive psychology and counseling use the concept of wellness to plan and implement interventions (Myers & Sweeney, 2005; Seligman & Csikszentmihalyi, 2000). The concept of wellness, according to Myers, Sweeney, and Witmer (1995) is:

> A way of life oriented toward optimal health and well-being, in which body, mind, and spirit are integrated by the individual to live life more fully within the human and natural community. Ideally, it is the optimum state of health and well-being that each individual is capable of achieving. (p. 252)

The indivisible self represents a wellness model helpful to understanding clients. It is based upon a holistic and strengths-based approach. Myers and Sweeney (2005) developed an assessment tool to measure individual wellness. For the purposes of this text, we present the concepts that explain their wellness model. The model incorporates three levels of factors to describe the many ways individuals exhibit well-being. The mid-level includes five factors that describe important aspects of human life (Myers & Sweeney, 2005).

The Creative Self   The creative self helps each of us define our unique place or perspective. This uniqueness becomes obvious as we relate to others and as we describe our personal experiences. Five factors, of thinking, emotions, control, work, and positive humor, comprise the Creative Self. This aspect of wellness represents the interrelationship between emotions, physical health, and cognition. In addition, a sense of control over one's life; humor; emotional, cognitive, and physical expression allowing us to retain a positive orientation under adversity; and work provide meaning to individual lives.

The Coping Self   Leisure, stress management, self-worth, and realistic beliefs comprise the coping self. The primary focus of the coping self is to help individuals survive, and in fact thrive, during and through life's challenges. The theorists view leisure as a creative outlet for coping, while a sense of self-worth and assuming realistic beliefs provide a cognitive orientation for mastering difficult situations. Finally stress management, or handling of life's problems, provides the foundation for positive growth and development.

The Social Self   Myers and Sweeney (2005) characterize the social self as relationships and connections with friends and family. Hence, friendship and love are the factors that enhance the value of life and longevity. These two factors counter feelings of alienation, isolation, and separation from others, while providing well-being over the life span.

The Essential Self   The focus of the essential self centers around the search for meaning(s) for individual lives and includes present contributions and legacy. It encompasses meaning. Factors associated with the essential self are spirituality, gender identity, cultural identity, and self-care. While spirituality represents the search for meaning, gender and cultural identity affect the worldview and an individual's perceptions of his or her place. Self-Care includes an active commitment to wellness and well-being and recognizes individual responsibility in making positive choices to achieve meaning.

The Physical Self   For individuals to reach wellness, the physical aspects of the human body need good nutrition and exercise. Both of these factors support present good health and longevity. Next let's look at an additional way to look at client strengths.

DEFINING STRENGTHS   Defining the strengths of clients is an important consideration and is included in assessing the nature of problems. In human services, client strengths refer to the positive characteristics, abilities, and experiences of the client. It is important to understand the nature of the strengths that clients have. This information, paired with an identification of problems they are experiencing, provides the helper with information that can help the client grow and change. The concept of building on strengths can help clients approach their problem areas by using their past successes.

Clients come to the helper with strengths. These represent the activities, characteristics, and achievements of the individuals, families, or communities who need help and support. Usually it takes the professional time to help clients identify past successful behaviors and situations; once identified, the clients can be more hopeful about solving their current problems.

Another positive focus of identifying strengths is asking the clients to take a new perspective on their difficulties. Although it is important to ask, "What brings you here today?" or "Tell me about your current situation," the conversation expands as clients have the opportunity to recall how they have solved problems in the past and what successes they have had at home, at school, in relationships, and at work. Helping clients set an agenda that builds on successes establishes a positive tone to the helping relationship and the work to be done.

There are several ways to apply the indivisible self model of wellness as a way to view individuals and their strengths. Before we describe how to use the wellness and strengths approach to describe the nature of the problems the homeless face, let's look at the prevalence and characteristics of this population. Accurate statistics describing the homeless are difficult to obtain; the very nature of the problem makes counting difficult. In many cases, **homelessness** is a temporary circumstance rather than a permanent condition. It is estimated that 671,000 people are homeless on any given night, and 1.2 to 2 million people experience homelessness during one year. The numbers of homeless continue to increase reflecting the economic downturn (SAMSHA, 2011).

People are homeless for any number of reasons. One is that the technological society in which we live has eliminated many unskilled and semiskilled jobs; the downsizing of many companies, the closing of factories, and the outsourcing of the production of goods to countries with cheaper labor have been the direct cause of job loss. In fact, within the context of the economic recession, employment-related problems such as unemployment and low wages represent the primary reason why individuals become homeless. A second reason is urban renewal or **gentrification,** which many municipal governments promote as a way to revitalize the downtown areas of cities. This movement has brought a decrease in low-cost housing, displacing individuals without providing any alternative affordable homes. The changing structure of the American family has also contributed to the growth of this population. Since the nuclear family is more isolated than in previous generations, such events as divorce and the death of a spouse have forced individuals (and in some cases, whole families) to adapt to a lower level of survival.

Veterans and those with mental health issues receiving community-based services are also vulnerable populations. Families with young children are among the fastest-growing segments of the homeless. Although some are without family and friends, many have relatives or other social ties, but they believe those in their support network would not "take them in" for more than a day or two. Urban schools are struggling to provide educational opportunities for homeless children. The schools are faced with the challenge to educate during a time when children do not have a stable home and do not know where they will be living from day to day. There are also a growing number of teens who are homeless and not living with a parent or older adult.

Children in homeless situations are vulnerable. These children live in poverty and have a higher percentage of risk for domestic abuse, live with one or more parents with substance abuse problems, have developmental delays, and experience mental health problems such as anxiety and depression. They also face barriers to attending school because they may lack transportation, records from previous school, immunization records, and clothing (National Center on Family Homelessness, 2013). The following story illustrates one teen's experience. Kisha became homeless when her parents threw her out of the house with only the clothes on her back.

> Kisha lived in four different places from January until March of last year. Over the years she has lived in a variety of housing that includes a VW bus, a tent, an apartment, a temporary housing shelter, a sleeping bag under a bridge, and a cardboard box in an alley. She has lived alone, with her mom, with her grandmother, with friends, and with a couple of other teens who she met on the streets. She is tired of moving from place to place, but she can't find anyone who will be able to help her for a long period of time. People don't mind helping her out for a while, but then she gets embarrassed that she is staying there and taking charity and sometimes they get tired of her living with them. She has attended three schools in the past four months and she wants a stable home so that she can go to school. She does not want the other teens to know that she has no home.

Now we will look at Kisha in terms of the indivisible self wellness model and a strengths approach. As you answer the following questions about Kisha, you will begin to notice how useful the model is to determine client strengths.

- What are Kisha's strengths related to her creative self?
  - Does she use thinking, emotions, control, work, or positive humor to handle her situation?
- What are Kisha's strengths related to her coping self?
  - Does she use leisure, stress management, self-worth, or realistic beliefs to handle her situation?
- What are Kisha's strengths related to her social self?
  - Does she use friendship or love to handle her situation?

BOX 5.2   INTERNATIONAL FOCUS

Communities in Crisis—Reaching the Vulnerable

The following excerpt illustrates the effects of war, poverty, disasters, and violence on women and children throughout the world. As you read about UNICEF, consider the following questions:

1. What problems do people experience?
2. How are they related to Maslow's hierarchy of needs?
3. What do you think the impact is developmentally and situationally?

Countries in Crisis:

Reaching the Vulnerable

The devastation wrought by emergencies is particularly harsh for children and women. In the last decade alone, more than 2 million children have died as a direct result of armed conflict, and more than three times that number have been permanently disabled or seriously injured. An estimated 20 million children have been forced to flee their homes. More than 1 million children have been orphaned or separated from their families. HIV/AIDS, rampant in war-affected countries, has orphaned more than 13 million children. The majority of displaced persons and refugees are children and women.

UNICEF's mission is to provide special protection for the most disadvantaged children: victims of war, disasters, extreme poverty, all forms of violence and exploitation, and those with disabilities. The human dignity of children and their families is often the first casualty of a crisis. During an emergency UNICEF focuses on meeting the basic needs of women and children as well as protecting their fundamental rights.

Reaching the most vulnerable during humanitarian crises is our greatest challenge. During many emergencies, safe access to vulnerable populations is often delayed because of armed combat, nonexistent roads and bridges, land mines, or weather conditions. Sometimes access is simply denied by those in control. The consequences are usually devastating, leaving entire communities deprived of the most basic assistance and protection. Most of those who die in wartime, for instance, do not die as a direct result of violence but from the loss of basic health services, food, safe water, or adequate sanitation. This is especially true for children. The countries with the highest rates of preventable deaths among children are countries which have experienced protracted periods of armed conflict: India, Nigeria, China, Pakistan, the Democratic Republic of Congo, and Ethiopia.

Discrimination based on ethnicity, gender, health status, or age keeps people from having a voice in decision making. Vulnerability is often exacerbated when war or natural disasters cut people off geographically. These factors—isolation, lack of voice, discrimination—make it imperative that we reach affected children as quickly as possible. Not only must we meet their basic needs, we must also protect their fundamental human rights and take the necessary steps to restore their dignity.

Source: http://www.unicef.org/emerg/index.html

- What are Kisha's strengths related to her essential self?
  - Does she use spirituality, gender identity, cultural identity, or self-care to handle her situation?
- What are Kisha's strengths related to her physical self?
  - Does she use nutrition or exercise to handle her situation?
- Can you summarize the factors that describe Kisha's overall wellness?

To improve your understanding of how human service helpers understand this complex client group—the homeless—think of some homeless people in your community. As this group becomes more numerous and more visible, you may see them sleeping beside buildings or rummaging through garbage cans. Think of an individual you have seen, and describe his or her physical appearance. How old do you think this person is? How do you imagine this person spends an average day? Where in your community does this person stay at night? How might this individual fit into the categories of the homeless as described? Identify five problems that this homeless individual has. Which problems are represented in Maslow's hierarchy? Which problems relate to the strengths model?

ENVIRONMENTAL INFLUENCES   The homeless population also emphasizes the importance of an individual's environment on one's history, living situation, and current problems. Understanding the influences of the environment in which clients exist is another helpful way to understand them. One type of environmental influence could be the results of rapid **societal change** described earlier. Other environmental influences could include specific locations in which a client lives, friends and family who influence the client, groups to which the client belongs, and activities in which the client engages. These dimensions are part of the environment that influences a client's life.

Studying the impact of influences on the client allows the helper to better understand the reality of a situation. With an improved knowledge of the environment, the helper can also assist clients with adaptation to, or alteration of, their environments. Several theorists have contributed to the understanding of how the environment affects the individual. Bronfenbrenner (1979) first presented his ideas concerning influence to explain how children grow and develop. Later, he and others used his theory to explain difficult environmental situations such as child abuse and violence.

One way to consider a client's environment is to think of it in layers (see Figure 5.2). The further the distance the factors are from the individual, the less influence they have. In other words, those factors or individuals closest to the client are considered primary influences, or have a stronger impact than those that are not so close.

The most immediate and earliest influences on individuals as children are family (those who interact with the child), school peers and teachers, day care or child care workers as elsewhere, and social and sports organizations. Family influence includes parent interactions, child care situation, presence of or absence of the mother or father or both, and age and gender of siblings. These are key variables that determine the world of the child. At times, primary influences are complicated by divorce or blended families. Physical characteristics of the environment also contribute a direct influence and can include living space and television, computers, and reading materials.

TABLE 5.4 SUMMARY POINTS: HOMELESSNESS

- Basic survival, security and safety, and recognition and acceptance are needs.
- Homelessness results for a variety of reasons.
- The very nature of homelessness makes a count of the numbers of homeless difficult to obtain.
- Families with young children, dually diagnosed individuals, and teenagers comprise large groups of the homeless.

Global

Social
Institutions

The Family

The
Individual

Copyright © Cengage Learning®

FIGURE 5.2 ENVIRONMENTAL INFLUENCES

A middle layer of influences, or secondary influences, is represented by the neighborhood, social organizations, and faith-based organizations in which the individual is involved. The beliefs, common roles, and norms of the community also exert an influence. For example, the neighborhood may play a significant role in the individual's life, including location (rural, suburban, urban), playmates, sense of community (involved, friendly, or isolated), traffic patterns (quiet or busy streets), and play areas. The interactions within the secondary environment are also influences. For example, a child who lives at home and attends school is influenced by both. A child who is home-schooled experiences different influences.

The factors with the least influence in the life of a child are those such as international, regional, or global changes. For example, children in the 1950s grew up with threats of nuclear holocaust, spending time in school practicing civil-defense drills and stocking community bomb shelters with food and water. Children of the 1960s became part of a well-known rebellious generation, the baby boomers, who both protested and fought in the Vietnam War. Certain factors in this increasingly global environment will help define the children of this new millennium and shape what they believe. Such factors include increased violence in homes, schools, and the workplace; unemployment; migration to the cities; fear of substance abuse and AIDS; threat of terrorism; and environmental issues.

CASE STUDY

This case study helps you understand how to use the concept of environmental influences and defining strengths to think about client problems. Don Regalis is a helping professional working with welfare clients. Notice how he describes Sue Ellen Draper and his work with her.

SUE ELLEN DRAPER

Don Regalis has worked with Sue Ellen Draper, a welfare client, for the past six years. She is classified under the "hardship exemption" rule which means that she may receive benefits longer than the two-year minimum support allowed by the state. Hardship in Sue Ellen's case refers to her documented domestic abuse. Sue Ellen has four girls: Sharon, age 10; Suzie, age 8; and twins, Sarah and Sindy, age 5. Sue Ellen has always lived in this sparsely populated rural county. Welfare has been part of her family history. Her mother, Sarah McCall, raised Sue Ellen and her five brothers, Darin, Donnie, David, Drew, and Doug, on welfare. Sarah's husband lived in the home from time to time. Sarah depended on both welfare and food stamps to feed and clothe the children. For years, with few services available for welfare clients in this small community, Sarah pieced together a living that combined taking in washing, using church donations, and accepting government help to provide for her children.

Don Regalis first met Sue Ellen when her twins were born. She has never been married. Her father threatened to harm her daughter Sharon, so she moved out of the house. Sarah McCall suggested that Sue Ellen apply for assistance.

Throughout the years, Don Regalis has considered environmental factors as important to an understanding of his clients. The following example illustrates how he thinks about Sue Ellen Draper and her environment.

SUE ELLEN DRAPER: THE INDIVIDUAL

- Sue Ellen is of childbearing age, slender, and attractive.
- She is a confident homemaker.
- She lacks assurance to work outside the home.
- She is able to think through difficult issues.
- She excels at accounting tasks.
- She is willing to share her skills.
- She has mechanical aptitude and ability.
- She lives in poverty.

According to Don Regalis, Sue Ellen Draper's environment includes her family, neighborhood, school, and her physical environment.

SUE ELLEN DRAPER: THE FAMILY

- Sue Ellen was the youngest in the family and the only girl.
- Her mother focused on her to the exclusion of her brothers.
- She grew up with a father who was absent most of the time.
- She learned from her family that school was not important.
- She learned that the role of mother and homemaker was important.
- The home she lived in was small.

The larger environment in which Sue Ellen Draper lived also affected her development. Don Regalis believes that the culture of her rural environment has had its influence.

SUE ELLEN DRAPER: THE SOCIAL INSTITUTIONS

- There were strong influences of neighborhood and school, which is where Sue Ellen spent a majority of her time.
- Sarah McCall's work (washing) and gregarious nature established interactions with many of the neighbors.
- She had multiple interactions with her neighbors, since she both worked for and socialized with them.
- Sue Ellen had an active interaction within her neighborhood, helping with her mother's small business, drinking coffee with neighbors in their kitchen, providing meals and recreation space for neighborhood children, and participating in large-group summer play.
- School had the "feel" of the neighborhood.
- Teachers continually associated Sue Ellen with her five older brothers.
- Many were also acquainted with her mother.
- One math teacher, in particular, was especially encouraging to Sue Ellen and two of her brothers.

As he works with her, Don Regalis continues to gain information about Sue Ellen Draper's environment. This information helps him think about the problems she faces and the needs she has.

If you review the notes of Don Regalis, you will see that he has begun to identify several strengths of Sue Ellen Draper and her family. Note that she is described as a confident homemaker, is able to think through difficult situations, excels at accounting tasks, is willing to share her skills, and has mechanical aptitude and ability. One strength that she learned from her family is that homemaking is important. Her neighborhood environment provided her with social opportunities; she has good relationships with her neighbors; and her math teacher has been supportive. Sue Ellen can probably provide Don Regalis with additional information about her strengths. He can help her assess her emotional makeup, behavior, life skills, and other areas of functioning to assess the strengths upon which they can build during problem solving.

THE FEMINIST PERSPECTIVE   This perspective first articulated the political, social, and economic rights of women while challenging the existing power and hierarchy. The charge of feminism was to present views of life and its experiences from a female point of view and to eradicate the domination of men over women. At the foundation, the feminist perspective focused on specific rights such as access to education, property ownership, protection from domestic violence and sexual harassment, and equal pay for equal work.

A focus on the concept of power helps provide a foundation for understanding the feminist perspective. Power is implicit and explicit in human culture. According to sociologists, power and hierarchy occur when individuals become labeled as a group based upon socioeconomic factors. These economic, social, and political dimensions usually result in unequal treatment (Ferrante, 2011). The power aspects of identity are formed within the variables of the group level and the individual level (Sue & Sue, 2013). Although a part of our personal ideas about power and hierarchy stem from individual experience, power is directly related to how society views groups, not individuals. Social stratification carries from one generation to the next. For example, if a culture values the contributions of its elderly members, this honoring may continue over time; likewise, if infant girls have less value than infant boys, the practice of female infanticide may be common practice. In addition, within all cultures, there exist power differentials and dominance and oppression, but salient characteristics that inform the social stratification may vary. In Western culture, male-dominated power structures pervade while in several societies in Asia, Africa, the Americas, and Oceania more equal or female power structures exist (Goettner-Abendroth, 2012). Finally, reliance on power dimensions to define who we are, where we belong, who others are, and where they belong manifests itself in both behaviors and beliefs. What this means for us as helping professionals is our thoughts and values, as well as actions, translate into acts of power and control. Implicit in our professional responsibilities to help others lies a subtle statement about what we "have" and what they "have not."

To use the feminist perspective to understand clients, helpers, and the context in which the help occurs, reread the case study about Sue Ellen Draper. The following questions will help you think about Sue Ellen's case from this viewpoint.

- List the instances where Sue Ellen experiences power, authority, or control.
- List the instances where Sue Ellen does not experience power, authority, or control.
- How could helping grant Sue Ellen power?
- How does helping contribute to Sue Ellen's powerlessness?

CLIENTS AS INDIVIDUALS, GROUPS, AND POPULATIONS

This chapter thus far has presented approaches to identifying problems through understanding human needs. This section examines three ways to think about the term *client*, using a brief client history to illustrate different perspectives about client identity.

In many cases, the client will be an individual. In fact, most of us will think about each of our clients as one person. This means working one on one to define problems, assess possible interventions, and provide services. In the following case history, you will read one person's account of her life. Think about her as your client. As you read, make note of the facts you learn about her and her situation. What are her problems? Using the perspectives discussed in the previous section, apply what you have learned to help you understand her situation.

When I was 12 years old, my mother and her boyfriend left me with my grandmother and never returned. Momma told me they would be gone for the weekend and would pick me up on Monday. That was four years ago. My grandmother tried to do right by me, but she is old and can't get around very well. After Momma left, I was angry, hurt, and sad. How can a mother leave her child and never want to see her again? I managed to finish the school year, but my grades were down and I was absent a lot. The guidance counselor at my school talked to me about the importance of staying in school and working hard. That might be important to kids who have a family, but I was alone. School was just a place for other kids to make fun of me and call my mother names. When kids laughed at me, I wanted to die. I couldn't take it. I started fighting back. I was suspended from school for "consistent and persistent, disruptive behavior." It wasn't my fault that I had to fight. I only went off when kids picked on me or laughed at me. Why am I the one getting suspended?

Over the summer vacation, I met Victor. He was really nice to me. He was in a gang. He told me the gang would protect me from anyone who tried to mess with me. The school couldn't make that promise. Me and Victor started off as friends, but we got closer. I had sex with Victor on my 13th birthday. He said it would be really special. It wasn't. It hurt like hell. Not only that, but I got pregnant. Victor said not to worry, the gang family would be the baby's family. I really didn't want to get involved with the gang, but I felt like I didn't have any choice now with the baby coming. Victor was right about being protected. Once I joined the gang, nobody bothered me or laughed at me anymore. I moved out of my grandmother's house and lived with Victor. I guess Granny didn't care because she never came after me.

Things were good for a while. Soon after I got pregnant, Victor changed. He was distant and not around at night anymore. Even though I was Victor's girlfriend, I had to have sex with all the guys in the gang. Having sex with all the gang bangers in one night is called "pulling a train." They "pulled trains" on me until I got big with the baby. Victor stopped having sex with me, but he said he still loved me and wanted to be with me and the baby. I didn't believe him. I knew he was sleeping with a lot of other girls. I wanted to go home to Granny's but Victor went crazy when I talked about leaving. We had a huge fight. Victor covered my mouth with his hand while he held a knife to my stomach. He cut a "V" on my arm with a knife and said if I left he would do more than "scratch me on the arm" next time.

I didn't have to go to school because I was pregnant. The school sent a teacher to our apartment once a week to help me keep up. I told her she was wasting her time. I didn't want to go back to school, but she came every week. She also made arrangements for me to see a doctor for prenatal care check-ups at the health department. They gave me free food vouchers there to buy cereal, cheese, and milk. Victor liked it when I came home with the food vouchers. He used them to get weed. That was OK with me cause I liked to smoke pot. I was getting high as often as I could. When I was stoned, I could forget about all the shit in my life.

One night I was with Victor at a party. His fellas were getting too wild. They wanted Victor to be the shooter at a drive-by. He didn't have to do it, but I could tell he was not going to back down from a challenge. Victor didn't even say goodbye to me. I somehow knew I would never see him again. None of those guys came back. They shot up the wrong 'hood. The boys they wanted to pop found out they were planning a drive-by and were waiting for them. Victor shot up the crack house but when they tried to drive away, their car crashed into the curb. Before they could turn around, the other guys started shooting up the car. They shot Victor. I don't know how many times. Then they pulled Victor and his crew out of the car and crushed their faces with baseball bats. The police came too late. Victor was dead. I guess I should have been more upset. It really seemed more like a dream.

That was four years ago. I had my baby, but he was very small and sick when he was born. I named him Victor and call him Little Vic. We live in a group home for single teen mothers. I get a lot of help from the houseparents. They take good care of me and my little boy. I go to school here and want to get my GED. Little Vic has something called "developmental delays" and goes to a special school for special needs children. My life is not great but it's getting better.

If we think about clients as individuals, then there are several clients in this situation. The young woman who is sharing her story is a client and is, in fact, currently receiving services to help her with her education, housing, and parenting. Her son, little Victor, is also a client with special needs that may be both physical and mental. He is attending a special school. At some point, Victor, the father, may have been a client, but he is now dead. In any case, these individuals have needs and problems that they are unable to address alone. If they became our clients, we would use the concept of the whole person introduced earlier in this chapter to assess their needs and problems, think about the perspectives previously described that would help us understand their situations and consider ways to access the services that are needed.

Another way to think about this case is to consider a broader definition of client—groups as clients. Examples of such groups may be a couple, a family, or several individuals who share a similar situation or problem. In this case history, we might think of Granny, little Victor, and his mother as a family unit that might be a client. It is also possible to think about Victor's **gang** as a client group that needs human services. If we focus on the gang as a potential client group, then we would need to understand the gang culture, which might include the structure of gangs, the ways of identifying gang members, and why and how children and teens join gangs.

We can also think of larger groups as clients—neighborhoods, cities or counties, problem populations, or geographic regions. In this case history, we might consider gangs as a client group that is a community or a national or societal problem. For example, the United States has seen rapid proliferation of youth gangs since 1980. Their presence is felt in communities in several ways, including their dress, language, colors, and music. Perhaps of greatest concern though is the increase in violence and crime. Assaults and batteries, drug-related crimes, auto thefts, home invasions, drive-by shootings, graffiti, and an increase in truancy and school dropouts are associated with gangs. One response to community needs is the National Youth Gang Center, which is funded by the U.S. Department of Justice's Office of Juvenile Justice and Delinquency Prevention. The center assists state and local jurisdictions in the collection, analysis, and exchange of information on gang-related demographics, legislation, literature, research, and promising program strategies. See Box 5.3 for more information about gangs.

BOX 5.3   EXPLORING THE WEB FOR MORE INFORMATION

Find out more about the Office of Juvenile Justice and Delinquency Prevention on the Internet using "Office of Juvenile Justice and Delinquency Prevention" as a search term.

Please note, as you think about your role as a human service professional, that your work with clients is not restricted to individuals, families, and groups. It may also include others such as your employers and society at large. Human service professionals are employed within a social service delivery system and work for a specific organization or agency. Chapter 8 introduces this work environment and helps you understand your place in it. Society as a client emerges from human service professionals' explicit and implicit commitment to bettering the lives of others on a social scale. For example, a commitment to educate all children or eradicate poverty may guide your work in advocacy, outreach, and mobilizing, roles that are introduced in Chapter 6.

GETTING HELP

Having discussed *what* problems clients face and *who* the clients are, we now address the question of *how* clients get help. The answer is not simply that clients experience problems and then find the appropriate human service agency, because people do not always use the services they need.

Questions that are often raised about the help-seeking process are, "Why don't people use available services? Why don't they ask for what they need if it is not available?" These are questions we continue to ask today. A discussion of the conditions under which clients enter the human service system, the barriers clients experience as they enter the system, and clients' perspectives on human services immediately before and after receiving assistance will provide answers to these questions.

INTERNET EXERCISE

See this text's website at *www.cengagebrain.com* for video exercises. Choose Chapter 5, then Videos.

Lee Ann is a rehabilitation professional who has worked with clients who have mental, physical, and emotional disabilities that are handicaps to employment. In this segment, she describes some of the barriers her clients have encountered during human service delivery. After you watch this segment, answer the following questions.

1. *How do you think human service professionals themselves can become the problem for the client?*
2. *List the barriers Lee Ann discusses.*
3. *How do these barriers affect service delivery?*
4. *What does Lee Ann think the most significant barrier is?*

WAYS OF GETTING HELP

As stated, people do not experience problems and automatically go directly to the appropriate human service agency. Individuals can become involved with the human service delivery system in several ways, including self-referral and referral by other professionals. Clients can also be forced to receive services or can receive services inadvertently as members of a larger population. The Internet has made it possible for clients to find services on their own using search engines and Internet service directories. Social networking also provides access to services.

REFERRAL   **Referral,** a common method of getting help, includes self-referral and referral by others. Those individuals who initiate help themselves may experience a more productive helping relationship than individuals who are forced into a helping situation. Individuals may voluntarily seek assistance from human service agencies because they are desperate and confused. They have experienced a traumatic event or are in a situation so intolerable that they can no longer ignore it. Self-referral typically occurs when clients have tried every way they know to cope, to no avail, and have no other ideas about how to address their problems. Some potential clients have heard about services from their friends and neighbors or through television, radio, or billboard advertising and know exactly what their problem is and where to go. Others in desperate condition stop at the first agency available, regardless of its function, hoping that someone will be able to refer them to the right service.

Another type of referral is from another professional to a human service agency. Ministers, physicians, mental health workers, and other helping professionals often see an individual who needs assistance for problems beyond their expertise. The referring professional first assesses the client's complex situation and then refers this person to one or more additional human service agencies. For such a referral to be successful, the referring professional must help the potential client clarify problems and begin to provide some alternative solutions. (Referral may be one of those solutions.) This action may preempt the next professional's work, but it assures the client that the referring professional is not just "passing the buck." The referring professional should also provide the potential client with as much information as possible about the agency to which the referral has been made. If the client is somewhat reluctant to go to another professional for help, more assistance from the referring professional will increase the probability that the referral will be successful.

INVOLUNTARY PLACEMENT IN THE SYSTEM   Another way of getting into the human service system is to be placed in the system by others. **Involuntary clients**—referred by schools, prisons, courts, marriage counselors, protective services, and the juvenile justice system—are potentially difficult to work with because they have not chosen to receive services. The service to which they are referred usually offers only part of the treatment they are to receive. Their cooperation and participation in that service is often monitored, and decisions about subsequent treatment (including release from treatment) are partially based on their observed attitudes and progress. This creates some pressure on the clients to treat the referral seriously.

One example of the use of involuntary referral of clients is the case of child abuse. The decision to allow a child to remain in, or return to, a home may be contingent on agreement by one or both parents to receive counseling services. For another example, the juvenile court may order involuntary services for first offenders. Depending on the crime and the circumstances, judges often sentence juveniles to receive counseling, to perform tasks in the social services, or to assume other responsibilities related to their crimes. A third example involves individuals

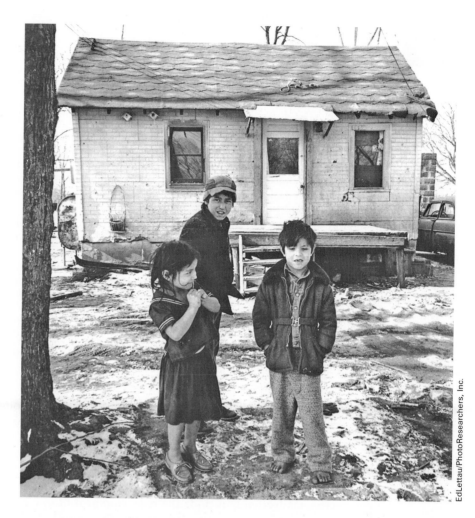

EdLettau/PhotoResearchers, Inc.

incarcerated for crimes. Much of their time in prison is programmed by others, and they have little say over their treatment.

Involuntary clients and voluntary clients may feel very differently about human services. Someone else has decided that the involuntary clients need assistance; they have not admitted that they need help and probably would not have chosen the human services they are receiving if they had decided to seek help on their own. They are often embarrassed or angry that someone else has decided what they need and has sent them to receive the services in question. Since they have not chosen the assistance, they may also feel trapped. Their alternatives are much more limited than those of voluntary clients. If they do not like the treatment or the helper, they may have little ability to change the helping situation.

INADVERTENT SERVICES   Another way of entering the human service system is to be part of a larger population that is targeted for services. In this situation, receipt of services does not depend on the individual's need or ability to qualify for the

---

BOX 5.4   GETTING HELP: *LOCATE SERVICES*

If unsure where to go for help, talk to someone you trust who has experience in mental health—for example, a doctor, nurse, social worker, or religious counselor. Ask their advice on where to seek treatment. If there is a university nearby, its departments of psychiatry or psychology may offer private or sliding-scale fee clinic treatment options. Otherwise, check the Yellow Pages under "mental health," "health," "social services," "suicide prevention," "crisis intervention services," "hotlines," "hospitals," or "physicians" for telephone numbers and addresses. In times of crisis, the emergency room doctor at a hospital may be able to provide temporary help for a mental health problem and will be able to tell you where and how to get further help. Listed next are the types of people and places that will make a referral to, or provide, diagnostic and treatment services.

- Family doctors
- Mental health specialists, such as psychiatrists, psychologists, social workers, or mental health counselors
- Religious leaders or counselors
- Health maintenance organizations
- Community mental health centers
- Hospital psychiatry departments and outpatient clinics
- University- or medical school–affiliated programs
- State hospital outpatient clinics
- Social service agencies
- Private clinics and facilities
- Employee assistance programs
- Local medical or psychiatric societies

Source: The National Institute of Mental Health, 2012. Getting help: Locate services. Retrieved from http://www.nimh.nih .gov/health/topics/depression/men-and-depression/getting-help /additional-resources-for-getting-help.shtml

---

services, and the client does not have to ask for them. Although inadvertent services can often help the client, they also have their limitations. Ideally, before services are provided to a large population, the consumers using the services are consulted. However, some of the clients receiving the services may not have had any input about the type of service provided or the manner in which it is delivered. In such cases, the services provided may seem useless to the client. Services that clients receive inadvertently include the redevelopment of low-cost housing; neighborhood crime-watch programs; shelters for the homeless, AIDS victims, or the elderly; and emergency help for disaster areas.

Many clients who need help do not receive the services they need, nor do they seek them for a variety of reasons. **Barriers** that clients experience are discussed next, including how they view the problem, the cost of the resources, and the reluctance to use friends as helpers. Reading a description of these barriers may be frustrating, because the problems are presented from the client's point of view, without any discussion of how helpers can overcome such client barriers. We have chosen to separate client barriers from helper responses to retain the focus on the client. Subsequent chapters will provide a human service response to such barriers.

BARRIERS TO SEEKING HELP

In discussing barriers, one of the first factors to consider is how the client views the problem. If the client considers the problem too difficult to solve, too overwhelming to consider, or too embarrassing to admit, then the person is less likely to seek help. Clients who perceive the problem in these ways may consider the process of seeking help a burden or a waste of time. From the client's perspective, the problem cannot be solved even by experts.

If the client is embarrassed at having the problem, seeking help means admitting to others that there is a problem. The very nature of many problems in living involves a reluctance to admit to having problems. Spouses in troubled marriages may be reluctant to talk about their difficulties because parents and significant others have warned them about the trouble this could cause them. Abused children, spouses, and parents keep the abuse quiet because making an accusation would cause great disruption and because they, the abused, feel that the situation is ultimately their fault. Men in this society are less likely to seek help than women experiencing similar problems because men are socialized to solve problems on their own.

Another barrier is the individual's perception of the human service professional. Such helpers are viewed as strangers and experts—two categories that establish immediate barriers for those in need. The helping process requires the individual in need to talk about personal issues and concerns with someone unknown. For many individuals in our society, the stranger evokes distrust and suspicion. The expert commands respect but also fear. The client initially sees the expert as an "accomplished" person who has little in common with individuals who have overwhelming problems. Fears of the stranger and the expert are barriers that prevent individual clients from seeking services and from trusting workers in the initial stages of the helping process.

Cultural factors sometimes prohibit seeking help. In some ethnic groups and in some areas of the country, there is a strong prohibition against sharing problems or concerns with people outside the family. In Appalachia, for example, problems remain within the family, or in some instances, the extended family. For an individual to seek help means embarrassment, ostracism, or both to the individual and the family. For Asian cultures the concept of losing face is important; many individuals do not seek help because they do not want to bring shame to the family. In many cultures the help that is offered is not the help that they need. For example, within the African American culture, religion and spirituality is an important source of help. Often traditional Western ways of helping do not embrace the cultural support of the client.

Three barriers are directly related to available client resources: money to pay for the services, transportation to reach the place of service delivery, and the time and distance involved in traveling to receive the services. For the disabled, architectural barriers may present additional problems. Many clients may be ready and willing to seek assistance but cannot determine a way to surmount the problems of paying for services or of finding time and transportation to receive them. One solution to the inability to pay is to provide services to poorer clients on a realistic sliding scale. Transportation is a difficult problem for rural clients who live miles from the nearest population center. Equally vulnerable are clients who live in smaller cities without mass transportation or in larger cities with expensive mass transportation. Other clients cannot use services because they work long hours or are caring for children or an elderly parent. Unless service hours are extended and family care relief is provided, services may be inaccessible (from the client's perspective) even if they are affordable and nearby. What makes these barriers particularly frustrating for the clients is that they add one more set of problems to an already troubled situation.

The psychological costs of seeking help are also serious barriers. Some clients view help as effecting an immediate loss of their freedom; they fear that helpers will demand changes in their behavior, lifestyle, and work habits. They do not want to lose what little freedom they have. Clients also fear that they will ultimately have to assume responsibility for their problems, and this may frighten them. When clients admit that they need help and seek assistance, they are also afraid that they will be considered inadequate. When a person seeks help, it is a signal to others that the individual cannot solve problems alone and that his or her efforts have failed. To admit such "failure" is very difficult. Sometimes there is considerable pressure from peers not to seek help, especially if the peers see themselves as having a similar problem. Finally, clients resist seeking help because they fear being indebted to a human service worker or agency. Asking for and receiving help means giving the worker the power of a caregiver. Clients feel pressed to live up to the worker's expectations, and they fear disappointing the worker if little or no change takes place in their lives.

BARRIERS TO FRIENDS AS HELPERS   The barriers are very real to individuals who are experiencing problems in living and choose not to seek help. Besides being reluctant to seek the help of professional workers, such individuals often hesitate to seek out informal help from family and friends. This reluctance stems from their own fears and fear of the reactions of others. Some of the barriers to seeking help from significant others are similar to the barriers to seeking professional services. Telling friends about their problems may cause a loss of face; reputations and good appearances may suffer if others know about the problems. People want others to think well of them. It is a common worry that once others know about their problems, then they will lose friendships or respect. People also fear that the disclosure will be a burden to those who have been told—that the problems might upset the listener or place him or her in an uncomfortable situation. To impose on friends might violate the "rules" of the friendship.

TABLE 5.5   SUMMARY POINTS: BARRIERS TO HELP

- Client's perspective of the situation
- Embarrassment
- Reluctance to admit to having a problem
- Perceptions of the helper
- Cultural factors
- Cost of services
- Transportation
- Time
- Fear

Another reason individuals do not ask their friends for help is that they do not find them helpful. Many friends do not know how to respond appropriately, offering only advice, authoritarian "shoulds," and clichés. Many friends also cannot be trusted. What the individual experiencing problems considers confidential may be considered public information by the friend. Most potential clients do not want their problems to be common knowledge in their own environment.

THE RELUCTANT CLIENT   **Reluctance,** in its many forms, may have its positive characteristics, although many experienced helpers believe that establishing a bond with a client is easier if the client wants and seeks help. Client reluctance is to be respected. Reluctance is often self-protective, designed to maintain personal integrity. Part of the helping process requires clients to admit there is a problem, to share information about themselves and their environment, and to engage with the helper to change their behaviors and then evaluate the change. This process requires an inner strength that potential clients may lack at the beginning of the process.

THE CLIENT'S PERSPECTIVE

People often decide to use the human service system with preconceived ideas or expectations about what will happen. Sometimes their expectations are confirmed; other times, they lead to misunderstandings. One reason client expectations are important is the emphasis many agencies and helping professionals place on client satisfaction.

CLIENT EXPECTATIONS

To understand clients, we must know what each expects from both the human service system and the service professional and how each person perceives that same system after receiving help. Today's clients are focusing more than ever on the

---

| BOX 5.5 | GETTING HELP |

One Client's Perspective

I needed help, and I had mixed feelings. I felt guilty needing help. It probably had something to do with the way I was raised. If you're strong enough, you shouldn't be having emotional problems. The barriers to getting help were mostly internal. I didn't feel like it was okay to be as angry or depressed as I was. I felt I should just snap out of it. There's a family history of breakdowns. I really don't know if it's hereditary. Some people thought that was an excuse.

I had one doctor who put me on so many medications I gained weight until I weighed over 200 pounds, which was just making me more depressed. I had to go for a physical, and the doctor said one of those medications shouldn't even be mixed with the others. That added to the depression, so I took myself off everything and I lay down to die. And my husband would have allowed it. It seemed like the depression was in cycles, too. I'd be depressed and I'd want to die, and then I'd get angry. When I got angry the last time, I was the one who called the doctor and said I needed help.

quality of care they will receive. The following discussion of client perceptions before and after receiving services is based on the results of several studies of client perception of the juvenile justice system, family services, protective services, and services to unmarried mothers. Although the information was collected from clients requiring different services, the results are surprisingly similar.

First, many clients imagine that the helper will have an unbiased attitude toward them and will have experience in working with the problems they are experiencing. The helper will understand the problems because he or she will have the client's point of view. Clients might also expect the helper to listen, help them decide what to do, and help them do whatever needs to be done. Clients also expect the helper to assist them in dealing directly with the environment.

Clients may also have clear expectations about the helper's behavior. For example, a client may expect the helper to tell him or her what to do. Helping professionals should be able to understand what clients say, provide them with necessary information, and offer an opinion of their own if it differs from the clients' opinions. In other words, the helper is expected to take a very active role in the helping process.

Clients also have ideas about what they expect from the helping process. First, clients want to resolve the problem they are facing, and they may expect quick solutions. Often, results are defined as change—either in themselves or in other people, and these changes are described in concrete terms. For example, a client may identify lack of resources and the need for tangible goods and services as the problems. Clients may also be reluctant to define something as a problem if they think it cannot be resolved.

CLIENT EVALUATIONS OF SERVICES

Clients today are much more sophisticated in the area of client satisfaction. They are acquainted with issues of access and quality of services, and many of them provide feedback to agencies and service providers by filling out satisfaction surveys and questionnaires after they have received services. Because of the current climate of accountability, clients are more vocal about what they expect and what will satisfy them.

Clients' views of services after the process are often consistent with their prior expectations. The most positive outcomes are the practical improvements in their lives, such as better living conditions, food, and clothing, as well as intangible improvements, such as increased self-confidence, assumption of new roles, acquisition of new skills, and solution of their problems in living. Helper activities that may be helpful are the ones that go beyond talking.

Clients often want workers who will help them get something, take them somewhere, talk with someone for them, see someone with them, and refer them. Many clients consider the outcomes of the helping experience to be very positive, view helpers as helpful and fair, and believe that things will be better for them after the service than before the service. Many will also perceive at least some improvement or the potential for improvement in their situations.

BOX 5.6	A CLIENT SPEAKS

About Being a Client

When I chose to be a client, I didn't think there was any hope for me as far as my disease of alcoholism was concerned. I thought that I didn't have a choice, that I would end up one day dying as an alcoholic. And I didn't know anything about AA or about treatment centers. One day I stumbled on this information from another alcoholic who was still practicing his disease, and he told me they had a treatment program for veterans. At that point, I was in school, I was trying to get some education to better myself, and I was sick and tired of trying to fight this disease on my own. I wasn't getting anywhere with it. I might go two or three days, but then the next thing I know I'm back out there again.

When exams came around, I got test anxiety, and just to relieve that pressure I would take a drink, saying to myself, "I'm just gonna take a couple of drinks." But I would drink until I'd get sick. So I called the hospital and they set up an appointment. I really didn't know what to expect when I got there. I was kind of fearful. I thought it was a place where you go to dry out and get back on your feet and then they send you back out. But it was not that way. They educated us about the disease of alcoholism and that people were beginning to accept it as a disease, and that there was hope for the alcoholic. I started to feel a little better, because until then I didn't think there was any hope for me. And I found out that I had a choice. I had a choice to drink, or to go to AA meetings to get help.

About Barriers to Getting Help

I think the biggest barrier was myself. I don't think it's anything out there, because wherever I go, there I am, and I still have those same problems. The world is not gonna change; you can't change other people, places, and things.

About Human Service Professionals

The majority of the helpers are compassionate people and are very understanding. The ones that I find are not understanding are the ones that have not experienced this disease. They don't know what alcoholism is all about. People who have been through alcoholism understand, and they can see through all your cunning, manipulative ways.

About Getting Help

I think the biggest thing for any person seeking help, or anyone who is in an institution, is to break out of the denial stage. I think that is the biggest downfall for everybody, for any client. That was my biggest problem for years. I knew I had a problem, but I would not admit it. I always said, "No, it was just circumstances, I was at the wrong place at the wrong time," or "I just had one beer too many." The key is awareness; today I'm aware of what my downfalls are, and what I need to do to make life better. If you really and truly want to do something about your problem, you have to be totally honest with yourself, because you can't be honest with other people until you start being honest with yourself. In my case, I needed to stop being passive and start being assertive and not letting people control my feelings.

The factors linked to client satisfaction and client dissatisfaction follow.

SATISFACTION

1. Client satisfaction is linked to the client's perceptions of the helper. Specifically, clients are more satisfied with the services they receive if they perceive the helper as having similar values, if the helper accurately perceives their needs, and if they perceive the helper as an expert with experience in the problem area.

2. Clients also want to have a good relationship with their human service professional. For them that means that the helper spends time with them, listens to

their problems, and provides emotional support. This includes being called prior to appointments and receiving follow-up contacts.

3. Clients want to participate in the process of helping, especially if they are long-term clients. They want to have input into the decisions about their treatment. They also base their satisfaction on the amount and accuracy of the information that they receive.
4. Satisfaction is also linked to the helper's ability to solve problems and the amount of change that clients think occurs during the helping process.
5. A supportive environment also makes a positive difference.

Conversely, clients who are dissatisfied can be described as follows:

DISSATISFACTION
1. Dissatisfaction arises when clients want material assistance from the helper, but the helper wants to focus on personal and interpersonal problems. This may lead to a clash between the helper's and the clients' expectations.
2. Receiving unwanted help and advice may lead to dissatisfaction.
3. Clients may experience dissatisfaction when there is a lack of clarity about the problem and what the intervention or plan will be to resolve it.

KEY TERMS

barriers	gang	involuntary clients	situational problems
client	gentrification	problems	societal change
developmental process	hierarchy of needs	referral	whole person
environment	homelessness	reluctance	

THINGS TO REMEMBER

1. The term *client* may refer to an individual, a small group such as a family, or a larger population such as the residents of a geographic area.
2. The definitions of problem suggest that "problems in living" can have two components: a description of the problem and a course of action for resolving the problem.
3. A way of defining human problems is Abraham Maslow's hierarchy of needs, which begins with the most basic of physical human needs and ends with the need of individuals to become self-actualized.
4. A model of wellness or strengths describes how different aspects of an individual—creative, coping, social, essential, and physical—help individuals deal with challenging circumstances.
5. Learning about environmental influences and client strengths provides a way to examine client needs.
6. The feminist or power perspective allows helpers view the constraints and control that clients experience.
7. Individuals can become involved with the human service delivery system in several ways, including self-referral, referral by other professionals, or involuntary placement.
8. Self-referral occurs when individuals have tried every way they know to cope, to no avail, and have no other ideas about how to address their problems.

9. Ministers, physicians, mental health workers, and other helping professionals often see an individual who needs assistance for problems beyond their expertise, and after assessing the client's situation, refer the client to one or more additional human services agencies.

10. Client expectations fall into three categories: to find a cure or straighten out a situation, to define results as change in themselves and change in others, and to describe what changes should occur as concrete rather than general or abstract.

11. From the clients' perspective, positive outcomes are the practical improvements in their lives, such as better living conditions, food and clothing, and intangible improvements, including increased self-confidence, assumption of new roles, acquisition of new skills, and solution of their problems in living.

12. Clients' satisfaction is linked to their perceptions of the helping professional and of the relationship, the helper's ability to solve problems, and the amount of change the clients thought occurred during the helping process.

13. Conversely, clients who expressed dissatisfaction did so because they wanted material assistance from the helper or they received unwanted advice and help.

SELF-ASSESSMENT

- What are the strengths and limitations of the different ways to categorize problems?
- Explain the problems of homelessness based upon the developmental, situational, and human needs perspectives.
- What are the barriers to receiving services and how might a human service professional counter them?
- What are the possible sources of client reluctance?
- What expectations do clients have of human services?

WANT TO KNOW MORE?

There are several resources you can tap to learn more about specific client populations and some of the other concepts introduced in this chapter. Check them out!

Additional Readings: Focus on Clients

Butterworth, D. A., & Wikstrom, P. O. H. (2007). *Adolescent crime: Individual differences and lifestyles*. Canada: Butterworths Books.
    This text explores the results of the Peterborough Youth Study to explore the relationship between individual and contextual factors that influence adolescent crime.

Farrington, P. (2012). *From juvenile delinquency to adult crime: Criminal careers, justice policy, and prevention*. New York: Oxford University Press.
    In this text, the author details the contexts that prevent juvenile offenders from achieving rehabilitation. He provides models of care that could alter this trend.

Garland, S. (2009). *Gangs in the Garden City: How immigration, segregation, and youth violence are changing America's suburbs*. New York: Nation Books.
    In this text, the author details the historical, economic, and cultural influences of increased gang activity in the U.S. suburbs. Vignettes help humanize the gang problem.

Harrison, K. (2003). *Another place at the table*. New York: Tarcher/Penguin.
    This book is Harrison's personal account of foster parenting needy children and providing an emergency care "hotline" for foster children. In addition to abandoned infants, runaway teens, disabled preschoolers, and children with psychiatric problems, Harrison also deals with lawyers, social service providers, and therapists who are involved in the lives of foster children.

Hearn, E., & Milne, M. (2008). *Our new home: Immigrant children speak*. Olympia, WA: Orca Book Publishers.
The authors tell the stories of children from diverse regions of the world who have left their homes and moved to another country.

Hopkins, J. E. (2011). *The broken*. Amazon.com. Retrieved from http://www.amazon.com/Broken-J-E-Hopkins/dp/1460942116/ref=sr_1_10?s=books&ie=UTF8&qid=1350665244&sr=1-10&keywords=foster+care
The author describes the professional and personal life journey of a helping professional committed to treating abused children.

Lahiri, J. (2003). *The namesake: A novel*. Boston: Houghton Mifflin.
This novel is the story of Gogol, a second-generation immigrant who can never quite find his place in the world. His family leaves their tradition-bound life in Calcutta to be transformed into Americans, and Gogol is raised as an American boy.

Morales, A. T., Sheafor, V. W., & Scott, M. E. (2007). *Social work: A profession of many faces*. Boston: Allyn & Bacon.
The focus of this book is the various groups of people who need help, including children, older adults, women, disabled people, and members of minority racial and ethnic groups.

Case Study

If you would like to learn more about the application of the concepts discussed in Chapter 5, read about Alphonse in Chapter 5 of *Introduction to Human Services: Cases and Applications*, the companion text to *Introduction to Human Services*. The case of Alphonse takes you into the world of a teenage gang member. You will read about his life and his interaction with the social service system from his perspective.

REFERENCES

Bronfenbrenner, U. (1979). *The ecology of human development*. Cambridge, MA: Harvard University Press.

Erikson, E. (1963). *Childhood and society*. New York: Norton.

Ferrante, J. (2011). *Seeing sociology*. Pacific Grove, CA: Cengage.

Garfield, J. L. (2012). *Meaning of life: Perspectives from the world's great intellectual traditions*. The Great Courses. Retrieved from http://www.thegreatcourses.com/tgc/courses/course_detail.aspx?cid=4320

Goettner-Abendroth, H. (2012). *Matriarchal societies*. New York: Lang.

Mangione, H. (2011). *Negotiating culture: Immigrant mothers' parenting beliefs*. Retrieved from http://dspace.sunyconnect.suny.edu/bitstream/handle/1951/52177/Heather%20MangioneThesis.pdf?sequence=1

Myers, J. E., & Sweeney, T. J. (2005). The indivisible self: An evidence-based model of wellness. In J. Myers and T. Sweeney (Eds.), *Counseling for wellness: Theory, research, and practice*. Alexandria, VA: American Counseling Association.

Myers, J. E., Sweeney, T. J., & Witmer, J. M. (1995). *The wellness evaluation of lifestyle*. Palo Alto, CA: MindGarden.

National Center on Family Homelessness. (2013). *Home*. Retrieved from http://www.familyhome lessness.org/children.php?p=ts

Natural child column. (2012). *The benefits of sleeping with your baby*. Retrieved from http://www.naturallifemagazine.com/0710/cosleeping.htm

Pew Research. (2012). *Baby boomers retire*. Retrieved from http://pewresearch.org/databank/dailynumber/?NumberID=1150

SAMSHA. (2011). *Current statistics on the prevalence and characteristics of people in the United States experiencing homelessness*. Retrieved from http://homeless.samhsa.gov/ResourceFiles/hrc_factsheet.pdf

Seligman, E. P., & Csikszentmihalyi, M. (2000). Positive psychology: An introduction. *American Psychologist, 55*(1), 5–14.

Sue, D. W., & Sue, D. (2013). *Counseling the culturally diverse*. Hoboken, NJ: John Wiley.

Upton, P. (2011). *Developmental psychology*. Kindle book. Learningmatters.com. Retrieved from http://www.amazon.com/gp/reader/0857252763/ref=sib_dp_kd#reader-link

U.S. Department of Health and Human Services. (2009). *Summary. Child maltreatment: 2007*. Retrieved from http://www.acf.hhs.gov/programs/cb/pubs/cm07/summary.htm

Willis, R. (1999, November). Looking for sense in a senseless crime. *Counseling Today, 16*.

CHAPTER 6

THE HUMAN SERVICE PROFESSIONAL

Rachel Epstein/Photo Edit

After reading this chapter, you will be able to:

- Write a description of the five commonly accepted human service values.
- List four characteristics or qualities of helpers.
- Distinguish among the three categories of helpers.
- Identify the other helping professionals with whom a human service professional may interact.
- List the three areas of job responsibilities for human service professionals.
- Provide examples of the roles included in each of the three areas of professional responsibilities.

Helping means assisting other people to understand, overcome, or cope with problems. The helper is the person who offers this assistance. This chapter's discussion of the motivations for choosing a helping profession, the values and philosophies of helpers, and the special characteristics and traits helpers have assists in establishing an identity for the helper. We also define helpers as human service professionals, as well as introduce other professionals with whom they may interact. An important key to understanding human service professionals is an awareness of the many roles they engage in as they work with their clients and with other professionals.

In this chapter you will meet two human service professionals, Beth Bruce and Carmen Rodriguez. Beth is a counselor at a mental health center and has previous experience working with the elderly and adolescents. Carmen is a case manager at a state human service agency. She has varied responsibilities related to preparing clients for and finding gainful employment.

WHO IS THE HELPER?

In human services, the helper is an individual who assists others. This very broad definition includes professional helpers with extensive training, such as **psychiatrists** and psychologists, as well as those who have little or no training, such as volunteers and other **nonprofessional helpers**. Regardless of the length or intensity of the helper's training, his or her basic focus is to assist clients with their problems and help them help themselves (Chang, Scott, & Decker, 2013; Okun & Kantrowitz, 2008).

The human service professional is a helper who can be described in many different ways. For example, effective helpers are people whose thinking, emotions, and behaviors are integrated (Cochran & Cochran, 2006). Such a helper, believing that each client is a unique individual different from all other clients, will greet each one by name, with a handshake and a smile. Others view a helping person as an individual whose life experiences most closely match those of the person to be helped. The recovering alcoholic working with substance abusers is an example of this perspective. Still another view of the helper, and the one with which you are most familiar from your reading of this text, is the **generalist** human service professional who brings together knowledge and skills from a variety of disciplines to work with the client as a whole person.

Your understanding of the human service professional will become clearer as this section examines the reasons why individuals choose this type of work, the traits and characteristics they share, and the different categories of their actual job functions.

MOTIVATIONS FOR CHOOSING A HELPING PROFESSION

Work is an important part of life in the United States. It is a valued activity that provides many individuals with a sense of identity as well as a livelihood. It is also a means for individuals to experience satisfying relationships with others, under agreeable conditions.

Understanding vocational choice is as complex and difficult a process as actually choosing a vocation. Factors that have been found to influence career choice include individuals' needs, their aptitudes and interests, and their self-concepts. Special personal or social experiences also influence the choice of a career. There have been attempts to establish a relationship between vocational choice and certain factors such as interests, values, and attitudes, but it is generally agreed that no one factor can explain or predict a person's vocational choice. Donald Super, a leader in vocational development theory, believes that the vocational development process is one of implementing a self-concept. This occurs through the interaction of social and individual factors, the opportunity to try various roles, and the perceived amount of approval from peers and supervisors for the roles assumed. There are many other views of this process, but most theorists agree that vocational choice is a developmental process.

How do people choose helping professions as careers? Among the factors that influence career choice are direct work experience, college courses and instructors, and the involvement of friends, acquaintances, or relatives in helping professions. Money or salary is a small concern compared with the goals and functions of the work itself. In other words, for individuals who choose helping as their life's work, the kind of work they will do is more important than the pay they will receive.

There are several reasons why people choose the helping professions. It is important to be aware of these motivations because each may have positive and negative aspects. One primary reason why individuals choose helping professions (and the reason that most will admit) is the desire to help others. To feel worthwhile as a result of contributing to another's growth is exciting; however, helpers must also ask themselves the following questions: To what extent am I meeting my own needs? Even more important, do my needs to feel worthwhile and to be a caring person take precedence over the client's needs?

Related to this primary motivation is the desire for self-exploration. The wish to find out more about themselves as thinking, feeling individuals leads some people to major in psychology, sociology, or human services. This is a positive factor, because these people will most likely be concerned with gaining insights into their own behaviors and improving their knowledge and skills. After employment, it may become a negative factor if the helper's needs for self-exploration or self-development take precedence over the clients' needs. When this happens, either the helper becomes the client and the client the helper, or there are two clients, neither of whose needs are met. This situation can be avoided when the helper is aware that self-exploration is a personal motivation and can be fulfilled more appropriately outside the helping relationship.

Another strong motivation for pursuing a career in helping is the desire to exert control. For those who admit to this motivation, administrative or managerial positions in helping professions are the goal. This desire may become a problem,

TABLE 6.1   SUMMARY POINTS: WHY INDIVIDUALS CHOOSE TO WORK IN HELPING PROFESSIONS

Help others	Contribute to another's growth
Self-exploration	Discover more about self
Exert control	Good in administration and organization
Positive role models	Inspired by help from others

however, if helpers seek to control or dominate clients with the intent of making them dependent or having them conform to an external standard.

For many people, the experience of being helped provides a strong demonstration of the value of helping. Such people often wish to be like those who helped them when they were clients. This appears to be especially true for the fields of teaching and medicine. Unfortunately, this noble motivation may create unrealistic expectations of what being a helper will be like. For example, unsuccessful clients do not become helpers; rather, those who have had positive helping experiences are the ones who will choose this type of profession. Because they were cooperative and motivated clients, they may expect all clients to be like they were, and they may also expect all helpers to be as competent and caring as their helpers were. Such expectations of both the helper and the client are unrealistic and may leave the helper frustrated and angry.

When asked about making the choices, many helpers describe the process as a journey. Regardless of their primary or secondary motivation, they see individuals and experiences in their lives leading them to become helpers. For some the journey begins early in their lives while others appear to have discovered the field as adults. Consider your own journey to becoming a helper; think about your motivations and the people and experiences that led to your study of the human services. See Table 6.1.

VALUES AND HELPING

Values are important to the practice of human services because they are the criteria by which helpers and clients make choices. Every individual has a set of values. Both human service professionals and clients have sets of values. Sometimes they are similar, but often they differ; in some situations, they conflict. Human service professionals should know something about values and how they influence the relationship between the helper and the client.

Where do our values originate? Culture helps establish some values and standards of behavior. As we grow and learn through our different experiences, general guides to behavior emerge. These guides are **values**, and they give direction to our behavior. As different experiences lead to different values, individuals do not have the same value systems. Also, as individuals have more life experiences, their values may change. What exactly are values? Values are statements of what is desirable— of the way we would like the world to be. They are not statements of fact.

Values provide a basis for choice. It is important for human service professionals to know what their own values are and how they influence relationships with coworkers and the delivery of services to clients. For example, professionals who value truth will give the client as much feedback as possible from the results of an employment check or a home-visitation report. Because human service delivery is a team effort in many agencies and communities, there have to be some common values that will assist helpers in working together effectively. The following are the most commonly held values in human services: acceptance, tolerance, individuality, self-determination, and confidentiality.

The next paragraph introduces Beth Bruce, a human service professional with a variety of experiences. In this section, her experiences are used to illustrate the values that are important to the human service profession.

> Beth Bruce is a human service professional at the Estes Mental Health Center, a comprehensive center serving seven counties. She has been a counselor at Estes for the past eight months and has really enjoyed her first year's work in mental health. Her first job was as a social service provider in a local nursing home, where she worked for two years. She then worked with adolescents as a teacher and counselor at a local mental health institution before joining the Estes staff.

Let's see how human service values relate to Beth Bruce's experience as a human service professional.

Acceptance is the ability of the helper to be receptive to another person regardless of dress or behavior. Professionals act on the value of acceptance when they are able to maintain an attitude of goodwill toward clients and others and to refrain from judging them by factors such as the way they live, or whether they have likable personalities. Being accepting also means learning to appreciate a person's culture and family background.

> One of the most important values that Beth Bruce holds is accepting her clients for who they are. She has worked with the elderly, teenagers, and now people with mental illness. These populations are different, but they retain one important quality for her: They are all human beings. Her acceptance of others was put to the test at the nursing home when she encountered a staff who were mainly from Kenya, Ruanda, and Tanzania, all places unfamiliar to her. Sometimes it was difficult for her to understand their lilting accents. What she learned though was that these women were gentle, patient, and natural caretakers who were beloved by the patients.

The second value of human service work is **tolerance:** the helper's ability to be patient and fair toward each client rather than judging, blaming, or punishing the client for prior behavior. A helper who embodies this value will work with the client to plan for the future, rather than continually focusing on the client's past mistakes.

> Beth works with a friend and coworker who is not very tolerant of people with mental illness. Several times, this coworker's intolerance of client behavior has caused problems for the client. Just yesterday, a problem arose with Ms. Mendoza, a 26-year-old woman with schizophrenia who is currently receiving day treatment and lives in a group home. She refused to see her parents when they came to see her at the day treatment center. Mr. Martin, Beth's coworker, forced Ms. Mendoza to see them because he believes that family is very important and that parents have a right to see their children. Now the parents are upset because Ms. Mendoza threw a chair at them.
>
> Ms. Mendoza is upset with Mr. Martin for making her see her parents, and Mr. Martin is angry with his client because he feels he was right to insist that she see them.

| BOX 6.1 | AMANDA NALLS—EXPERIENCING IRAQ AS A MILITARY OFFICER |

Inshallah. Throughout my two tours in Baghdad, Iraq as an Army officer, I heard this Arabic expression more times than I can count from native Iraqi citizens, Arabic contractors, and, eventually, from Army soldiers. Literally translated as "as god wills," it is used to suggest that something in the future is uncertain, which, in retrospect aptly described the situation in Iraq for both its citizens and the American military forces.

My experiences in Iraq were not unlike those of many of the American soldiers: we spent long hours working (sometimes 18 hours a day) and looked forward to the occasional call home and letters from friends and family. The long months of staff work were often punctuated by memorial services for fellow soldiers who were unlucky enough to encounter enemy fire, improvised explosive devises, or suicide bombers while conducting their daily missions in the field. The daily routine for many officers in my situation was alternately boring, thrilling, and mentally exhausting.

Amidst the daily grind of paperwork, mission tracking, and planning for casualty evacuation, there were moments that I will not soon forget. As my unit's public affairs officer, I was able to help plan several "special" events for our soldiers. Each month, for example, a handful of soldiers were able to take a much-needed rest from missions and tour the palaces located in the Baghdad International Airport Complex where we were stationed. The highlight of the trip was a stop at the Al-Faw Palace, one of the eight presidential palaces used for hunting and recreation by the Baathist Party members, as well as by Saddam Hussein and his family. The tours provided an opportunity to teach the soldiers about Iraq's history and its culture, which, hopefully, allowed them to better identify with the Iraqi people that they were there to help.

Medical Capability Missions, or MEDCAPs, were another event that provided me with an opportunity to see Iraq and its citizens in a different light. During my time in Iraq, MEDCAP missions were conducted in conjunction with the Iraqi Army; both American and Iraqi medics and doctors spend a day at a particular site treating local citizens and providing much-needed antibiotics and medical advice. During one such mission, I had the opportunity to serve as a "patient administrator;" my job entailed meeting Iraqi citizens at the entrance to the site, determining (with the help of a translator) their ailment, and assigning them to one of the medical professionals for treatment. I met a wide variety of individuals that day. One woman brought her two-year-old son and requested help on how to get him to stop eating rocks. Families came seeking treatment for shrapnel and gunshot wounds, and children wandered in off the street hoping for a piece of candy from the medics. One family in particular stood out as being particularly unique; both teenage daughters spoke fluent English and were looking forward to attending school in Alaska the following month. Each individual I met helped put a face on the effort we were making to help Iraqi citizens achieve a free and peaceful nation.

Although my experiences in Iraq were often frustrating and exhausting, they were also incredibly rewarding. Few other times in my life have I gotten to be a part of something truly worthwhile and make a lasting impact on the world. The opportunities I had to meet with and work alongside Iraqi citizens helped me to better understand a culture vastly different from my own, and allowed me to use my helping skills in ways that most helping professionals do not have the chance to. Although the future of Iraq and its people truly is *inshallah*, I look back on my time in the Army and my contributions to the Iraqi people with pride and with the hope that one day they too will enjoy many of the freedoms that Americans experience on a daily basis.

Source: Amanda Nalls (2010). Used with permission.

Individuality is expressed in the qualities or characteristics that make each person unique, distinctive from all other people. Lifestyle, assets, problems, previous life experiences, and feelings are some areas that make this person different. Recognizing and treating each person individually rather than stereotypically is how helpers put this value into practice.

When Beth first started working with the elderly, she had had little contact with older individuals. What she knew about them she had learned from her grandparents. She thought of the elderly as lively and quick-witted like her grandmother or quiet and shy, living in the past, like her grandfather. During her first months at the nursing home, the clients she encountered continually surprised her. They represented a broad range of human attitudes, behaviors, and experiences. She learned to distinguish between the generalizations she had made about the elderly and the information she now possessed based on her experiences at the nursing home.

Deciding for oneself on a course of action or the resolution to a problem is self-determination. The helper allows clients to make up their own minds regarding a decision to be made or an action to be taken. The helper facilitates this action by objectively assisting clients to investigate alternatives and by remembering that the decision is theirs. In some cases, clients are limited by their situations or their choices. For example, a prison inmate may have restricted alternatives from which to choose recreational activities; however, it is the inmate's right to choose from the available alternatives.

When Beth worked with teenagers, she was constantly aware that their use of social media was important to them. Even though she frequently cautioned them about its abuses, she realized they needed to take responsibility for their sites and their postings.

The last human service value is confidentiality. This is the helper's assurance to clients that the helper will not discuss their cases with other people—that what they discuss between them will not be the subject of conversation with the helper's friends, family, or other clients. The exception to this is the sharing of information with supervisors or in staff meetings where the client's best interests are being served.

Lucas, a 15-year-old with whom Beth worked at the mental health center, confessed to her that he has been smoking marijuana just about every day and is afraid he can't quit. Beth reminded him of their very first meeting when they discussed confidentiality and its limits. So she said their next meeting would involve both Lucas and his parents. She would also share with them the reason for the meeting.

You should consider the following questions as you think about the meaning of these values in your own life and practice.

• What kinds of client behaviors would be the most difficult for you to accept? How would you meet the challenge of working with these clients?
• When was the last time you felt uncomfortable sharing information about another person? How did you resolve the situation?

As you think about these five values in relation to yourself as a future human service professional, consider the possibility of working with many different clients. As you think about the following list of clients, place a check beside those clients who would be difficult for you to work with. Which values might present problems or conflicts for you? Try to respond honestly, not what you think would be socially or professionally desirable.

1. _____ A man with religious beliefs that cause him to refuse treatment for a life-threatening illness.

2. _____ A same-sex couple who want to resolve some conflicts they are having in their relationship.

3. _____ A man who wants to leave his wife and two children in order to have sexual adventures with other women.

4. _____ A young woman who wants an abortion but is seeking your help in making the decision.

5. _____ A person who has severe burn scars on the face, shoulders, arms, and hands.

6. _____ A man or woman from a culture where the male is dominant and the female is submissive.

7. _____ A person who does not want to work.

8. _____ A man who strongly believes the only way to bring up his children is by punishing them severely.

9. _____ A woman who wants to leave her husband and children in order to have a career and independence but is afraid to do it.

10. _____ A person who is so physically attractive that you cannot concentrate on what the person is saying.

11. _____ A person who speaks no English and makes no effort to do so.

Values are the groundwork for creating a philosophy of helping, which in turn provides a basis for working with people. A philosophy of helping embodies beliefs about human nature, the nature of change, and the process of helping. As individuals grow and develop and as their values change, their helping philosophy and style also develop. An example is the way Beth Bruce's values translate into her philosophy of helping, which influences her human service practice.

> Beth believes that all human beings are good and that all behavior is directed to the good. She thinks that violence to others, cruelty, and self-abuse are all behaviors that the perpetrators consider to be positive ways to meet their personal needs. She also believes that people have the capacity to change, if only they believe they can change. Hence, the helper's responsibility is to develop clients' belief in themselves and help provide alternatives for change, practical assistance, and support. Because of these views, Beth has high hopes for her clients, and she believes that her major responsibility is to educate and motivate them. She is frustrated when she works with clients who have tried to hurt others, and she is puzzled when those clients do not want to change. In spite of her frustration, she has maintained her belief in the goodness of human beings.

CHARACTERISTICS OF THE HELPER

To be an effective helper demands the use of the helper's whole self, not just the professional segment alone. This requirement creates difficulty when one tries to generalize about the values and characteristics that helpers ought to have. Ideas differ widely about what helpers should be like and what they bring to their work with others. In this section, you will read about some of these ideas. You will also be encouraged to think about the qualities you possess that might be important to your work as a helping professional, as well as qualities you may want to develop more fully to increase your effectiveness. Box 6.2 outlines how a mental health professional thinks about helping and the helping process.

| BOX 6.2 | A PRACTITIONER'S VIEW OF HELPING |

Working in community mental health provides me with opportunities to interact with clients in their home environment. Seeing my clients where they live helps me gain perspective on how their daily life affects their overall sense of well-being. As a mental health professional, I believe that the "systems" we find ourselves in have an impact on how we view the world around us. From a systems perspective, I can understand how the external environment my clients experience affects their level of stress, their basic needs, and their emotional state.

In addition to understanding each client in his or her own unique system, I have found that the most important aspect of helping is the relationship. Each of us is a social creature, and we need connection with others. For my clients who are chronically and persistently mentally ill, being calm, consistent, and somewhat transparent has been therapeutically valuable. By approaching each relationship from a non-judgmental perspective, I give my clients the opportunity to teach me how to best help them. In order for a person to take risks towards change, there must be a firm foundation (i.e., relationship) on which to land.

One of the most important lessons I've learned from working in community mental health is that I cannot expect people to change or grow at a rate or in the way I would like for them to change or grow. Learning how to keep my own values in check has allowed me to become a better helper. I constantly strive to understand each client in his or her system, and provide a solid place in which risk-taking can occur. However, I cannot take risks for my clients; I can only support their growth.

Source: Ellen Carruth, PhD, Mental Health Crisis Specialist, Seattle, WA. Used with permission from the author.

Individuals learn attitudes and behaviors as they respond to their circumstances. Some responses may even be unconscious. Through the learning process, a person internalizes these attitudes and behaviors and they become a pattern in his or her life. A major influence on how an individual reacts to these needs is culture. Families, schools, and peers are among the agents who communicate ways of behaving and help determine what an individual considers to be acceptable and unacceptable behavior in different situations. An increasing body of research supports the concept that the personal characteristics of helpers are largely responsible for the success or failure of their helping. In fact, numerous studies concluded that these personal characteristics are as significant in helping as the methods helpers use (Corey, 2012).

A number of researchers have examined these characteristics, and we studied this work to identify the traits that seem to be universal in effective helpers. The helping person should be able to hear the client and then use his or her knowledge, skills, values, and experience to provide help. To do this, the helper should be self-aware, objective, professionally competent, and actively involved in the enabling process. In a review of a number of research studies, Okun and Kantrowitz (2008) concluded that certain qualities, behaviors, and knowledge on the part of the helper most influence the behaviors, attitudes, and feelings of clients. Self-awareness, honesty, congruence, the ability to communicate, knowledge, and ethical integrity are also included in their list.

Effective helpers have definite traits. One way to discuss what these traits are is to use a framework that suggests two sets of attitudes: one related to self and the other to how one treats another person (Brammer & MacDonald, 2003). Personal

TABLE 6.2   SUMMARY POINTS: VALUES THAT GUIDE PRACTICE

Acceptance	Maintain goodwill and refrain from judging
Tolerance	Be patient and fair
Respect for individuality	Respect differences, avoid stereotypes
Self-determination	Help clients make decisions
Confidentiality	Will not disclose client information

congruence, empathy, cultural sensitivity, genuineness, respect, and communication are considered important traits.

All the characteristics mentioned are important ones for helpers. Many other perspectives can be studied, but this brief discussion shows that certain characteristics tend to be common to most studies. In preparing this text, we have reviewed a number of perspectives. Our guiding question was "What characteristics are important for the beginning human service professional?" We identified the following qualities as important: self-awareness, the ability to communicate, empathy, professional commitment, and flexibility. Each of these is discussed in depth to help you understand what the quality is and why it is important for entry-level practice.

SELF-AWARENESS   Most authorities in the helping professions agree that helpers must know who they are because this self-knowledge affects what they do. Developing **self-awareness** is a lifelong process of learning about oneself by continually examining one's beliefs, attitudes, values, and behaviors. Recognizing stereotypes, biases, and cultural and gender differences are part of the self-awareness process. So is our desire for acceptance and client success; "needing" our clients to like us and to do well may be a sign of trouble, however. Self-awareness, then, is a particularly critical process for helpers because it assists them in understanding and changing their attitudes and feelings that may hinder helping. The importance of self-acceptance is underscored by the helper's use of self in the helping process.

Beth Bruce's awareness of self expanded greatly when she began to work in the field full time. As she began to learn about the culture and beliefs of others, she developed a keener sense of who she was. It seemed that as she developed the patience to work with her first clients, she also became more patient with herself.

ABILITY TO COMMUNICATE   Helpers' effectiveness depends in part on their ability to communicate to the client an understanding of the client's feelings and behaviors (Okun & Kantrowitz, 2008). Listening, a critical helping skill, is the beginning of helping and is necessary for establishing trust, building rapport, and identifying the problem. Careful listening means being "tuned in" to all the nuances of the client's message, including verbal and nonverbal aspects of what is said as well as what is not said. Such focused listening enables the helper to respond with thoughts and feelings to the client's whole message.

Beth Bruce's ability to communicate was challenged when she began her work with adolescents at the hospital. These young people were aggressive, belligerent, and violent. She worked hard to listen, gain their trust, and provide them honest,

TABLE 6.3   Summary Points: Characteristics of Effective Helpers

Self-awareness	Helper understands self
Ability to communicate	Being "tuned in" to client's message
Empathy	Understand experience from client's perspective
Responsibility and commitment	Devoted to well-being of others
Flexibility	Ability to shift one's perspective

constructive feedback. One of the most important skills Beth learned was to listen to the client's entire statement before formulating a response.

Empathy   **Empathy** is acceptance of another person. This quality allows the helper to see a situation or experience a feeling from the client's perspective. This may be easier for helpers who have had experiences similar to those of their clients. For example, this may explain the understanding that recovering alcoholics have for other alcoholics, widows for the recently bereaved, and parolees for the incarcerated. It does not mean, however, that helpers whose experiences are different cannot express the unconditional acceptance of the client that is a characteristic of empathy.

When Beth worked with her elderly clients, they used to tell her, "You will not really understand until you are older." Beth used her communication skills to reflect feelings and content of her clients in order to demonstrate her understanding of their plight.

Responsibility and Commitment   Feeling a responsibility or commitment to improve the well-being of others is an important attribute of human service professionals. This includes attending to the needs of clients first and foremost. It also means a commitment to delivering high-quality services that reflect evidence-based practice. In other words, human service professionals act in the best interests of clients and do so to the best of their ability. One way that helpers do this is by following a code of ethics or a set of ethical standards that guide professional behavior or conduct. Among other things, codes of ethics in the helping professions spell out what the client has a right to expect from the helper. Honesty may be one expectation of the client—a belief that the professional will be honest in answering questions or in practicing only what he or she is trained to do.

Beth has been troubled by ethical dilemmas throughout her work experience. Fortunately her values have guided her practice and her supervisors have praised her responsible actions. Several examples of ethical codes and standards are presented in Chapter 9.

Flexibility   **Flexibility** is a multifaceted trait that allows human service professionals to shift their perspectives on the nature of helping, their view of the client and the client's problems, and their preferred interventions. Professionals are willing to reconsider, modify, or abandon their approaches to helping when they encounter difficult or unusual situations. Continually seeking new ways of understanding or other options for providing support to the client, helpers who are flexible understand the complexities of human service work. Sometimes it is challenging for new professionals to be flexible in their approaches to work responsibilities because of their limited experience and inability to consider alternatives. Flexibility is an increasingly important characteristic as human service professionals work with individuals representing different ethnic and cultural groups.

Just as self-awareness helped Beth Bruce be more aware of herself, as she worked with others from different cultures, she has increased her knowledge and understanding of other cultural norms. Her work with African Americans, Cubans, Haitians, and a new wave of Russian émigrés continually expands her perspectives on family, gender roles, the role of spirituality in individual health and development, and the meaning of work. She keeps an open mind in each encounter as she listens for cultural values that differ from her own.

TYPOLOGY OF HUMAN SERVICE PROFESSIONALS

Besides understanding who the human service professional is in terms of characteristics and values, the student of human services should also know the professional categories that describe such helpers. The human service profession includes several levels of helpers who may be classified in a variety of ways. Two considerations present in most categorizations are educational preparation or training, and competence. Specialists, human service professionals, and nonprofessionals are discussed next.

CATEGORIES OF HELPERS

Generally, individuals who provide human services fall into one of three categories that are defined by preparation, what they know how to do, or both. Specialists are helpers who are characterized by certification from professional groups, licenses by governing bodies, and degrees from educational institutions. Examples of professionals in this category are social workers, nurses, ministers, and counselors. The second group consists of **human service professionals** who perform some of the traditional counseling functions but also engage in broader roles, such as those of advocate and mobilizer. Peers and volunteers are a third broad group that encompasses those with little or no training in helping as well as those with extensive training. Often training and orientation is offered to prepare these individuals for their responsibilities working with clients and providing indirect administrative services. These three categories are discussed in the next sections.

THE HUMAN SERVICE PROFESSIONAL

Human service professionals are generalists who have education and training at the undergraduate level and job titles such as psychiatric technician or aide, social and community service manager, youth street-outreach worker, day care staff, probation officer, case manager, and church staff. They possess the knowledge, values, and skills to perform a number of job functions in most human service settings. Because of their generalist orientation and preparation, human service professionals understand how their functions fit with client goals and agency goals. For example, a helper trained to conduct interviews, write social histories, and develop a treatment plan should be able to perform those responsibilities with a client who is elderly, young children, or those who have mental disabilities or emotional disorders.

In a move toward professionalization, the National Organization for Human Services in collaboration with the Council for Standards in Human Service Education and the Center for Credentialing and Education (CCE) offer a certification in human services called the Human Service-Board Certified Practitioner (**HS-BCP**). Certification indicates that the individual meets 11 core human service content areas. To learn more about certification, go to the CCE website.

The *Occupational Outlook Handbook*, 2012–2013 edition, includes a range of entries that describe human service professionals. Among them are counselors, probation officers and correctional treatment specialists, social and human service assistants, and social workers. According to the descriptions of these occupations, probation officers and correctional treatment specialists, substance abuse counselors, social and human service assistants, and social workers fit within the definition of those performing human service work (Bureau of Labor Statistics, 2012).

According to the *Occupational Outlook Handbook*, those who work in the field of corrections usually have a bachelor's degree in social work, criminal justice, or a related field. The primary job responsibilities include working in probation, in parole, or at correctional institutions. When describing the field of social and human service assistants, the *Occupational Outlook Handbook* states, "Social and human service assistants help people get through difficult times or get additional support. They have a wide array of job titles, including human service worker, case work aide, and family service assistant" (Bureau of Labor Statistics, 2012). The *Occupational Outlook Handbook* suggests that these professionals work under the supervision of other helping professionals such as nurses, physical therapists, psychologists, and others. The jobs vary, as do the responsibilities and type of supervision. Job opportunities in these two categories are growing rapidly.

The category titled "social workers" also describes opportunities for both social workers and human service professionals, especially those graduating from four-year human service programs. Those in direct service "help people solve and cope with problems in their everyday lives while clinical social workers diagnose and treat mental, behavioral, and emotional issues" (Bureau of Labor Statistics, 2012). The various areas of responsibility include counseling, child welfare, family services, child or adult protective services, mental health, substance abuse, criminal justice, occupational counseling, and work with the aging. Job opportunities for social workers and professionals from related fields will increase through the next decade.

OTHER PROFESSIONAL HELPERS

As a human service professional, you will be working with a variety of other professional helpers who have specialized training and experience. This category includes individuals who have graduate-level training in helping theory and skills and who often have supervised clinical experience; however, the training and

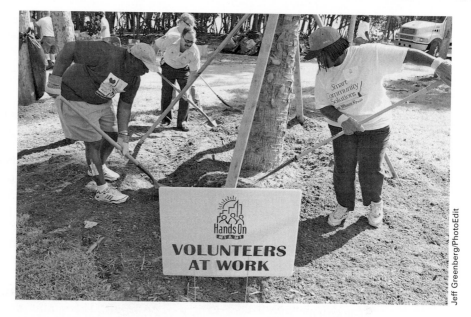

VOLUNTEERS AT WORK

Jeff Greenberg/PhotoEdit

credentials of these individuals may vary. This section, adapted from the *Occupational Outlook Handbook*, 2012–2013 edition, identifies the nature of the work and the training of these individuals so that you will be familiar with them.

PHYSICIANS **Physicians** perform medical examinations, diagnose illnesses, treat injured or diseased people, and advise patients on maintaining good health. They may be general practitioners or specialists in a particular field of medicine. Physicians are required by all states to be licensed. It usually takes about 11 years to become a physician: four years of undergraduate school, four years of medical school, and three years of residency. Those who choose to specialize usually spend three to five years in training and another two years in preparation for practice in a specialty area.

One example of a specialist with whom you will likely be in contact is a psychiatrist. Concerned with the diagnosis, treatment, and prevention of mental illness, psychiatrists may be found in private offices and institutional settings, courtrooms, community-center care facilities, and specialized medical areas such as coronary and intensive care units. They frequently act as consultants to other agencies. Psychiatrists are medical doctors who have an additional five years or more of psychiatric training and experience and are qualified to use the full range of medical techniques in treating clients. These include drugs, shock therapy, and surgery, in addition to counseling and behavior modification techniques.

PSYCHOLOGISTS   Although their training and the kinds of treatment they use are different, **psychologists** are sometimes confused with psychiatrists. Psychologists study the human mind and human behavior, including physical, cognitive, emotional, and social aspects. An individual may specialize in any of several areas within psychology, including clinical, counseling, developmental, industrial organizational, school, and social psychology. Each specialty focuses on a different aspect of human behavior. For example, the developmental psychologist is concerned with the behavioral changes people experience as they progress through life. Clinical psychologists, on the other hand, may work in hospitals, clinics, or private practice to help individuals with cognitive or emotional issues adjust to life, and to help medical and surgical patients deal with their illnesses and injuries. They may use interviews, diagnostic tests, and psychotherapy in their work.

Psychologists may practice with a master's degree or a doctoral degree. A master's degree prepares the person to administer and interpret tests, conduct research, and counsel patients. The doctoral degree usually requires five to seven years of graduate study and is often required for employment as a psychologist. A doctorate in psychology and two years of professional experience are generally required for licensure or certification; although requirements may vary from state to state, certification is necessary for private practice.

SOCIAL WORKERS   The focus of **social workers** is helping individuals, families, and groups cope with a wide variety of problems. The nature of the problem and the time and resources available determine the methods used, which may include counseling, advocacy, and referral. Social workers also function at the community level to combat social problems. For example, they may coordinate existing programs, organize fund-raising, and develop new community services. Social workers may also specialize in various areas. Medical social workers are trained to help patients and their families cope with problems that accompany illness or rehabilitation. Those who specialize in family services counsel individuals to strengthen personal and family relationships. Corrections and child welfare are other popular areas of study and employment. School social workers work with parents, guardians, teachers, and other school officials to ensure students reach their academic and personal potential.

Preparation for the field of social work occurs at two levels. The baccalaureate level (BSW) is the minimum requirement, followed by the master's degree in social work (MSW), which is usually required for positions in mental health and for administrative or research positions. Training generally includes courses of study focusing on social work practice, social welfare policies, human behavior, and the social environment. Supervised field experiences are also necessary.

The National Association of Social Workers (NASW) awards certification in the form of the title ACSW, which stands for the Academy of Certified Social Workers. All states and the District of Columbia have some licensure, certification, or registration requirement, although regulations vary.

COUNSELORS   One of the largest categories of professional helpers is **counselors**. Although their exact duties depend on the individuals or groups with whom they work and the agencies or settings in which they are employed, counselors help people deal with a variety of problems, including personal, social, educational, and career concerns. Examples of the different types of counselors are school and college counselors, rehabilitation counselors, employment counselors, marriage and family therapists, and mental health counselors. Employment for counselors is expected to increase by 37% between 2010 and 2020 (Bureau of Labor Statistics, 2012). Two types of counselors with whom you may interact as a human service professional are mental health counselors and rehabilitation counselors.

The *mental health counselor* works with individuals who are dealing with problems such as drug and alcohol abuse, family conflicts, suicidal thoughts and feelings, stress, depression, problems with self-esteem, issues associated with aging, job and career concerns, educational decisions, and issues of mental and emotional health. Their work is not limited to individuals, however; it may involve the family of the individual. These counselors often work closely with other specialists such as psychiatrists, psychologists, clinical social workers, and psychiatric nurses.

The *rehabilitation counselor* helps people deal with the personal, social, and vocational effects of their disabilities. Disabilities may be social, mental, emotional, or physical, calling for the services of counseling, evaluation, medical care, occupational training, and job placement. Rehabilitation counselors also work with the family of the individual when necessary and frequently with other professionals such as physicians, psychologists, and occupational therapists.

Positions as a counselor usually require a master's degree in a counseling discipline or a related area. This preparation frequently includes a year or two of graduate study and a supervised counseling experience. Licensure and certification are available; requirements vary, depending on the specialty. The National Board for Certified Counselors (NBCC) and the Commission on Rehabilitation Counselor Certification (CRCC) are two national certifying bodies. There are also certifying boards in each of the 50 states.

Human service professionals could assume the responsibilities of social workers or counselors, or be given this title, even though they might not be specifically certified as such. The variation in the needs of agencies and the competencies of individual helpers makes it difficult to establish rigid categories for function or title. However, having the title or performing the job of a mental health counselor is definitely not the same as being nationally certified. Some states and agencies will only hire helpers with national certification, whereas other sites have more flexible hiring categories.

NONPROFESSIONAL HELPERS

Community caretakers, natural helpers, and volunteers are examples of nonprofessional helpers who provide basic human service functions. You may, in fact, be a member of one of the following groups or be a recipient of their services.

Community caretakers, such as police and clergy, provide essential community service. Professionals in their own fields, they are involved in some aspects of human service work. For example, many of the clergy counsel members of the congregation and others from the community. Police officers work with victims of crime or abuse in many instances.

Hairdressers and bartenders are examples of *natural helpers*. Their primary job function is to cut hair or to mix drinks, but in performing these tasks, they find themselves listening, responding, and discussing alternatives to problem situations in which their customers may find themselves.

TABLE 6.4   SUMMARY POINTS: OTHER PROFESSIONAL HELPERS

Physicians	Licensed medical professionals who provide general medical services or specialty services
Psychologists	Study human behavior to understand individual thoughts and actions
Social Workers	Help individuals, families, and groups cope with problems
Counselors	Help people deal with a variety of issues

Another category of nonprofessionals who are helping human services respond to today's challenges is **self-help groups**. These are laypeople from all walks of life who come together to create a mutual support system to meet their own needs. Members share a common problem, they consider themselves peers, and they organize separately from human service organizations. The purposes of such groups include helping with chronic problems or general problems in living, raising consciousness, securing political rights, and providing support for behavioral changes. Over half a million groups like Alcoholics Anonymous (AA) and Mothers Against Drunk Driving (MADD) are currently providing support for people with similar problems.

Volunteers, another example of nonprofessionals in human services, are people who give their time and talents free of charge, have a sense of social responsibility, and have little concern for monetary gain. People volunteer for many reasons, among them to work with people, to meet people, to gain job references, or to help others. In 2011, 63.4 million Americans or 26.3% of the adult population age 16 and older contributed 8.1 billion hours of volunteer service worth $173 billion, using Independent Sector's 2011 estimate of the dollar value of a volunteer hour ($21.79). "To find information like this, perform an Internet search for 'volunteer hour value.'" Often, during a time of economic recession, volunteering declines. The fact that rates have held steady during the recent economic downturn is a positive sign. Nonprofit organizations striving to meet the needs of individuals and families across the country are also affected economically but find some relief in using more volunteers to achieve their goals.

Another impetus for the increase in volunteerism is the passage of the Edward M. Kennedy Serve America Act signed by President Obama on April 21, 2009. Its purpose is to encourage Americans from grade school students to retirees to volunteer by dedicating over $5.7 billion over five years to this cause. The act also vastly expands AmeriCorps from 75,000 volunteers to 250,000 (AmeriCorps, 2012; Milligan, 2009). These volunteers receive a living allowance of approximately $12,000 for 10 to 12 months of work during which they staff programs for low-income groups, veterans, the environment, health care, and education.

The nonprofessionals described here have been welcomed by professionals. Perhaps the most immediate reason for their acceptance is that all agencies face financial constraints at one time or another, and this can lead to a shortage of professionally trained helpers. Additionally, some agencies may have an uneven distribution of human service professionals with respect to race, social class, and place of birth; nonprofessionals may fill these gaps.

HUMAN SERVICE ROLES

At this point in Chapter 6, you have some idea about the identity of the human service professional and the relationship of this individual with other helping professionals and nonprofessionals. An examination of their roles further defines the human service professional.

The many human service roles to be introduced provide the framework for the helping process. In performing the various roles, the human service professional is continuously focused on the client; this client focus provides the common thread to connect the roles. Although the roles of human service professionals are constantly evolving, the helper remains a Jack (or Jill) of all trades, or, in human service terms, a generalist. The generalist knows a wide range of skills, strategies, and client groups and is able to work effectively in a number of different settings. Engaging in a variety of roles enables the human service professional to meet many client needs. What exactly do these helpers do?

Many professionals have attempted to answer this question. The Southern Regional Education Board (SREB) conducted a study in the late 1960s to define the roles and functions of human service professionals. As a result of this analysis, SREB identified 13 roles that human service workers could engage in to meet the needs of their clients, agencies, or communities (Southern Regional Education Board, 1969). These 13 roles include administrator, advocate, assistant to specialist, behavior changer, broker, caregiver, community planner, consultant, data manager, evaluator, mobilizer, outreach worker, and teacher or educator.

In a more recent study, the U.S. Department of Education funded the Community Support Skills Standards Project to define the skills that human service personnel need to work in the field. The result of the work was a set of 12 competency areas of work in human services. These emerged from a job analysis and are reflected in the project's report as competency areas. The areas are as follows: participant empowerment; communication; assessment; community and service networking; facilitation of services; community living skills and supports; education, training, and self-development; advocacy; vocational, educational, and career support; crisis intervention; organizational participation; and documentation (Community Support Skill Standards Project, 2012). Each competency area has several skill standard statements that describe job function in that area.

The National Organization for Human Services, in concert with the Council for Standards in Human Service Education, also defines the human service professional and summarizes the work of these helpers. In a document that defines the human service worker, commitment to others in need is emphasized. The document states:

> "Human services worker" is a generic term for people who hold professional and paraprofessional jobs in such diverse settings as group homes and halfway houses; correctional, mental retardation, and community mental health centers; family, child, and youth service agencies; and programs concerned with alcoholism, drug abuse, family violence, and aging. Depending on the employment setting and the kinds of clients served there, job titles and duties vary a great deal. The primary purpose of the human service worker is to assist individuals and communities to function as effectively as possible in the major domains of living (National Organization for Human Services, 2012).

TABLE 6.5   HUMAN SERVICE ROLES

Providing Direct Service	Performing Administrative Work	Working with the Community
Cultural Broker	Cultural Broker	Cultural Broker
Behavior changer	Broker	Advocate
Caregiver	Data manager	Community and service networker
Communicator	Evaluator	Community planner
Crisis intervener	Facilitator of services	Consultant
Participant empowerer	Planner	Mobilizer
Teacher/educator	Report and grant proposal writer	Outreach worker
	Resource allocator	

To better understand the varied roles that are assumed by the human service professional, we used the results of these studies to categorize three areas of responsibility: providing direct service, performing administrative work, and working with the community. In the following sections, we examine these three categories and the roles that represent each area of responsibility. (See Table 6.5.)

PROVIDING DIRECT SERVICE

Providing direct service to clients is a responsibility with which many beginning professionals are familiar. This work represents the development of the helping relationship and the work that helpers do in their face-to-face encounters with their clients. Many roles, such as behavior changer, caregiver, communicator, crisis intervener, participant empowerer, and teacher or educator, are included in the category of direct services. The following illustrate many of these roles and how human service professionals perform them.

Behavior changer—carries out a range of activities planned primarily to change clients' behavior, ranging from coaching and counseling to casework, psychotherapy, and behavior therapy.

> Sun Lee Kim is a substance abuse counselor at a drug and alcohol inpatient clinic at a local hospital. Sun Lee, one of the staff group leaders, facilitates a reality therapy group each day. The purpose of this group is to encourage participants to change their communication behavior, first in the group and later in the wider context of the facility. Peer support and pressure are used to facilitate this behavior change.

Caregiver—provides services for people who need ongoing support of some kind, such as financial assistance, day care, social support, and 24-hour care.

> Jim Gray works in foster care. His major responsibility is to provide support to families with foster children. One of his favorite activities is to visit foster homes to determine

the success of the foster care situation and provide emotional and practical assistance to the families. In addition to his visits, he also maintains contact by calling or texting.

Communicator—is able to express and exchange ideas and establish relationships with a variety of individuals and groups, including clients, families, colleagues, administrators, and the public.

Dal Lam works with AIDS patients in a self-help center established by a regional hospital in a rural desert area. His responsibilities require him to communicate orally and in writing with different populations. He prefers face-to-face meetings with individuals who test HIV positive and those with AIDS. E-mails are often most effective with medical staff and insurance providers. His prevention work takes him to the elementary schools, local high schools, civic meetings, and churches.

Crisis intervener—provides services for individuals, families, and communities who are experiencing a disruption in their lives with which they cannot cope. This intervention is short term, focused, and concrete.

Christy Holston works in a sexual-assault crisis center and is a victim advocate. She receives four or five new clients a week, mostly women, who are dealing with issues of sexual assault, attempted rape, or rape. Some of her clients call through the hotline immediately after being assaulted, others are referred through the emergency room at the hospital, and others call to ask for help many years after the crisis.

Participant empowerer—shares with clients the responsibility for the helping relationship and the development and implementation of a plan of action. This helper ultimately encourages clients to care for themselves.

Judy Collins is a case manager for young adults who are developmentally disabled. In the First Steps program, she works with clients to move from group-home living to apartment living. She coordinates daily living training, vocational assessment and training, and first employment. Her clients participate fully in the case management process and are called "co-case managers." There is a graduation ceremony when these clients become their own "case managers."

Teacher or educator—performs a range of instructional activities, from simple coaching to teaching highly technical content, directed at individuals or groups.

Dr. Washington Lee, a physician, and Ned Wanek, a human service professional, work in a family planning clinic. They spend two mornings a week teaching classes to women and men about the reproductive system and alternative methods of family planning. In addition, they counsel individuals, provide physical exams, plan educational media, and talk to schools and community groups about family planning.

PERFORMING ADMINISTRATIVE WORK

Performing administrative work is another important responsibility for many human service professionals. In addition to providing direct services to clients, many helpers are involved in managerial activities as they supervise or oversee processes or projects. As they work with clients, they assume administrative responsibilities such as planning, linking clients to services, allocating resources, and evaluating. The specific administrative roles are broker, data manager, evaluator, facilitator of services, planner, report and grant writer, and resource allocator.

Broker—helps people get to the existing services and helps make the services more accessible to clients.

Maria Giovanni's caseload at the Office for Student Services consists primarily of students with physical disabilities. One of her functions is to make sure these students have their classes scheduled in accessible buildings on campus and are able to get around campus to their classes and school events. To achieve this goal, Maria may have to help students reschedule classes or arrange for parking. She is also "on call" to assist these students in getting other services they might need.

Data manager—gathers, tabulates, analyzes, and synthesizes data and evaluates programs and plans.

Roosevelt Thompson is part of the staff of a local day care center. Although he assists the child care staff when needed, his actual responsibilities are business oriented. The day care center is privately owned but partially funded by the city. Its clients include children referred to the center from the courts for temporary care as well as children of working parents. His concern is to see that the center maintains an appropriate balance between referred and regular paying clients to maintain its financial stability. He continually gathers information, inputs data, and projects the financial needs of the day care center.

Evaluator—assesses client or community needs and problems, whether medical, psychiatric, social, or educational. Assesses standards of care that reflect evidence-based practice.

Karen Tubbs leads a community planning organization established to assess the community's needs in the event of a national disaster. In her coastal region, disaster means the threat of damaging winds, rain, and numerous hurricanes. Its meetings are part of a complex process of planning for and developing resources to begin providing human services should a hurricane strike their region. She and her team study the protocols used in other regions of the world and determine what planning and service delivery actions were most effective.

Facilitator of services—brokers (links the client to services) and then monitors the progress the client makes with the various helping professionals. This helper also uses the problem-solving process when services are deficient or inappropriate.

Louisa Gonzales works in a group home for young children who need a short-term safe haven. During the time the children are in the home, Louisa spends many hours coordinating their care with schools, child-care agencies, the health department, and the welfare department. Many times, without her services, these children would get lost in the system and would receive substandard care.

Planner—engages in making plans with both short-term and long-term clients in order to define accurately their problems and needs, develops strategies to meet the needs, and monitors the helping process. Planners also help develop programs and services to meet client needs.

Ruth Strauss works with families who are planning for the long-term care of aging parents. This requires careful attention to the needs and priorities of all involved. She has better luck with her families when she uses a very structured planning and decision-making model. With this model, everyone in the family has a clear understanding of the problems and the goals and can monitor the success of the plan. She also serves on a program development team that creates new programs for families.

Report (documentation) and grant proposal writer—records the activities of the agency work. This can include intake interview reports, social histories, detailed treatment plans, daily entries into case notes, requests for resources, rationale and justification for treatment for managed care, and periodic reports for managed care. The role of writer also involves preparing proposals for funding from local, state, and federal agencies and organizations.

> Lisa Wilhiem is a social worker in a local hospital emergency room. She is the intermediary for clients who will potentially need longer-term care. It is her responsibility to coordinate the initial requests for services to the managed care organizations or insurance companies via e-mail. Although she spends several hours of her day with patients and the medical care staff, a majority of her time is spent at her computer documenting how the patient entered the health care system and what the current needs of the patient are. She is currently applying for two federal grants and one state grant that support innovative intake and discharge processes for emergency room care.

Resource allocator—makes recommendations on how resources are to be spent to support the needs of the client. These recommendations are made once priorities are set and prices for services are determined.

> Hoover Center, a psychiatric facility for adolescents, is developing a new program that will individualize the treatment of its clients. In the past, there was a standard treatment for all clients regardless of their problems. Because of the pressures from managed care and the limited resources available for the Center, the decision has been made to ask each client's case manager to establish priorities and determine how the resources per client are to be spent. The case manager will submit a plan that will be approved by the supervisor and then submitted to the managed care organization for review and final approval.

WORKING WITH THE COMMUNITY

Many professionals are also very involved with their community as they develop collegial networks and work on behalf of their clients to create and improve services within the local area and beyond. The roles of advocate, community and service networker, community planner, consultant, mobilizer, and outreach worker are those which the helper assumes responsibility in the community context.

Advocate—pleads and fights for services, policies, rules, regulations, and laws on behalf of clients.

> José Cervantes is a lawyer for a legal aid clinic in an urban area. His clients, referred by the courts, are individuals who need legal services but cannot pay for them. Most of his cases involve marital separation, divorce, custody of children, and spouse and child support. Besides handling individual cases, José works with politicians, judges, and other lawyers to develop a legal system that is sensitive to the needs of his clients.

Community and service networker—works actively to connect with other helpers and agencies to plan for providing better services to the community and to clients, share information, support education and training efforts, and facilitate linking clients to the services they need.

> Ian DeBusk has been working for the public schools for the past 20 years. Early in his career he worked with in-school suspension programs, and today he supervises school counselors in 15 high schools, 12 middle schools, and 32 elementary schools. One of his responsibilities is to help his counselors find the services their students need. He has established two listservs. One is for the school counselors he supervises and a second one is for his network of colleagues in the criminal justice system, child welfare services, health department, and vocational rehabilitation agency, to name just a few. These two listservs help him connect and remain current.

Community planner—works with community boards and committees to ensure that community services promote mental health and self-actualization, or at least minimize emotional stress on people.

> Hector Gomez is director of the local department of human services. As director, part of his responsibility is to provide leadership in human services to the city and county. He spends many evenings attending board meetings with other members of the community discussing funding and future planning for human services.

Consultant—works with other professionals and agencies regarding their handling of problems, needs, and programs.

> Three members of a pediatric language lab serving young children with communication disorders have formed a consulting service as part of their job responsibilities with the lab. The focus of the service is to educate teachers and day care staff about communication disorders and help them work with children in their own facilities. The consulting activity will enable the lab to expand the impact of its services.

Mobilizer or community organizer—helps to get new resources for clients and communities.

> Just last week James Shabbaz, a psychiatric social worker at a research hospital, discovered that the funding for the newly formed hospice service was not being renewed. The support services provided to family members of dying patients will be difficult to replace. James has decided to schedule a meeting with hospital staff and members of local churches to assist him in thinking about alternative support for these family members.

Outreach worker—reaches out to identify people with problems, refers them to appropriate services, and follows up to make sure they continue to their maximum rehabilitation.

> Greg Jones from the local mental health center travels into rural sections of a three-county area to follow up on patients who have been released from the regional mental health facility. His primary responsibilities are to provide supportive counseling, assess current progress, and make appropriate referrals. He also alerts them to services and agencies using Facebook and Twitter.

Each job in the human service field represents a unique combination of roles and responsibilities. The following list shows the way in which roles and responsibilities can be configured.

HOME HEALTH CARE COORDINATOR
- Broker
- Data manager
- Evaluator
- Facilitator of services
- Report (documentation) and grant proposal writer

PAROLE OFFICER
- Broker
- Data manager
- Planner
- Report (documentation) and grant proposal writer

MENTAL HEALTH CASE MANAGER
- Behavior changer
- Caregiver
- Crisis intervener
- Data manager
- Evaluator
- Facilitator of services
- Report (documentation) and grant proposal writer
- Resource allocator

CHILD CARE PROFESSIONAL
- Advocate
- Behavior changer
- Communicator
- Report (documentation) writer
- Teacher or educator

FOOD BANK ORGANIZER
- Communicator
- Community and service networker
- Community planner
- Mobilizer or community organizer
- Outreach worker

WORKING AS A CULTURAL BROKER

All human service professionals assume the role as a **cultural broker** whether they provide direct service, assume a leadership role, or focus on community-based issues. In this role, according to the National Center for Cultural Competence (NCCC) (2012), the cultural broker commits to help clients negotiate the cultural divide that influences access and effective use of services. NCCC outlines the following competencies necessary for professionals to perform the role of cultural broker.

- Assess and understand their own cultural identities and value systems;
- Recognize the values that guide and mold attitudes and behaviors;
- Understand a community's traditional health (mental health) beliefs, values, and practices and changes that occur through acculturation;
- Communicate in a cross-cultural context;
- Interpret or translate information;
- Advocate with and on behalf of children, youth, and families;
- Negotiate health, mental health, and other service delivery systems; and
- Manage and mediate conflict (National Center for Cultural Competence, 2012).

The National Center for Cultural Competence provides this example of a human service professional, Ms. Helen Dao, serving in the role of cultural broker.

> One of the providers serving a child with severe epilepsy and her family expressed frustration that the family had not followed up on scheduled appointments and evaluations recommended by the care team. When working with the family Ms. Dao learned that they were concerned about out-of-home care and that the appointments were all associated with residential placement. It was simply unacceptable, not at all in keeping with the family's values, to have the member cared for outside the family circle in a nursing home or other facility. The family chose not to inform the provider of their belief system because they did not want to be disrespectful. Ms. Dao was instrumental in this situation because she was able to bridge the gap between both the provider and the family by 1) clarifying the reasons why the appointments were needed and missed; 2) setting an example of how patients and providers can have a dialogue to discover their respective beliefs and practices that are immersed in culture; 3) identifying cultural beliefs and practices about respecting professionals who are in positions of authority; and 4) mediating a compromise between the family's values and practices vs. recommendations by the medical community. (NCCC, 2012)

In summary, as you learn more about human services and meet human service professionals, try to determine the roles they are performing and the responsibilities they assume as they work with clients, their colleagues, and the community.

FRONTLINE HELPER OR ADMINISTRATOR

Helpers may generally be categorized as having either frontline or administrative responsibilities. Using only these two categories may oversimplify the actual responsibilities of a given helper, but the categorization is useful when you are visualizing what human service professionals actually do. The schedules that follow outline the typical day of a **frontline helper** and that of an **administrator**.

FRONTLINE HELPER: WOMEN'S CASE COORDINATOR (SHELTER FOR BATTERED WOMEN AND THEIR CHILDREN)

8:00 a.m. Use this time to finish what needs to be completed from the previous day if planned activities were interrupted by an emergency with a client. Check both voice and e-mail messages. Read the progress notes in the case files. See clients at about 8:30 a.m.—set up the appointments a day in advance. See each client two or three times each week, depending on their schedules. Be prepared for a crisis and a new client.

10:00 a.m. Go to court for orders of protection. This can last all day, depending on how many cases are on the docket. Go to court with a client for her hearing or to file for an order of protection.

11:00 a.m. If back from court, see clients or do paperwork. Return telephone calls and e-mails.

12:00 noon. Go to the dining room to eat with clients.

1:00 p.m. Run errands with clients; go to their homes for clothing or important documents. Get a police escort for entering the home.

3:00 p.m. Attend staff meetings once a week (usually lasting a couple of hours). During these meetings, discuss each case and service issues.

5:00 p.m. Update case notes. Set up appointments for the next day. Make telephone calls and check e-mails.

ADMINISTRATOR: DIRECTOR, SOCIAL SERVICES

8:00 a.m. Attend morning meetings to coordinate staff activities. Prioritize week's projects.

9:00 a.m. Check client vacancies; plan for number of admissions. Make telephone calls. Check e-mails. Gather information, review referrals, and schedule meetings and follow-up activities.

10:00 a.m. Meet with families, phone hospitals for possible admissions, meet with clients.

11:00 a.m. Meet with head administrator. Make plans, revise schedule for afternoon. Check telephone calls and e-mails.

12:00 noon. Eat at desk or with clients. Catch up on mail, read reports, write letters.

1:00 p.m. Discharge planning for clients. Meet with part-time staff. Reprioritize based on morning's activities.

2:00 p.m. Meet with other professionals, such as bookkeepers and nurses; contact services outside agency for information, planning, and referrals.

3:00 p.m. Complete referral book and complaint log. Make sure all tasks and written correspondence are completed. Be available to see clients and families. Follow up on a crisis encounter by a case manager. Client is in jail.

| **BOX 6.3** | EXPLORING THE WEB FOR MORE INFORMATION |

Check out the following terms on the Web to find out more about helper roles.

- volunteer
- human service professional
- psychologist
- psychiatrist
- social worker
- case manager

4:00 p.m. Answer telephone calls. Check e-mails. Finish reports due that day. Visit with clients and families.

5:00 p.m. Complete paperwork. Plan for the next day. Answer telephone calls, call people at home. Check e-mails.

7:00 p.m. Evening visit with family or client in hospital, read mail, work on big projects to improve services, attend professional meetings.

As you can see by reading these examples, both professionals perform more than one role. Although frontline helpers and administrators sometimes have similar responsibilities, each has a different focus. The frontline helper focuses on caring for the client; the administrator's primary focus is on planning and organizing services. Both have valuable responsibilities in human service delivery and share the ultimate goal of helping clients.

INTERNET EXERCISE

See this text's website at *www.cengagebrain.com* for video exercises. Choose Chapter 6, then Videos.

Mike is a clinician at a community mental health center. He works primarily with children and adolescents. In this segment, Mike describes his typical day at work. After listening to Mike, answer the following questions.

1. *Compare Mike's morning and afternoon. How are they alike and different?*
2. *How does Mike handle documentation?*
3. *What challenges does Mike encounter throughout the day?*

In the next segment, Deirdre, who directs a residential mental health program, describes her typical Monday.

1. *Identify the people Deirdre interacts with during the day.*
2. *Describe Deirdre's administrative responsibilities.*
3. *What challenges does she encounter in a typical day?*

As you think about both of these segments, answer the following questions.

1. *How do the days of a clinician or frontline human service professional and an administrator differ? How are they similar?*
2. *Compare their activities and responsibilities.*
3. *Which role most appeals to you? Why?*

CASE STUDY

The following case study provides an example of a human service professional who is involved with many of the issues encountered by helpers. As you read the case study, consider the helper's motivations, roles, values, and characteristics. Are there any potential sources of frustration for the helper? What are her expectations?

Carmen Rodriguez has worked as a case manager for a state agency in the American Southwest for the past four years. She considers herself a human service professional; with most of her clients, the focus of her work is much broader than just vocational counseling. She describes her job as follows.

MEET CARMEN RODRIGUEZ

I have been a case manager for the past four years. In my position, I work with clients to assist them in preparing for and finding gainful employment, housing, and support. Often, clients have needs beyond those that the agency provides. As a case manager, part of my responsibility is to help with those needs as well.

One of the aspects of my work that I like a lot is the variety of clients I encounter. They are of different ages and from varied backgrounds. I work with many Mexican Americans and Native Americans. My clients are both males and females, and they have various problems. Rarely do I see a client who only needs housing or only needs a job. Usually I work with a client everyday for a period of six to eight weeks. Because of this close contact, I feel that I get to know my clients well.

Clients come first with me. I constantly think about what I can do for them, and I want to help them in any way I can. Sometimes their circumstances seem so poor, but I know that if I work hard enough I can make their lives better.

Another rewarding part of my job is working with other professionals. We are all committed to meeting client needs, although at times we are limited by the purposes of our various agencies. We've found that we are much more successful working together. Listservs are a valuable support tool. In fact, ten of us from different agencies meet monthly for lunch to talk about our work and find out about other services that may be available. It's also a good time to find out about new legislation and regulations and the ways agencies are dealing with funding problems or new grants. Our group includes social workers, counselors, psychologists, and occasionally a physician or a psychiatrist. Often, these are the very professionals and agencies to which I refer clients for services that I'm unable to provide.

I guess it's pretty obvious how I feel about my work. It's rewarding and challenging, and I feel as if I learn something new each day. It may seem as if it's the perfect job, but it really isn't. There are some negative aspects to it, and probably the most frustrating is that in a bureaucracy things never seem to move as quickly as I want them to. For example, there is quite a bit of paperwork. Even with computers and servers, to receive an authorization for services requires going through several channels. This sometimes takes days, and since I work with the client on a daily basis, I get as impatient as the client.

The other aspect of my job that I sometimes find frustrating is that clients often do not do what I would like them to do. When you work with people, it's important to realize that you don't tell them what to do. Actually, we try to teach them to take responsibility for their actions, and this involves making decisions for themselves. When they make a decision that is not in their best interest or may lead to problems or failure, it's very difficult for me not to intervene. I want so much for my clients to succeed, but I've learned that they are independent individuals who must live their own lives. In spite of the frustrations, I hope to keep this job for several years. It offers many opportunities for professional growth and gives me a chance to make a difference.

Apply what you have read in this chapter by answering the following questions about Carmen Rodriguez.

- What motivates Carmen Rodriquez in her work?
- What do you think Carmen's philosophy is? What are her values?
- Identify the professionals with whom Carmen works.
- What human services roles does Carmen play?

KEY TERMS

acceptance

administrator

community caretakers

confidentiality

counselors

cultural broker

empathy

flexibility

frontline helper

generalist

human service professionals

HS-BCP

individuality

nonprofessional helpers

physicians

psychiatrists

psychologists

self-awareness

self-determination

self-help groups

social workers

tolerance

values

volunteers

THINGS TO REMEMBER

1. Helping means assisting people to understand, overcome, or cope with problems. A helper is one who offers such assistance.
2. The primary reason why individuals choose helping professions (and the reason most will admit) is the desire to help others. Related to this is the desire for self-exploration.
3. Values are important to the practice of human services, because they are the criteria by which human service professionals and clients make choices.
4. Acceptance, tolerance, individuality, self-determination, and confidentiality are important values for human service professionals.
5. Characteristics that are important for the entry-level human service professional are self-awareness, the ability to communicate, empathy, professional commitment, and flexibility.

6. One way of categorizing helping professionals is a three-level system: specialists, human service professionals, and nonprofessionals.
7. Human service professionals work with specialists, including physicians, psychologists, social workers, and counselors.
8. The broad range of job titles, duties, client groups, and employment settings in human services supports the generic focus of the profession.
9. Roles and responsibilities of human service professionals can be grouped into three categories: providing direct service, performing administrative work, and working with the community. Human service professionals assume the role of cultural broker as they perform the roles in all three categories.
10. Frontline helpers and administrators are two more categories of human service professionals that describe the complexities of their roles.

SELF-ASSESSMENT

- Describe the motivations for choosing a helping profession.
- How do values and a philosophy of helping relate to motivations for choosing a helping profession?
- List the helper characteristics that are important for the human service professional.
- What are the similarities and differences among human service professionals,

physicians, psychologists, social workers, and counselors?
- How does the *Occupational Outlook Handbook*'s entry on human service workers help you define them?
- What are the three primary areas of job responsibilities for human service professionals?

WANT TO KNOW MORE?

There are several resources you can tap to learn more about human service professionals. Check them out!

Additional Resources: Focus on Helpers

Blumberg, T. A. (2004). *No time for lunch: Memoirs of an inner city psychologist*. New York: Devora Publishing.
As a school psychologist for the Baltimore City Public Schools for almost 25 years, the author has worked with a cross-section of children—those who endured physical abuse, those who chose elective mutism, those who lived in fear, and those who created fear.

Corey, M. S., & Corey, G. (2010). *Becoming a helper*. Belmont, CA: Brooks Cole.
An overview of the helping process coupled with the skills and knowledge necessary to be a successful helping professional makes this a valuable resource for anyone considering a career in human services.

Emener, W. G., Richard, M. A., & Bosworth, J. J. (Eds.). (2009). *A guidebook to human service professions: Helping college students explore opportunities in the human service field*. Springfield, IL: Charles C. Thomas.
This book reviews 18 professions for those individuals who want to help others. Case management, clinical psychology, rehabilitation counseling, gerontology, and marriage and family therapy are included as well as discussions about motivations, ethics, and professionalism.

Grobman, L. M. (2005). *More days in the lives of social workers: 35 professionals tell "real-life" stories from social work practice*. Harrisburg, PA: White Hat Communications.
First-person narratives illustrate the variety of roles of social workers.

Jacob, J. (2007). *Our school: The inspiring story of two teachers, one big idea, and the charter school that beat the odds*. New York: Palgrave MacMillan.
The account of an inner city school in San Jose, California, that adopted a new approach to charter school education. The book captures the struggles, inspiration, and gutsy determination of teachers, students, and parents.

Case Study

If you'd like to know more about the work of a human service professional, read a firsthand account of a week in the life of a probation officer in *Introduction to Human Services: Cases and Applications*, the companion text to *Introduction to Human Services*. Allison has a human service degree and works in an intensive supervision program. This means that she works some evenings and conducts random home visits and curfew checks. As you read about Allison and her work, you will better understand how many of the concepts introduced in this chapter occur in the "real world."

REFERENCES

AmeriCorps. (2012). Retrieved from http://www.nationalservice.gov/sites/default/files/documents/10_0421_saa_implementation.pdf

Brammer, L. M., & MacDonald, G. (2003). *The helping relationship: Process and skills*. Boston: Allyn & Bacon.

Bureau of Labor Statistics. (2012). *Occupational outlook handbook* (2012-2013 ed.). Retrieved from http://www.bls.gov/ooh.htm

Chang, V. N., Scott, S. T., & Decker, C. L. (2013). *Developing helping skills: A step by step approach*. Pacific Grove, CA: Cengage.

Cochran, J. L., & Cochran, N. (2006). *The heart of counseling: A guide to developing therapeutic relationships*. Pacific Grove, CA: Brooks/Cole/Thomson.

Community Support Skill Standards Project. (2012). Retrieved from http://www.collegeofdirectsupport .com/CDS50/content/CDSContent/csss.htm

Corey, G. (2012). *Theory and practice of counseling and psychotherapy* (9th ed.). Pacific Grove, CA: Cengage.

Milligan, S. (2009, April 22). *President signs $5.7 billion measure to boost volunteerism.* New York: New York Times Company. Retrieved from http://www.boston .com/news/nation/Washington/articles/2009/04/22

National Center for Cultural Competence. (2012). *National Center for Cultural Competence: Promising Practices.* Retrieved from http://nccc .george town.edu/documents/NCCC_PP_Cultural %20Brokers.pdf

National Organization for Human Services. (2012). *The human service worker: A generic job description.* Retrieved from http://www .nationalhuman services.org/hsworker.html

Okun, B. F., & Kantrowitz, R. E. (2008). *Effective helping: Interviewing and counseling techniques* (7th ed.). Pacific Grove, CA: Brooks/Cole.

Southern Regional Education Board. (1969). *Roles and functions for different levels of mental health workers.* Atlanta, GA: Author.

THE PRACTICE OF
HUMAN SERVICES

Jim Commentucci/Syracuse Newspapers/The Image Works

Questions to Consider

- What is the nature of the helping process?
- What communication skills facilitate the process?
- How can knowledge of the working environment be useful in understanding human service delivery?
- What important ethical and professional issues must human service professionals be prepared to face?

Part III focuses on the practice of human services and the context in which it occurs. Chapter 7 explores the helping process, introducing the skills helpers need to do their jobs well. The chapter concludes with a section on brief therapy and crisis intervention. Chapter 8 addresses the environment of the human service system. It begins with an examination of components such as mission and goals that help define the nature of the organization. The chapter then covers the referral process, the challenges human service professionals face in their day-to-day work, and the ways of using the system to assist clients and the community at large. As community organizers, human service professionals are able to extend their work to meet the needs of a wider audience and to serve as advocates for those in need. Part III concludes with Chapter 9 which presents ethical considerations for the human service professional and describes practical applications of ethical principles. The purpose of Part III is to refine the definition of human services (developed in Parts I and II) by examining the helping process in actual practice. As you read the three chapters in this section, think about the questions above.

THE HELPING PROCESS

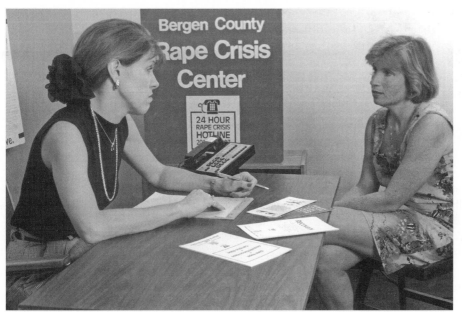

CHAPTER 7

Rhoda Sidney/PhotoEdit

After reading this chapter, you will be able to:

- Distinguish helping relationships from other relationships.
- Recognize the skills essential for the development of a helping relationship.
- Demonstrate how a helper listens and responds to a client.
- Describe challenging clients.
- Summarize the goals of motivational interviewing.
- Identify the phases of a crisis and the skills necessary for crisis intervention.
- List the four stages of resolution-focused brief therapy.

Helping can take many forms, such as gathering information from the client and other sources, looking for assistance, deciding how to solve a problem, and talking about feelings. Yet it is always guided by two questions: (1) What is helpful? (2) How can the needs of the client be met? In human services, assistance to the client occurs through the *helping process*. As they engage in this process, human service professionals must remember that clients are responsible for themselves and make their own decisions. Giving advice or telling someone what to do does not encourage responsibility or promote self-help, which are goals of the helping process.

The effectiveness of the helping process depends greatly on the skills of the helper, which is the focus of this chapter. The helper's ability to communicate an understanding of the client's feelings, clarify what the problem is, and provide appropriate assistance to resolve the problem contributes to the effectiveness of the process. Of course this help occurs within the multicultural context, emphasizing the uniqueness of the individual and recognizing individual strengths. The nature of the helping relationship, the skills of helping, group work, and the challenges of difficult clients will be explored in this chapter. A look at special human service methodologies such as motivational interviewing, crisis intervention, and resolution-focused brief therapy will provide descriptions of the helping process.

To illustrate some of the important concepts in this chapter, you will read about three individuals. We first renew our acquaintance with Carmen Rodriguez, the helping professional you met in Chapter 6. Then, you will read about Michiko, an international student from Japan, who struggles with living in a new environment. Finally, you will read about Joan, a wife abandoned by her husband, who needs support and assistance during this crisis and help after the crisis event has been resolved.

THE NATURE OF THE HELPING PROCESS

The helping process occurs in both formal and informal settings. In this chapter we will explore the helping that occurs in formal settings, for example offices, institutions, agencies, street corners, and any other setting where human service professionals deliver services to clients. As noted in Chapter 5, the term *client* can refer to an individual, a small group such as a family or a street gang, or a larger group such as a neighborhood or a geographic area.

THE HELPING RELATIONSHIP

The cornerstone of helping, the medium through which help is offered, is the **helping relationship**. The helping process takes place within the context of a relationship that

FIGURE 7.1 THE HELPING PROCESS

differs from others in that one person sets aside personal needs to focus on the needs of the other (or others), refraining from expressing opinions or giving advice.

Each participant brings to the relationship different perspectives and experiences (see Figure 7.1). Both the client and the helper bring attitudes, values, feelings, and experiences, which may be similar or may be different. In addition, the client brings needs, problems, and expectations about what will happen, as well as personal and environmental strengths. The helper comes with knowledge, training, and skills to assist with the problems of the client. Matching clients with helpers is often random, but there is considerable evidence that compatibility between the two is important for an effective helping relationship.

Because the helper has the knowledge and expertise that the client is seeking, much of the initial responsibility for establishing the relationship rests with the helper. The importance of the characteristics and values of the helper are discussed in Chapter 6. A growing body of research shows their importance in establishing and maintaining the helping relationship. The following questions (adapted from Rogers, 1958) may help you increase your self-awareness in relation to your own helping skills:

Can I be perceived as trustworthy, dependable, and consistent?

Can I express myself well enough that the client understands what I am saying?

Can I experience attitudes of warmth, caring, liking, interest, and respect for the client?

Can I separate my needs from those of the client?

Am I secure enough myself to allow the client to be separate and independent from me?

Am I able to see the world as the client does?

Can I identify the cultural uniqueness of the client?

Can I accept the client as he or she is?

Can I help the client see his or her strengths?

As you begin to grasp the concept of the helping relationship and its importance to human service delivery, you may be asking yourself how it differs from other relationships. Several characteristics make it unique. First, helping relationships are formed for a recognized and agreed-upon purpose; they are goal oriented. Second, a helping relationship is time bound, which means it usually occurs over several sessions (depending, of course, on the nature of the problem); the relationship ends when the purpose has been accomplished. Third, the helping relationship carries authority. In this sense, the word *authority* has a very different meaning from the one with which you are probably familiar. The helper's authority consists of the knowledge and skills that enable him or her to work with the client toward resolving the problem. The client maintains authority by working with the helper to establish the direction and nature of the help. Finally, this relationship is for the client. The focus is always on the client's problems and concerns within the context of client strengths and the client's cultural context.

Among the most poignant illustrations of helping and the helping relationship was the work of Mother Teresa and the Missionaries of Charity. As you read about Mother Teresa in Box 7.1, think about how the characteristics of the helping relationship apply.

STAGES OF THE HELPING PROCESS

Usually the agency or organization with which a helper works shapes the focus, the services, and the duration of the helping process. For example, vocational rehabilitation agencies are concerned with the work histories of clients, any disabilities that may prevent them from being employed, and their vocational capabilities and aspirations. Finding low-income housing, arranging adoptions, and processing applications for food stamps are not part of their services. Regardless of the focus of an agency and its services, you will find that the stages of the helping process are similar. They will include components of the problem-solving process such as identifying the problem, setting goals to resolve the problem, and determining and applying strategies designed to help the client reach those goals.

PREPARATION   Before the client arrives, the helper will want to attend to several matters. One is the physical setting. Are there any barriers that will prevent or make it difficult to establish a relationship with the client? For example, many clients will perceive a desk as a symbol of authority, which may seem a barrier to them when the helper sits behind it. It may also be unwise to seat the client facing a window. Activities outside may distract clients and prevent them from focusing on what is happening in the office. Sounds from electronic devices may provide additional distractions. Does the physical setting ensure confidentiality? Promising the client that all matters discussed will remain between the two of you means nothing if the setting is such that any discussion may be overheard by others.

Most agencies require extensive paperwork on clients. How will you handle note taking, filling out forms, and recording information? These decisions are best made before the client arrives. They can be handled in several ways; each helper must choose his or her own best method. For example, some helpers prefer taking notes while interviewing the client because it enables them to get all the facts while the client is present. Others say that taking notes while the client is talking is too difficult for them. They find that they miss important gestures and facial expressions. Others believe computers greatly assist the note taking while others view technology as a hindrance to relationship building.

The same is true of filling out forms. Some agencies require forms to be completed before the client sees a human service professional. In such cases, the helper may have little choice. If there is no such policy, the helper may choose to have the

BOX 7.1   INTERNATIONAL FOCUS: MOTHER TERESA AND THE MISSIONARIES OF CHARITY

Mother Teresa received God's call to serve the poorest of the poor in 1946. Her work began in Calcutta, India, in a small way by caring for one sick and dying person she found on the streets there. Until March 1997, she was head of the Missionaries of Charity, a religious order she formed with the Vatican's blessing in 1950. The numbers of sisters and brothers in this order now total more than 4,000 worldwide.

They live what they teach, not owning more than the poor they serve. Mother Teresa won many awards, including the Nobel Peace Prize, the Pope John XXIII Peace Prize, and India's Jawaharlal Nehru Award for International Understanding.

She founded hundreds of homes throughout the world, including four in Calcutta: Shishu Bhavan (the children's home); Prem Nivas (the center for leprosy patients in Titagarh); Nirmal Hriday (the home for the dying and destitute); and Prem Dam (the home for TB sufferers and individuals with mental disabilities). As late as 1995, Mother Teresa was expanding her list of concerns. She was working with AIDS patients and fighting against abortion and prostitution, and for battered women. She traveled worldwide to advocate for the less fortunate and to enlist the support of others in the causes that she championed (Negri & Kramer, 1995).

Mother Teresa died on September 5, 1997. The Catholic Church is considering her for sainthood.

Mother Teresa accepting honorary U.S. citizenship in 1996.

client complete necessary forms before their meeting, or the helper may wish to assist the client in completing the forms, using this opportunity to establish rapport with the client and begin developing a helping relationship. Finally, before the client arrives, the helper reviews the information about the client that is already accessible. What records are available? Is additional information needed? Based on the information available, what is the best way to approach the client? Has the helper made arrangements to have uninterrupted time with the client?

What follows is one client's description of an initial visit to a Social Security office. As you read it, pay attention to the physical setting, the workers, and the climate. What messages do those seeking services receive?

> The first thing I noticed when I entered the double glass doors of the Social Security office was the back of everyone's head. There were rows of people sitting in metal folding chairs facing a blank white wall that had a door in the middle of it. All kinds of people were there—young, old, White, Black, Hispanic, a couple of mothers with babies, some with disabilities. On the left side of the room was a counter with a glass partition. Three women were behind the counter. I watched the person who entered in front of me. He approached the counter and one woman told him, in a rather loud voice I thought, to take a number and sit down to wait his turn. I took number 38 before she could yell at me.
>
> As I sat there facing the blank white wall, I had a chance to observe how the agency operated. As each professional was ready for a client, she simply yelled the number. The person then approached the counter, and there was an exchange of information, which I could plainly hear. In some cases, the individual then approached the door in the middle of the blank white wall. A buzzer sounded, unlocking the door, and the person entered. I suppose there were other workers behind the door, but I only made it to the counter. When number 38 was called, I found out I needed to write a letter to the regional office. The local office could not help me with my problem.

THE CLIENT ARRIVES   When the client enters the office, a climate of respect and acceptance is established if the client is greeted with a smile, a handshake, and an introduction. Remember that clients come with problems, often feeling vulnerable, and sometimes in pain or discomfort. A helper who takes charge of the initial meeting will help the client feel at ease by giving the client time to adjust to the new situation. The use of "ice breakers" or "door openers" allows the client to become accustomed to the setting and the helper: "Did you have any trouble finding the office?" or "Parking is sometimes a problem here. I hope it wasn't for you."

Since the helping relationship is time bound and goal oriented, the helper will at some point need to inquire about the client's problem. Many clients will be eager to share their problems. Others will be reticent about discussing problems that are personal and painful; they may test the helper by sharing less important problems first. The helper can initiate problem identification in a number of ways: "Let's talk about why you're here," "Tell me what's going on," or "I'm wondering what's on your mind." In addition, the helper works with the client to identify personal and environmental strengths: "Tell me about a time when you solved this type of problem successfully," or "What do you consider your best characteristic?" These are relatively nonthreatening ways of focusing on the client and the problem. Another way to do this is to have focused dialogue. After greeting the client, the helper and client can fill out the intake form together. This is a humanizing way to complete the form, and it does not require asking so many questions. Some forms include questions that build on strengths, such as, "What do you enjoy?" "What do you do well?" "Who do you go to for help?" or "What have you learned from your family and friends?"

During this initial stage, the helper can provide the client with information about the agency. For example, the client may want to know exactly what services the agency can provide. Other questions might concern the cost of the services, the criteria for eligibility to receive services, and the responsibilities of clients. In turn, the helper will probably have additional questions for the client: Does the client have any insurance? How did the client hear about the agency? Did someone refer the client here? What expectations does the client have for the agency and the helper? At this time, the helper establishes a tone of cooperation and collaboration to establish a foundation for rapport and trust between client and helper. This occurs when the client believes that the helper understands his or her world. Even though rapport develops over time, helpers in this initial stage of the helping process provide a positive and realistic setting in which the helping occurs.

EXPLORING THE PROBLEM   Chapter 5 discussed different perspectives on client problems. As the helper and the client begin to explore the problem, the helper should keep those perspectives in mind. The human service concepts of the whole person and the multidimensionality of problems will also guide this phase of the helping process (see Box 7.2). Once the problems are identified, it is time to move to the next stage.

INTERVENTION STRATEGIES   During this stage, the helper and the client set goals and determine how those goals will be reached to resolve the problem. This means addressing the current status of the problem, the client's aspirations and desires, and the client's personal and social resources and strengths. Should the helper find that the client's problem calls for expertise or experience that the helper does not have, the helper should refer the client to another professional who has the necessary knowledge and skills. Another reason for referral at this point arises if, once the problem has been identified, the helper has such strong feelings or biases

---

BOX 7.2   CARL ROGERS AND CLIENT-CENTERED THERAPY

Carl Rogers, American psychologist and educator, was born on January 8, 1902, in Oak Park, Illinois. He attended the University of Wisconsin and graduated in 1924 with a degree in history. He then attended Union Theological Seminary in New York City and began to study for the ministry. He soon became influenced by a number of psychologists affiliated with Columbia University and transferred there to receive both his master's and doctoral degrees.

Rogers was initially concerned with environmental and institutional solutions to the problems of children, which he described in *The Clinical Treatment of the Problem Child* (1939). Later, he became interested in the psychotherapeutic process and gradually formulated the approach associated with his name—client-centered therapy. Client-centered

therapy, or nondirective counseling, had a controversial beginning but proved to be a successful psychotherapeutic model. In *Counseling and Psychotherapy* (1942), Rogers maintained that the client knows better than anyone else what the problem is; with the help of a permissive, caring counselor, the client can find a solution to the problem. In client-centered therapy, the helper does not direct, give advice, or offer solutions and interpretations. The primary technique is "reflection of feelings." When the client speaks or acts, the helper responds by communicating perceptions of what the client means and feels. Through this "mirroring," the client can think more clearly about problems and feelings.

Source: From Taylor (1985).

TABLE 7.1   SUMMARY POINTS: HELPING STAGES

- Physical setting, paperwork, and review of information occur before the client arrives.
- When the client arrives, the helper greets the client, inquires about the problem, and provides information about the agency.
- Concepts of the whole person and the multidimensionality of the problem guide problem exploration.
- Intervention may involve referral, service provision, or both.
- Termination that is positive occurs when the needed services are provided and the objectives obtained.

about the situation that he or she is unable to work objectively with the client. Referral will be discussed in detail in Chapter 8.

Depending on the problem, strategies may be as simple as providing a one-time service such as pregnancy testing or as complex as working with a client who has been injured in a car wreck and is permanently disabled. In the latter case, problems may include the client's loss of ability to work at a previous job, difficulties of the client and the family in adjusting to the client's disability, and barriers in the home to the client's mobility. These issues must be addressed if the client is to adjust to his or her new reality. Each strategy used supports client strengths and helps the client negotiate his or her own environment. The role of cultural broker, introduced in Chapter 6, brings cultural considerations during interventions.

The final stage of the helping process is **termination**. The relationship between the helper and the client may end in several ways. The most positive conclusion is when the needed services are provided and both participants are satisfied that the objectives have been reached. Unfortunately, not all terminations are so positive; services may be interrupted by either the helper or the client before the objectives have been reached. For example, the client moves from the area; the helper is transferred, promoted, or leaves the agency; or the client refuses to return for services.

In the case study that follows we visit Carmen Rodriguez, whom we met in Chapter 6. Here she discusses how she deals with many of the concepts discussed in this section.

> One aspect of my work that makes it challenging is that I perform a variety of functions. For example, I always begin my work with a client with an interview. During this initial contact with the client, I try to establish rapport. I believe that each helping encounter represents a multicultural experience. I tell the client throughout the process, I am interested in learning how gender, race, ethnicity, and other factors influence client values and experiences. Then, I explain our work together and what the schedule is like at our agency. It also helps clients know what is expected of them. One of the best ways I've found to get this relationship off on the right foot is to talk to the client as someone I really want to get to know. I do have some background information on the client (usually an intake form and a financial statement), and I briefly skim it before I see the client. When I meet with the client the first time, I always stand up and invite him or her in with a handshake and a smile. My greeting changes if this traditional Western greeting does not seem to be appropriate. I leave the folder in a drawer, because I can concentrate on the client totally if I'm not distracted by reports.

After the initial meeting, I read the client's folder carefully. At that point, I usually ask myself the following questions: What do I know about this client? What are the presenting needs or problems? What strengths does the client possess? I always focus on the client's strengths as a way of boosting confidence and building on past successes. What do I know about this client's culture? Finally, what additional information would be helpful to best serve this client?

For the protection of the client, the agency, and the human service professional, it is necessary to maintain written case notes and documentation of services. This can be very time-consuming. I've noticed that each professional handles this task differently. What works for me is reserving the last 30 minutes of the day for updating files. I realize that these notes are important—the client may be transferred, I may change jobs, or I may be out sick—but some days it's a real chore to pull all the files and condense what's necessary into two or three sentences. Our computer software continues to change. Switching to new systems always requires additional time and effort.

I hope to continue in my job for several more years, but eventually I would like to go back to school for further training. I want to develop my counseling skills to work with clients as individuals or groups in a more specialized way. My current position as a case manager gives me practical experience and allows me to explore my career options by working with a variety of clients and professionals.

AN INTRODUCTION TO HELPING SKILLS

Communication is the foundation for all interpersonal relationships. Exchanging messages to understand another's perceptions, ideas, and experiences is especially important in helping relationships. Helping others will be difficult if we do not understand their problems or concerns.

In this section we introduce basic helping skills. We begin by focusing on the client's message, which means perceiving both the verbal and the nonverbal messages of the client. Next, we focus on the helper's communication by identifying the skills necessary for effective listening and responding. Finally, we discuss what the helper needs to know about cultural differences.

Communication involves sending a message to another person with the conscious intent of affecting the receiver's behavior. This process is illustrated in Figure 7.2. When the receiver interprets the message the way the sender intended, **effective communication** has taken place. When one person interprets the message differently from the way it was intended, the result is communication failure, the most common source of misunderstandings in interpersonal relationships.

The message that a person sends can be verbal or nonverbal. Both of these messages occur within a cultural context, and a message within one culture is not necessarily the same message in another culture. The most common example of a **verbal message** is the spoken word: "Hello, how are you today?" The smile and

FIGURE 7.2   COMMUNICATION

handshake or hug accompanying that verbal greeting are **nonverbal messages**. The skillful helper is able to "hear" the client's behavior (the nonverbal message) as well as what is actually said (the verbal message) and is able to respond verbally and nonverbally to these messages (Okun & Kantrowitz, 2008). It sounds complicated, and it takes practice to communicate effectively. A good beginning is through an introduction to each component of the communication process.

NONVERBAL MESSAGES

Nonverbal behaviors (body language) include a person's posture, tone of voice, gestures, eye contact, and touch. Everyone communicates nonverbally within the context of their own cultural environment. Each of us engages in some nonverbal behavior that we are aware of and perform intentionally. For example, when meeting someone for the first time, most of us want to make a positive first impression, so we deliberately greet that person with a smile or some other pleasant facial expression. However, we also communicate unconsciously in a nonverbal fashion. You may recall a time when you visited the doctor's office for shots and afterward wondered at the soreness in your muscles. The tension, fear, or hurt you experienced during the visit caused you to tense your muscles.

In a normal two-person conversation, more than 65% of the meaning is carried nonverbally. This fact emphasizes the importance of nonverbal communication in a helping situation. Frequently, you may find that a client's nonverbal message will provide you with valuable clues about what the client is thinking or feeling—important ideas that the client is unable to verbalize. Table 7.2 lists some common nonverbal cues and their meanings.

Another area in which nonverbal cues are important is the expression of feelings. Feelings are most often communicated nonverbally, particularly by facial expressions and tone of voice. One difficulty with "hearing" the nonverbal expression of feelings is the ambiguity of the nonverbal message. A nonverbal behavior such as crying could be interpreted in various ways; one cannot determine just from the tears on a person's face whether the person is sad, hurt, or disappointed. In fact, the person may be scared or even very happy. Thus, we may think that nonverbal communication is a fairly straightforward process of sending and receiving messages, but it is actually a complicated mode of communication. Although they provide us with important clues about the person with whom we are conversing, nonverbal messages should be interpreted with caution. It is important to note that nonverbal messages vary from culture to culture.

Try this exercise: At some point today, select two people who are communicating with each other. (You may be in the library, a food-service area, or anywhere you choose.) For 10 minutes, observe the nonverbal communication of one of the participants. What behaviors do you observe? What possible interpretations can you make about the meanings of the behaviors?

VERBAL MESSAGES

Verbal messages consist of words spoken by a person, again within a cultural context. Such messages can be divided into a cognitive component and an affective component. The cognitive component consists of the facts of a message and reflects

TABLE 7.2 NONVERBAL CUES AND THEIR POSSIBLE MEANINGS

Cue	Meaning
Lifting an eyebrow	Disbelief
Lowering eyebrows	Uneasiness, suspicion
Lifting both eyebrows	Surprise
Eye contact	Interest, confidence
Winking an eye	Intimacy
Slapping forehead	Forgetfulness
Rubbing the nose	Puzzlement
Turning up corners of mouth	Happiness
Cocking head to one side	Friendly, human
Little or no head and/or hand movements	Cool, no emotion
Raised shoulders	Fear
Retracted shoulders	Suppressed anger
Square shoulders	Responsibility
Bowed shoulders	Carrying a burden
Shrugging shoulders	Indifference
Sitting with arms and legs crossed	Withdrawal, resistance
Clasping arms	Protection
Tapping fingers	Impatience
Fondling and touching inanimate objects	Loneliness
Leaning forward in a chair	Interest
Leaning back, arms uncrossed	Open to suggestion
Leaning back, arms crossed	Not open to suggestion
Postural change—facing away	Finished with interaction

the person's thinking processes. This is the realm in which we are most comfortable. A cognitive message addresses such matters as who, what, where, when, and why. Consider the following statements and try to pick out the cognitive messages.

> I left work at 5:00 p.m. today. The last client I saw was Raphael Santini, and I just can't seem to get him off my mind. He is making such an effort to find a job, but he's had no luck. I couldn't believe it when he showed up today. I hardly recognized him, and I guess he could tell I was surprised, because I couldn't think of anything to say for a moment. He looked great. His hair was clean and neatly combed, and his clothes were new. He was so proud of himself, and I was proud of him, too. I told him I was so pleased with the changes. I also felt good about myself, because some of my hard work with this client has paid off. I'm going to make some telephone calls and conduct an Internet search first thing in the morning to see what assistance I can find to help him locate a job. There's just got to be help for a motivated client like Raphael.

Some of the cognitive messages you probably identified were the speaker's leaving work at 5:00 p.m.; the appointment with Raphael Santini, who is trying to find a job; and the description of his neat, clean appearance. In the cognitive realm, facts are the focus.

The affective component, the feeling part of the message, may be expressed directly or indirectly. Many clients who are unsure about what they are feeling, or who are simply uncomfortable talking about feelings, may choose to express their feelings indirectly. This means that the individual may not name the feeling at all ("Stop driving so fast!"), or may describe it by telling what he or she feels like doing ("I feel like punching him in the nose"). One of the helper's main tasks may be to encourage the client to become aware of feelings and to learn to express feelings appropriately and directly: "I'm scared when you drive so fast," or "I'm angry at you for spoiling the surprise."

Review the statements about Raphael Santini. What feelings are expressed directly? In fact, there are very few, but they do include feeling "proud," "surprised," and "good." These feelings are named, and the reader clearly understands how the helper feels. Read the excerpt again, and consider the feelings that are being expressed indirectly. (It might be helpful to read it aloud.) You might identify such feelings as discouragement at Raphael's lack of success, exasperation at the job situation, disbelief at his appearance, and determination to find some type of assistance for Raphael. Determining exactly what the client (or, in this case, the helper) is feeling may be more difficult when feelings are expressed indirectly.

LISTENING AND RESPONDING

The way we listen and respond to the client is crucial in building a helping relationship. The first thing a helper must do before making any response to the client is to listen carefully to what the client is expressing, both verbally and nonverbally. Even though listening takes up more of a person's waking hours than any other activity and many people consider themselves good listeners, few of us actually are. This section will introduce listening behaviors and some helper responses that promote effective helping (see Table 7.3).

THE HELPER LISTENS   The kind of listening that helpers engage in is called **responsive listening** or **active listening**. These terms describe the behaviors of helpers as they attend to both the verbal and the nonverbal communication of the client. What makes this type of listening special or different from other listening behaviors is that helpers also attend to what is not said, that is, to the underlying thoughts and feelings of the client, which are not expressed in words. Two ways of considering responsive or active listening as helping behaviors are presented here.

Egan (2010, pp. 134–135) suggested several things helpers can do to communicate to clients that they are listening. These five behaviors are presented as a set of guidelines that helpers can follow to let their clients know they are physically present and actively involved in the helping relationship. You can easily remember the behaviors by thinking of the acronym SOLER.

S   Face the client *Squarely*. This is a posture of involvement. To face away from the client or even at an angle lessens the degree of involvement.

O   Adopt an *Open posture*. This is usually perceived as nondefensive. Crossing arms or legs may not communicate openness or availability.

TABLE 7.3   HELPFUL BEHAVIORS IN COMMUNICATING

Verbal	Nonverbal
Mirroring feelings	Making eye contact
Clarifying	Listening
Showing a sense of humor	Smiling
Providing support	Nodding one's head
Providing information that client needs	Leaning forward
Explaining helper's role	Maintaining a relaxed posture
Sharing information about oneself	Facing the client
Being nonjudgmental	Displaying facial expression
Asking few questions	Being punctual
Occasionally making appropriate use of gestures and touching	Maintaining a moderate rate of speech

L   *Lean toward* the other person. A natural sign of involvement, this posture is a slight forward inclination. Moving forward or backward can frighten a client or communicate lessened involvement.

E   Maintain good *Eye contact*. This is normal behavior for two individuals who are involved in conversation. It is different from staring.

R   Try to be relatively *Relaxed*. This means avoiding nervous habits such as fidgeting or tapping a pencil. Behaviors such as these can distract the client.

Remember that these are only guidelines. A helper's physical behavior may vary in accordance with the cultural identity of the client or what is comfortable for that particular helper.

Attending behavior is another way to let the client know the helper is listening. The goal of attending behavior is to encourage the client to talk about and examine issues, problems, or concerns. Attending behavior has four dimensions: three non-verbal components and one verbal component (Ivey, Ivey, & Zalaquett, 2011).

1. *Visual/eye contact*. If you are going to talk to people, look at them.
2. *Vocal qualities*. Your vocal tone and speech rate indicate clearly how you feel about another person. Think of how many ways you can say, "I am really interested in what you say" just by altering your vocal tone and speech rate.
3. *Verbal tracking*. The client has come to you with a topic of concern. Do not change the subject; stick with the client's subject matter.
4. *Body language: attentive*. Clients know you are interested if you face them squarely and lean slightly forward, have an expressive face, and use facilitative, encouraging gestures. In short, allow yourself to be yourself—authenticity in attending is essential (p. 65).

Engaging in these behaviors encourages the client to talk, reducing the amount of talk from the helper. Benefits include communicating interest and concern to the client and increasing the helper's awareness of the client's ability to pay attention. Attending behaviors also allow the helper to modify helping behaviors to work effectively with clients who may be racially, culturally, or sexually different.

The Helper's Response   Once the helper has heard the verbal and nonverbal messages of the client, it is time for the helper to speak. Remember that helpers' responses must be purposeful. Think about the characteristics of the helping relationship. This is not a casual conversation between two people but a goal-directed exchange. Therefore, the helper must know his or her intent before speaking.

The helper has several options at this point. For example, did the helper understand what the client said? Was the message clear? Does the helper need further information to grasp the message correctly? Questions such as these will assist the helper in determining the intent of his or her response. Let us examine some of these options.

First, suppose the helper does understand the client's message and decides that the most helpful response would be one that lets the client know this. To communicate that intent, the helper may choose to **paraphrase**, to make a statement that is interchangeable with the client's own words.

CLIENT: I've been able to complete five tasks today that were on my list.

HELPER: You've had a productive day today.

The helper may determine that more than a simple paraphrase is needed to help the client become aware of or clarify feelings. In this case, a helper statement that reflects both the feeling (or affective component) and the facts (or cognitive component) is helpful. For example:

HELPER: You're really pleased that you were able to accomplish what you set out to do today.

If the helper is confused about what the client said, perhaps because the client was relating a complicated incident, the helper should ask the client for clarification. To attempt a response that will make little sense to the client and will let the client know that the helper did not understand what was said is not helpful. Responses such as, "I'm not sure I understand ..." or "I'm confused about ..." are appropriate at this point. They also let the client know that the helper is interested enough to want to get the story right in order to be able to help.

Beginning helpers sometimes encounter situations in which clients are asking questions or seeking information that the helper does not know. Many helpers believe they should know everything and may feel embarrassed about being asked something they do not know. Unfortunately, they may attempt to answer "off the tops of their heads" or give an answer they believe may be correct. A better response in situations like this would be, "I do not have that information, but I do know where we can find it; let me check on that for you," or "I'm not sure about the eligibility requirements for that type of assistance, but I can refer you to someone who knows." Helpers are not supposed to have all the answers. The effective helper who wants to maintain a relationship with the client will enrich that relationship by being honest with the client.

Asking Questions   Another technique that beginning helpers should be wary of is **questioning**. Most of us consider ourselves skilled at asking questions and find it a natural form of communication in everyday life—particularly questions that begin with the words *who*, *what*, *where*, *why*, and *when*. For the beginning helper, the question is the most common method of eliciting information from the client, and many helpers find themselves resorting to questions frequently. Unfortunately, one question seems to lead to another, and too many questions can interfere with the helping relationship, causing the client to feel like a witness. An overreliance on questioning, and neglecting other kinds of responses, hinders the helping process. It also creates a dependent client who has no role other than answering questions. Most questions can be rephrased as statements that elicit the same information. For example, the question, "What was the last grade completed in school?" can be rephrased as, "Tell me about your school experiences." In addition to discovering the final grade completed, the helper may learn how the client felt about school, whether the client enjoyed learning, and what circumstances surrounded the end of the client's educational experience.

Now that you have been alerted to the pitfalls of questioning, let us explore the time when asking questions is appropriate and how one asks good questions. There are several situations in which a question is helpful. In the first situation, you can begin the interview with a question: "How would you like to begin?" or "Could you tell me a little about yourself?" A second situation occurs when specific information is needed. Asking for information to clarify ("How long have you been ill?") or to elicit examples of specific behavior ("How does that make you feel?") can provide the additional information necessary for complete understanding. Finally, questions can be useful to focus the client's attention. For example, a client who is digressing or rambling on about several problems may need the helper's assistance to focus. Such assistance can be provided by statements such as the following:

> You've mentioned several concerns that you have about your daughter. You're afraid she is using drugs, and you suspect she is not doing well in school. I guess I hear you expressing the most concern, though, about your inability to talk with her. Let's focus on that. What happens when you do try to talk with her?

Thus, there are times in a helping relationship when asking questions is appropriate and beneficial. How does one ask good questions? The helper might first want to consider how the question will relate to and promote the helping relationship (Egan, 2010). Having specific objectives in mind before asking the question will help in formulating a good question.

TABLE 7.4 SUMMARY POINTS: WHEN TO ASK QUESTIONS

- To begin the interview
- To obtain specific information
- To seek clarification
- To elicit examples of specific behavior
- To focus the client's attention

Both closed and open questions can facilitate the development of the helping relationship when the helper has specific intentions. *Closed* questions are those that elicit facts necessary to facilitate the helping process. "How old were you when your father died?" and "How many brothers and sisters do you have?" may provide important information regarding the client's family situation if the client is having difficulties at home. Closed questions that require a "yes" or "no" answer should usually be avoided, because they lead the beginning helper to ask more and more questions.

Open questions, on the other hand, are broader, allowing the client to express thoughts, feelings, or ideas. They contribute to building rapport with the client and also assist him or her in exploring a situation, a problem, or an interaction. For example, "How did you feel after talking it over with your parents?" asks for the client's view. On the other hand, "Did you feel better after talking with your parents?" can be answered with a simple "yes" or "no," which does not enhance the helping process.

In summary, questions can be useful tools in the helping process. As with other types of responses, the key to effective questioning is knowing the intent of the question before posing it to the client. Are you seeking factual information or asking the client to offer thoughts or opinions about the topic of discussion? Considering how the question will promote the helping relationship will assist the helper in determining the appropriate strategy.

This section has been a brief introduction to helping skills. As you pursue your education and training in preparation for work in the human services, you will increase your knowledge about these skills and refine your use of them so that you become an effective helper. One area that requires a mastery of communications skills is working with groups of individuals. By the end of the 1980s, groups were recognized as viable means of helping individuals in a variety of settings. Group work flourished during the 1990s and will continue to be a major strategy in the 21st century to provide direct service to clients as well as to collaborate with colleagues and community groups. An introduction to basic group concepts and the role of communication in group work follows.

WORKING WITH GROUPS

Groups are natural. Since the beginning of time, individuals have banded together for survival, security, tasks, and problem solving, thus making groups a critical mode for accomplishing what needs to be done. Think about your own life—your living situation, your work, and even your leisure time. Most of these activities take place in groups. In human services, individuals also band together to accomplish tasks. Membership may be voluntary. For example, individuals with similar problems or experiences, such as victims of incest or suicide survivors or children of alcoholics, may work together on their problems. Involuntary membership occurs when participating in a group is mandated by some authority. Joining a group for abusive parents or one for substance abusers may be a condition for probation. These human service–focused groups exist face to face and online. With the growth of social media, Skype, chat rooms, discussion boards, and weblogs (blogs), the possibilities of belonging to a group expand. Online communities represent one way that individuals form groups to address social problems. For example, organization-sponsored online communities, such as the support group established by the National Alliance on Mental Illness, have an articulated goal and a professional tone consistent with for-profit, nonprofit, and governmental organizations. In contrast, peer-initiated online communities, such as Breast Cancer Support, emerge from the ground up as the members themselves determine the goals for the community and provide the space for social interaction. Additional information about both examples may be found by searching the Internet for the National Alliance on Mental Illness and Breast Cancer Support.

In this section we will define groups, explore the skills necessary to work with a group, and consider the trends that will affect group work in the 21st century.

A **group** is a number of individuals who interact with each other. Groups have several characteristics (Jacobs, Masson, Harvill, & Schimmel, 2012). An important characteristic is the interaction that occurs among group members. They participate in group meetings and discussions, share resources, give and receive help, and influence each other. Sharing common goals and values is a second characteristic. The group may be formed for an agreed-upon purpose, or the group may establish its own goals once members meet. The group also develops its own values, identifying what is important to the group and translating it into behavior for individuals as members of the group and for the group as a whole. Groups also have a social structure. Roles define the formal structure of the group and influence how individuals act in the group. Different group members play different roles. Examples of roles include the leadership role, which may be a designated person or a shared role among members; the maintenance role, which sees to the well-being of the group by encouraging and compromising; the facilitative and building role, which helps everyone feel part of the group by initiating, seeking information and opinions, coordinating, and evaluating; and the blocking role, one that is aggressive, dominating, and antigroup. A final characteristic of a group is cohesiveness among members. Members perceive that they belong to a group, they are interdependent in some way, and they work together to keep the group going as well as focus on common goals.

Groups have their own dynamics that influence the group's development and its productivity. One important influence is the context or purpose for which the group was formed. For example, if a group is formed to help members deal with a chronic illness such as diabetes, the purpose guides many of the activities of the group. Group process also influences how the group functions. Conflicts, anxieties, validations, agreements, and hopefulness are all byproducts of meeting together. Group dynamics, or how members of the group behave with each other, can be directed by helpers who understand the conditions that help a group run smoothly. Groups do develop unwritten rules and often resemble a family unit.

Alcoholics Anonymous (AA) is an example of a well-known group that illustrates these characteristics. Although many self-help groups formed during the late 1960s, AA is one of the more enduring ones, established in the late 1930s by founders who realized the effectiveness of individuals meeting together and interacting in such a way to support change (Jacobs, Masson, Harvill, & Schimmel, 2012; The History of Alcoholics Anonymous, 2012). Interaction among members is the foundation of AA meetings; for example, members share experiences and information. They also have a common goal, which is to gain and maintain control of their lives by remaining sober. To that end, members encourage, coordinate, evaluate, support, and lead, both in regular meetings and outside meetings. These techniques are similar to those used in other self-help groups such as Parents without Partners and Weight Watchers. These organizations also use online groups to provide support to their members.

Groups are formed for reasons other than self-help. Today there are specialty areas in group work and a set of core competencies and standards that have been established for preparation for group work in these areas (Association for Specialists in Group Work, 2012). Identified specialty areas include task or work groups that are focused on accomplishing identified work goals, for example, task forces, planning groups, or community organizations. The teams described in Chapter 1 are examples of this type of group.

Guidance and psychoeducational groups are another type of group whose focus is education, prevention, or both. In these groups, information may be shared about AIDS, bereavement, or divorce. The goal is to prevent the development of psychological disturbances. Another type of group is counseling and interpersonal problem solving, whose focus is the resolution of problems group members face. Examples may be test anxiety, relationship difficulties, or career decision making. Psychotherapy and personality reconstruction groups are most often found in mental health facilities such as clinics or hospitals and include individuals who have serious psychological problems of long-term duration. Both abusers and victims of abuse may benefit from involvement in such a group.

What is the role of the human service professional in a group? In natural groups, such as a family or a street gang, human service professionals enter as outsiders and must make a place for themselves (Levine, 2012). They are present because a member is in trouble or there are significant problems in the group or both. In formed groups, that is, those that are organized for a specific purpose or goal, the human service professional may have responsibility for getting people involved and getting the group underway. Organizational issues such as meeting times and places, purpose, and group structure must be addressed by members before the real work of the group begins. At this point, the human service professional facilitates the work of the group toward its goal.

The foundation of all group functioning is communication skills. As stated earlier, interaction is key to the group's existence and involves the exchange of information and transmission of meaning. It is by means of effective communication that group members reach some understanding of one another, their goals, the division of labor, and other group tasks. Both verbal and nonverbal behaviors comprise effective communication and are every bit as complex in groups as they are in individuals. For example, silence may have many meanings: processing information, mulling over what was said, avoidance, or discomfort with the topic. Therefore, many of the points made earlier in the chapter about sending messages, listening, asking questions, and responding are critical for group work. In fact, the core skills identified by the Association for Specialists in Group Work (2012) include the communication skills to open and close group meetings, impart information, self-disclose, give feedback, and ask open-ended questions.

Groups are experiencing increased popularity at this time and focus on special populations. Examples are groups for individuals who are divorcing or are

BOX 7.3   A CLIENT SPEAKS

Life was not very good for me about 15 years ago. I just hit rock bottom. I was a builder and an engineer by training and had established an excellent environmental consulting firm. In fact, during my consulting activities, I was fortunate enough to meet several individuals who helped me become a commercial land developer. Over a period of five years I amassed a fortune; I had increased my personal wealth to such a degree that I owned three homes—one in New York City; one in Lisbon, Portugal; and one in Miami, Florida. My kids attended private school; my family belonged to a prestigious country club; I was able to buy a home for my parents.

All of a sudden my financial situation began to deteriorate as the business began to crumble. Because of depressed economic conditions and a recession, the land value dropped and individuals and corporations were no longer interested in land investments. Because of stressful times and other complicating factors, my wife asked me for a divorce. She kept our family home and gained custody of our three children. The two dogs stayed with her as well. It seemed that I would have to file for bankruptcy and face the losses (financially, socially, and professionally) alone. My lawyer, who was handling the fight to avoid bankruptcy, recommended that I join a men's therapy group sponsored by Consumer Counseling Centers of America.

At the first meeting, I was scared to death. A million times during the day I changed my mind about going. I drove up to the agency at 6:45 p.m. and decided once again that I would have to skip the 7:00 p.m. meeting. My hands were sweaty, I had a headache, my stomach hurt, and I had not had much sleep in months. I watched the participants enter one by one. My knees seemed to buckle as I stepped outside the car and headed for the door. The group met every week; this was an ongoing group that had been meeting for 10 years. I arrived awkwardly, sat in one of the chairs that formed a circle. I was asked to introduce myself and then I was welcomed by the other group members and the leader, a local psychologist.

The first night I talked was because I was challenged by one of the group members for coming, gaining from the group, and not really being willing to give. After I finally made my first contributions, I was able to participate in the meetings, although I never had a lot to say. One of the group rules was that we could not see each other socially. This was in part for confidentiality since we had to promise not to divulge the contents of the group discussion. We also could not acknowledge others who participated in the group. Another rule was that each person had to be honest when he spoke. There was no "B.S." allowed or tolerated.

It was amazing what I learned in the group. I made some incredibly good friends, people whom I would have never met in any other circumstance. A few I really did not like at all; we did not share many common values. The one thing that we did share was a tragic financial encounter. Some members were like me, caught in a very difficult financial situation due to the recession. Others, it seemed, had always been troubled by financial worries. I felt supported and understood.

divorced, adult offenders, overeaters, those with HIV/AIDS, adolescents, elderly living in institutions, unwed teenage fathers, and those who need support for any number of situations. This trend will continue. Most face-to-face groups provide support for a community or regional area; online group membership can include individuals across the United States and outside the United States.

SKILLS FOR CHALLENGING CLIENTS

Ideally, all clients of human services are motivated, cooperative, responsible, and like each of us; however, it is one of the challenges of this profession that not all clients fit that description. In your experience as a helper, you will likely meet clients who are different culturally or who are resistant, silent, overly demanding, or unmotivated. They may also be different from you in other ways, including background, religion, values, and life experiences. You need to know something about these client groups because they often elicit in the helper feelings of uncertainty, hostility, and resentment. They are particularly difficult for many beginning helpers to work with, and it is important to realize that the client's behavior is not necessarily the helper's fault.

CULTURALLY DIFFERENT CLIENTS

Shifts in America's population will make the country far more ethnically diverse than ever before. By 2050, the Hispanic population will grow to 24% of the population and Asians to 9%. Non-Hispanic Whites will be reduced to 53%. This shift reflects a change in immigration patterns and differences in birth rates, combined with an overall slowdown in the growth of the country's population. Latinos and Asians will grow fastest in number, whereas African Americans will nearly double in number by 2050. In addition, as described in Chapter 3, 56,000 refugees were resettled in the United States, including individuals from Burma, Bhutan, and Iraq (Russell & Batalova, 2012).

As these population shifts occur, it is increasingly likely that human service professionals will encounter clients whose cultural backgrounds differ from their own. In fact, it is important to consider each helping encounter as a multicultural experience. The key to working with clients who are culturally different is awareness of and sensitivity to these differences. In many places in the United States, there is a need to hire professionals who appreciate different cultures, especially when the client population is diverse. Helping professionals who are bilingual, bicultural, and/or African American or Latino are in demand. Sometimes getting people to accept help is difficult because accepting outside help is not part of their culture. Instead of saying to a Latino client, "You need counseling," a more acceptable phrase might be "Maybe you need someone to talk with." In some locales in the United States, many agency clients might be Latino and helping professionals are finding that they can no longer refer to them as Hispanic or Latino. Now, it is important to recognize that Latino includes people from Puerto Rico, Nicaragua, Colombia, and Honduras—and they are all different.

Helpers must realize that culture shapes body language. Few gestures and body movements have universal meaning. For example, Arabs tend to cling or huddle together, whereas Americans like their space. Postures also vary by culture. For example, within the Taiwanese culture demonstrating erect posture is a way to show respect to the other. In South America, specifically Argentina, one shows annoyance, fury, or rage by putting one's hands on one's hips (The Provider's Guide to Quality and Culture, n.d.). The direct eye contact that is so critical to standard American helping behavior may be offensive to people from Native American and Latino cultures. A helper with no knowledge of this may intend to communicate complete attention, but may be perceived by the culturally different client as disrespectful.

The beginning helper is cautioned against assigning too much meaning to a single gesture; instead, all means of expression—verbal, postural, facial, and cultural—should be considered. It is also wise not to generalize about cultural traits. Some Asian Americans may not like direct eye contact, yet some might.

The first step to a multicultural approach to human services begins with recognition that all people have in common the capacity for thoughts, feelings, and behaviors. Knowing about several cultures, understanding their similarities and differences, and being sensitive to any special needs and problems is a second step. A third step is developing an appreciation and acceptance of diverse world views.

Slavin, Gulanti, and Kuo (n.d.) described "The 4 C's of Culture" to guide helping professionals enter a culturally sensitive conversation with clients. This specific method helps human service professionals implement a multicultural approach.

1. What do you **call** your problem? *(Remember to ask "What do you think is wrong?" It's getting at the patient's perception of the problem. You should* **not** *literally ask, "What do you call your problem?")*
2. What do you think **caused** your problem? *(This gets at the patient's beliefs regarding the source of the problem.)*
3. How do you **cope** with your condition? *(This is to remind the practitioner to ask, "What have you done to try to make it better? Who else have you been to for treatment?")*
4. What are your **concerns** regarding the condition and recommended treatment? *(This should address questions such as, "How serious do you think this is?" "What potential complications do you fear?" "How does it interfere with your life, or your ability to function?" "Do you know anyone else who has tried the treatment I've recommended? What was your experience with it?")*

The following account, written by Michiko, a female foreign student from Japan, may help you to begin thinking about culturally different clients in light of the preceding three steps and the 4 C's of Culture.

MICHIKO

I am a foreign student from Japan who is studying at an American university. It has been more than a month since I arrived in the States, and still I am not making American friends. I usually hang around with my Japanese buddies, so that does not help either. I hardly have any time for socializing because of all of the assignments I have to do for class. I am tense and timid around people and feel uncomfortable most of the time because I do not know how to act in pleasing, acceptable ways. I miss my friends and family and often cry when I am alone.

I have two great needs. One is to feel accepted among Americans and to adjust to the American culture. The other need is for academic excellence, since I did not come all the way from Japan just to fool around. I would like to have American friends with whom I can talk and share experiences, who will like me the way I am. I find most of my classes large and impersonal and have hardly any hope of finding a friend there. I need someone who is interested enough to get past the language barrier to get to know me. As for the academics, my professors know that I am a foreign student and they will go out of their way to help me with any difficulties I might be facing. I appreciate the attention, but that is not enough. I need help with the report assignments because I am unfamiliar with formats in English writing. I also need to be advised on study skills, because even if I prepare well in advance for a test, the grades I get are Cs and Ds.

I have many fears. I am afraid being Japanese, a racial minority, makes me less desirable as a person worth knowing in the eyes of an American. I am in constant fear of saying wrong things at the wrong moments and acting weird in front of people. My language problem still persists. Conversational English is something I find difficult, and people must speak slowly and clearly for me. I am afraid this makes me boring to talk to and hard to discuss complex subjects with. The greatest fear of all is having to go back to Japan because I could not make it academically and socially at an American university.

The young woman in this case study is one among many culturally different clients. The three steps mentioned before this case are useful in understanding Michiko as a unique, worthwhile individual. Michiko has the capacity for thought, feeling, and behavior as she attempts to function successfully in a culture foreign to her. A helper would need to learn about the Japanese culture and the ways in which it differs from and resembles American culture. Michiko has established personal goals that focus on academic and social success and is frustrated by the barriers she is experiencing. To engage effectively in the helping process with Michiko, the helper would need to explore the relevant differences between American and Japanese cultures. For example, many Asian cultures are collectivist—the individual is less important than the group. Michiko may be fearful of not succeeding academically and socially because of the disgrace it would bring to her family.

The helper would also want to adjust his or her helping behaviors to the individual of a different culture and to assess appropriate strategies of intervention. In American culture, the individual is perceived as autonomous and separate from groups. Even though a person can be a member of many groups, no one group determines identity completely. In collectivist societies, however, the individual belongs to fewer groups, but the attachment is stronger; often the individual is defined by membership in a group. Taking this information into account, the helper would choose an intervention that would focus on Michiko in relation to her group rather than an intervention designed to promote independence.

THE RELUCTANT OR RESISTANT CLIENT

There are some distinctions between reluctant and resistant clients, but the principles for working with them are similar. The *reluctant* client is one who does not want to come for help in the first place and is more or less forced to come. Such clients may be found in schools, correctional settings, court-related settings, and employment agencies (Egan, 2010). The *resistant* client may come more or less willingly but fail to carry through or participate actively in the helping process. Some of the causes of clients' **reluctance** and **resistance** are having negative attitudes about help, seeing no benefits in changing, feeling that getting help means admitting weakness or failure, and seeing no reason for going for help in the first place.

Reluctant clients may be embarrassed or angry that they are there for help. In many cases, they are there only because the court or some other authority has said they must be. These feelings are compounded by their unfamiliarity with the agency or the process. To attempt to lessen the reluctance, the helper can explain the process to the client. Discussing matters such as confidentiality, time limits, and expectations (for the client as well as the helper) can help demystify the process. Also, the manner in which the helper relates this can allow the client to see him or her in a role other than that of interrogator or advice giver. The following case provides an example.

JOSEPH

Joseph came into my office with his mother and father. He sat in the chair with his arms folded. His feet did not touch the floor. He was swinging one foot and then another. He looked at his knees. I talked with his mother and father first for a few minutes and then asked them to be excused so that I could talk with Joseph alone. I am used to working with young children who do not want to see a counselor. When I work with them the first time, many say nothing during a 35- to 45-minute period. Some just sit and stare at me. Some stare at the floor. Others pretend to be asleep or sing quietly to themselves. On rare occasions, they try to damage the room, me, or themselves in some way.

Over the 20 years that I have worked with children, five of them have never talked with me, after weekly meetings for over six months to a year. Many of them will begin to relate to me after two or three weeks, mainly through games and drawing or watching short films or videos together. Some will finally talk with me and once they get started, they cannot stop. My foremost approach is to let them know that I care about them in whatever way I can. Even for those who never spoke, I was a consistent, caring presence in their lives for an extended period of time.

Resistance is slightly different from reluctance, because resistance can occur at any time in the helping process. Clients who come to the attention of human service agencies may initially feel threatened by the referral and application procedures. Resistance may also arise later in the helping process if the client feels threatened by the subject being discussed, by the helper, or even by the helping relationship.

What is resistant behavior? Missing appointments, rejecting the helper, and inattentiveness are examples of such behavior. Clients may try to protect themselves by denying the existence of a problem, claiming it is caused by other people or situations, or distancing themselves from it.

I feel that the counselor in my school has betrayed me. We have had a good relationship ever since I came to the high school. I have worked with her one-on-one to determine my school schedule. She has conducted groups in our high school. I have participated in ones on family life, balancing a checkbook, how to apply for a job, and how to maintain healthy friendships. Today I went to see her after basketball practice. I have not been feeling well. My coach is concerned and she asked me to go to see Ms. Sharpelli. You know what she asked me? "Do you think you might be pregnant?" I walked out without saying a word to her. Even though she might be right, I promise, I will never speak to her again.

The helper can use several strategies when working with a resistant client. First, recognizing and accepting the antagonism may defuse the situation. This type of action is very different from what the client might expect; a statement such as, "You probably don't want to see anyone like me" may minimize the threat to the client. Second, asking for the client's perceptions of the problem will communicate support for the client's feelings. This does not mean that the helper must accept or believe everything the client says, but it does communicate support and respect. Asking what the client wants to happen in this situation is a third strategy. It engages the client in the helping process and also emphasizes the worker's support and respect for the individual. In addition, it can provide the client with some sense of control over his or her life. Finally, for resistance that occurs later in the relationship, changing the pace or the topic may temporarily lessen feelings of threat.

INTERNET EXERCISE

See this text's website at *www.cengagebrain.com* for video exercises. Choose Chapter 7, then Videos.

In this segment, Shawn, a counselor, is working with Shelley, a client. Shawn explores why Shelley has come for help and discovers that she is resistant to help. Watch this segment and listen closely to Shawn's probes and responses.

1. *What behaviors alert you to Shelley's resistance?*
2. *What does she say to confirm your suspicions of resistance?*
3. *What does Shawn do and say?*
4. *How would you describe the effectiveness of his approach?*

Now, watch and listen as Shawn talks about resistance from a human service professional's view.

1. *How does Shawn recognize resistance?*
2. *What strategies does he use to counter it?*
3. *How does he deal with it on a personal level?*

THE SILENT CLIENT

Particularly challenging for the beginning helper is the silent client. The uncomfortable silence may cause the helper to believe that nothing is taking place; in fact, silence can have many different meanings. It is the helper's responsibility to evaluate what a silence means so he or she can decide how to respond. Silence can mean that the client is waiting for direction from the helper. In this case, the client may feel that it is the helper's place to determine the topic of discussion or the direction in which the relationship should move. A second meaning of silence can be that the client is pondering what has been said. Resistance (discussed previously) may also manifest itself as silence; a change of pace or topic may be necessary until the client is ready to deal with what is happening. Silence may also relate to culture, specifically cultural norms. For example, in some cultures women defer to men in conversation. In other cultures, the family speaks for the individuals in the family. Within cultures where individuals may bring shame to the entire family, a client's silence may be a way of protecting the family.

> Mr. Lopez and his wife were referred for counseling by their family physician. Mrs. Lopez is experiencing signs of dementia, and her deteriorating condition requires that Mr. Lopez be the caregiver. During the first session, Mrs. Lopez talked about her

TABLE 7.5   SUMMARY POINTS: STRATEGIES FOR RESISTANCE

- Recognize and accept the antagonism.
- Ask for the client's perception of the problem.
- Ask the client for solutions.
- Change the pace or topic.

son, Enrique, and how he is learning to tie his shoes. Mr. Lopez volunteered the information that Enrique is 24 years old, lives in a neighboring state, and is a computer analyst. Other than this comment, he sat silently.

In this case, Mr. Lopez may be silent for several reasons: despair over his wife's condition, confusion about her behavior, discouragement, or simply nothing to say. The helper will want to be sensitive to his behavior and to consider what he is feeling.

THE OVERLY DEMANDING CLIENT

Calling the helper at home, monopolizing time in the office, and scheduling frequent and unnecessary appointments are behaviors of an overly demanding client. Sometimes such clients become so dependent that they may want to be told what to do. When the client makes demands, the helper may become resentful of the time the client takes and frustrated with the unsuccessful nature of the helping process. For these reasons, the helper must deal appropriately with the client's behavior.

> I just called my case worker, Ms. Renfro, and she promised to come right over. I know that she usually goes to church on Sunday evenings, but I really need to see her. She is so good to me and tells me to call her whenever I need her. And she helps me all of the time. I have a regular scheduled appointment with her for 30 minutes every Tuesday morning, but I would not be able to get through a day without talking with her. Last Friday she called to tell me that she was going out of town next Tuesday and cancelled our regular Tuesday appointment. I have called her each day to urge her not to go.

Ms. Renfro will probably develop some resentment toward this client when her patience is exhausted. At some point, it will be in both their best interests for her to establish some boundaries for the relationship.

One strategy that may help with the overly demanding client is setting reasonable limits to decrease the client's dependence. Limiting client–helper contact to working hours only is one step toward decreasing dependence. A second step is to examine the helper's own need to be needed. Is the helper actually encouraging the demanding behavior of the client?

THE UNMOTIVATED CLIENT

Clients who are present because someone referred them or encouraged them to seek help may be unmotivated. They may not see the need for the service and may be showing up only because some authority such as their parents, the school, or the court is forcing them to attend. Unfortunately, the unmotivated client is often unwilling to change and only goes through the motions of the helping process. The helper may find that he or she is doing most of the work in the relationship and may come to feel resentful, frustrated, and even angry. Such clients may be classed as reluctant clients, and many of the same strategies previously suggested may be helpful in establishing rapport with them. A parolee is an example of a client who must have regular meetings with a parole officer.

> Many of my parolees come in to see me just because they have to. In fact, most of them come because it is one of the terms of their probation. They figure seeing me is not as

bad as being returned to prison. Each day I try to see at least seven of them; and I also try to make two or three visits to see them at their work site. Most of the conversations are predictable: "How are you doing?" "Fine, I guess." "Looks like your job is going well." "Yep." "Tell me a little about your family." "They are fine." "I got some information about a new skills course ..." "Oh." "Is there anything that I can do for you?" (The client offers no response and shrugs his or her shoulders.) For these folks I am just a person that they must see or suffer the consequences.

INTERVENTION STRATEGIES

Now that you have learned about the helping process, it is important to look at three intervention strategies human service professionals are using. **Motivational interviewing** focuses on the client by exploring internal or intrinsic motivation to change (Miller & Rollnick, 2002). **Crisis intervention** is a helping process that is used to respond to stressful events and emergencies. **Resolution-focused brief therapy** is used when limited time or resources require a short-term intervention.

MOTIVATIONAL INTERVIEWING

Motivational interviewing provides a methodology to encourage behavior change. According to Miller and Rollnick (2002), this approach encourages the development of internal (rather than external) motivation or desire for change. Within the context of a client-centered, safe environment, clients and helpers explore client ambivalence about change. Based upon the nature of the ambivalence, the helper matches treatment strategies to individual needs. The ultimate goal of the approach is to increase the desire for change. Professionals report positive outcomes using motivational interviewing with specific populations such as youth and adult probationers, individuals with substance abuse issues, and family interventions.

Three aspects of motivational interviewing establish a positive helping environment and address a client's motivation for change (Miller & Rollnick, 2002). First, using motivational interviewing, the helper engages the client in a special conversation about change and the change process. The role of the helper is collaborative; the helper sets aside his or her role as an expert and assumes the role of an equal partner in the change process. Second, the helper's goal is to draw from the client the ideas and feelings the client experiences about working to change his or her behavior. During this time of drawing out, the helper and the client assess client strengths. Third, during the motivational interviewing process the client retains the autonomy for choice and responsibility for actions. Helpers encourage clients to explore ways that might work for them to engage in a change process.

The techniques supporting the motivational interviewing approach include aspects of helping we described in this chapter and earlier chapters of the text. They include expressing empathy, providing support for self-efficacy, de-escalating resistance, and finding the discrepancies between where the client is and where the client wants to be (Miller & Rollnick, 2010). In addition, open-ended questions, affirmation (recognizing client strengths, reflections, and summaries all encourage the client-centered, positive atmosphere. Each of these strategies assists the helper in assessing the client's readiness (ready), importance (willingness), and confidence (able) to change. To learn more about motivational interviewing search the Internet using terms such as motivational interviewing, motivational interviewing techniques, and motivational interviewing questions. You will find in-depth information about goals and objectives of motivational interviewing, strategies and techniques, and skills and values needed to work with clients.

CRISIS INTERVENTION

Crisis intervention is a helping process that occurs at a much faster pace than other helping and incorporates many of the helping roles and skills that have been discussed in this chapter. You may find yourself engaged in crisis intervention when there is an emergency. For example, a crisis can be precipitated by suicide threats or attempts, the discovery of an unwanted pregnancy, abandonment, or natural disasters such as hurricanes or tornadoes. In this section, you will read a description of crisis intervention as a human service, including types of crises, the development of a crisis, the principles and skills of intervention, and the role of the human service professional in providing this service.

DEFINING CRISIS   Stressful events and emergencies are going to occur; individuals can probably handle some but may find themselves unable to cope with others. The inability to cope creates the potential for crisis. An individual's equilibrium is disrupted by pressures or upsets, and this imbalance results in stress so severe that the person is unable to find relief by using coping skills that have worked previously.

When identifying crises, we need to distinguish between the event or situation and the person's response. The crisis is the individual's emotional response to the threatening or hazardous situation rather than the situation itself. Thus, the crisis lies in the individual's interpretation or perception of an event; the same event does not lead to crisis for all people. What one individual can handle may be a crisis for another person.

Crises can be divided into two types: developmental and situational. A *developmental crisis* is an individual's response to a situation that is reasonably predictable in the life cycle. Chapter 5 explained that as individuals grow and develop, they undergo periods of major transition such as childhood to puberty, puberty to adolescence, and adolescence to adulthood. Stresses can occur at each phase. For many people, the stresses are normal developmental problems with which they are

---

BOX 7.4	EXPLORING THE WEB FOR MORE INFORMATION

Check out the following sources to learn more about crises and crisis intervention.

American Psychological Association

crisis group

crisis intervention

healing of nations

able to cope. For those who cannot cope, the stresses of these stages can have destructive effects, such as suicide attempts, rejection of others, and depression. Such reactions constitute a developmental crisis in those circumstances.

Situational or *accidental crises* do not occur with any regularity. The sudden and unpredictable nature of this type of crisis makes any preparation or individual control impossible. Examples are fire or other natural disaster, fatal illness, relocation, unplanned pregnancy, and rape. Hazardous situations such as these may cause periods of psychological and behavioral upset. A crisis may result, depending on the individual's personal and social resources at the time of the event.

The skills and strategies that helpers use to provide immediate help for a person in crisis constitute *crisis intervention*. This is short-term therapy that focuses on solving the immediate problem and helping the individual to reestablish equilibrium. Common practice areas of crisis intervention are childhood and adolescence, mental health problems, marital and family conflicts, emergency hospitalization, suicide prevention, and substance abuse.

How a Crisis Develops   Even a sudden or short-lived crisis has identifiable components that create a pattern of development. The case study that follows examines crisis in terms of its development. You may want to make note of the different roles the helper plays.

BEN AND JOAN MATTHEWS

Background. Ben and Joan Matthews and their three children (ages nine months, two years, and five years) left their trailer in rural Illinois to drive to Florida. Ben had lost his job because the factory where he worked for minimum wage closed down. He hoped to find a job in Florida working on some of the fruit farms. The hope for a job did not materialize in Florida, so they headed back to their trailer in Illinois and an uncertain future. Two of the children became ill, the car broke down twice, and Joan and Ben argued constantly about what they should do next. A couple of times, the arguments escalated into shouting matches that ended when Ben hit Joan.

By the time the Matthews were about halfway to Illinois, they had no money for food, lodging, or gas. They stopped at a fast-food restaurant so that everyone could use the bathroom and have a drink of water. Joan gathered the children together and headed into the restaurant. When they returned, Ben and the car were gone. Joan's cell phone was in the car so she cannot call Ben.

Crisis development has four identifiable phases. In the first, the person reacts to a traumatic event with increased anxiety. The individual then responds with problem-solving mechanisms to reduce or eliminate stress. Here is Joan's initial response:

Phase One. Joan thinks that Ben has gone to get gas, so she returns to the restaurant. Selecting an out-of-the-way booth, she and the children sit watching and waiting for his return. After an hour, Joan begins to feel desperate. Joan fusses with the children and tries to look natural and unworried.

In the second phase, the individual's problem-solving ability fails. The stimulus that caused the initial rise in anxiety continues. In this case, the source of Joan's anxiety does not change: Ben is still missing. Her initial attempts to deal with the situation fail, and her anxiety continues to increase.

reach Joan's mother. In other cases, the intervention may be more complicated, relying on the skills, creativity, and flexibility of the worker. During this phase, the helper must focus on reality and identify the clients' positive coping mechanisms and support systems. This may help clients deal with feelings that may have been suppressed (such as anger) or feelings that have been denied (such as grief).

The final step is the resolution of the crisis, in which the case worker and the client plan for the future, reinforcing the new ways of coping. The case worker also helps the client in planning for the future and preparing for any new crises that may arise. Here is how Joan's situation is resolved.

> Joan is finally able to reach her mother, who wires money for bus fare for Joan and the children. While they are waiting for the money to arrive, Joan talks with the helper, expressing her feelings about what happened and verbalizing her need for continued support. In response to Joan's need for support, the case worker gets the necessary information to refer her to a free counseling service at a mental health center near her home in Illinois.

As you reflect on the case study, what principles of intervention are illustrated? What roles did the helper play? What skills did the helper use in this situation? How would you describe the outcome? Finally, how is the helping process followed in this example?

At the conclusion of the crisis intervention, the client may need to continue with professional services. If the client shows little progress after the crisis intervention, the crisis helpers may recommend more traditional types of problem solving. If the help needs to be time-limited in scope, resolution-focused brief therapy might be recommended. The next section will explain how Joan benefited from receiving resolution-focused brief therapy from the counselor in Illinois.

RESOLUTION-FOCUSED BRIEF THERAPY

In response to the demands, guidelines, and funding constraints of managed care, brief therapy has emerged as a strategy to provide help that is limited in time and scope. This brief counseling intervention focuses on reaching specific outcomes in a relatively short time by making an immediate difference in the client's life, targeting behaviors that need to be changed and facilitating that change, and helping clients make new choices about thinking and behaving. Action is central to resolution-focused helping but takes place rather quickly. It now appears in treatment for chemical dependency, in children and youth services, and in mental health services.

Resolution-focused brief therapy is based upon client strengths with a focus on the present and the future. This orientation also advocates that small changes make a difference in the lives of clients. For success with each small change, clients begin to believe that they can effect change and continue to grow and develop on their own. The goals of the helping process are stated in positive, measurable terms, so that helpers and clients can measure the success of client progress.

There are several stages included in resolution-focused brief therapy (Ivey, Ivey, & Zalaquett, 2011). These stages are applied in the two resolution-focused brief therapy sessions Joan attends once she reaches Illinois.

1. *Relationship building is at the heart of this brief counseling process.* The helper establishes rapport and uses listening skills to focus on a precise description of the problem. The helper also assesses client strengths and examples of past successful problem solving.

   At the beginning of the first session Mark introduces himself to Joan and asks her to sit down. From a short intake interview he is able to ascertain information about the crisis Joan and her children experienced. He explains to Joan that his role is to provide a two-session helping experience that will focus on a specific problem she wants to address. Because they only have two sessions, he lets her know that he will ask questions and keep her focused on the present, the future, her strengths, and her positive attributes. Joan explains that she is devastated by all of the responsibility that she is assuming without Ben. She is able to identify her strengths as an ability to problem solve, a commitment to caring for her children, and knowledge of other resources in the area such as her family.

2. *The helper continues to identify client strengths* by asking the client to talk about a time when she experienced positive outcomes. During this phase the client does not have to describe the problem in detail; in fact, the focus is really on what successes the client has had so far in dealing with the problem. The helper wants clients to be able to relate their own problems to normal "problems in living." During this time the helper and the client continue to look for resources such as client characteristics and skills, support of family and friends, and support of community organizations and institutions.

   Mark discovers that Joan has previous experience working as a secretary, has computer skills, is close to her family, makes friends easily, and believes that she is a good mother. Joan explains that she has survived the last few days because she has refused to blame herself, she has focused on loving her children, and she knows that she can support herself.

3. *The helper and client establish specific goals* that the client wants to achieve and that the helper can help the client achieve. Here the helper wants to know what the client expects. It is time to write down these goals in concrete and measurable terms.

   Joan wants to talk about how badly she felt when she discovered that Ben had really left. Mark is empathetic but draws her back to the task at hand, setting one goal for herself. He states that he wants her to leave the helping session with a positive, action-oriented goal. Joan decides that she wants to begin searching for a job.

4. *The helper and the client begin to talk about how to reach the goal* and the helper continues to talk about client success. The helper also provides the client with "homework" or a specific intervention that the client can work on after the session. Role playing and other strategies help the client practice new behaviors and try to link these behaviors to past successes that have already been discussed.

   Because Joan knows that she and her children can live with her family for a time, she is assured that their basic needs will be met. Mark and Joan work through a short action plan to conduct a job search. They practice each part of the plan that includes collecting newspapers, looking in the Yellow Pages, enlisting the help of her parents and some of their friends, and posting a letter asking for help in her parent's newspapers. Joan leaves with her homework.

   She returns for her next session. She reports on her progress. Mark asks her about her strengths and what helped her in her tasks. She identifies additional strengths such as being able to ask for help and listening well to what others have to say. She decides that she wants to practice interviewing since she has three interviews in the next week. By the time Joan leaves Mark's session, she has identified the strengths she brings to interviewing well, they have practiced an interview, and Joan has identified two individuals she will ask to conduct mock interviews with her. The session concludes as Joan articulates a list of strengths that she brings to her new situation.

The helping process is fundamental to the work of helping others. Understanding the nature of the process, the difficult clients one might encounter, how to help clients in a crisis, and how to apply group work and resolution-focused brief therapy guides your work as a human service professional.

KEY TERMS

active listening

attending behavior

crisis intervention

effective communication

group

helping relationship

motivational interviewing

nonverbal messages

paraphrase

questioning

reluctance

resistance

resolution-focused brief therapy

responsive listening

termination

verbal message

THINGS TO REMEMBER

1. Helping is always guided by two questions: (1) What is helpful? (2) How can the needs of the client be met?
2. The effectiveness of the helping process depends on the helper's ability to communicate an understanding of the client's feelings, clarify what the problem is, and provide appropriate assistance to resolve the problem appropriate to the client's cultural perspective.
3. Formal helping takes place in human service organizations and agencies.
4. Before the client arrives, the helper should attend to matters such as establishing the physical setting, deciding how to handle the paperwork, and determining how to gather information about the client.
5. During the helping process, the human service professional and the client set goals and determine how those goals will be reached to resolve the problem.
6. The way a helper listens and responds to the client is crucial in building a helping

relationship with that person, "hearing" the client's verbal and nonverbal messages.
7. Attending behavior is a way to let the client know that the helper is listening.
8. There are four dimensions of attending behavior: eye contact, attentive body language, vocal qualities, and verbal tracking.
9. Beginning helpers should be wary of excessive questioning, which may hinder the helping process and make clients dependent.
10. The key to working with culturally different clients is awareness of and sensitivity to cultural differences.
11. Among the challenging aspects of human service practice is the reality that not all clients are cooperative and willing; helpers are likely to meet the resistant client, the silent client, the overly demanding client, and the unmotivated client.
12. Motivational interviewing is a promising new approach to helping clients enter and succeed in the change process.

13. Crisis intervention occurs at a very fast pace and incorporates many of the helping roles and skills.

14. Resolution-focused brief therapy is an intervention that provides focused, short-term, and concrete help to the client.

Self-Assessment

- What distinguishes the helping relationship from other relationships?
- Explain the purposes of each of the five stages of the helping process. What special attitudes, skills, and values do helpers need for each of the five stages?
- What special knowledge do helpers need to understand nonverbal messages? How can this understanding aid in the helping process?
- Why are verbal messages important? How does an understanding of verbal messages

help when working with culturally different clients? Reluctant or resistant clients?
- Describe how the helper might best listen and respond to the client.
- What special understanding do helpers need to work with culturally different clients and reluctant or resistant clients?
- Why is a crisis different from other problem situations?

Want to Know More?

There are several resources you can tap to learn more about helping. Check them out!

Additional Readings: Focus on Helping

Kanel, K. (2012). A *guide to crisis intervention*. Pacific Grove, CA: Cengage.
   The author presents the latest theories and techniques in crisis intervention. Case material from real situations illustrates theories and techniques.
Meier, S. T., & Davis, S. R. (2010). *The elements of counseling*. Pacific Grove, CA: Brooks/Cole.
   This book responds to the questions beginning helpers may have about the counseling process. It covers such fundamentals of counseling as explaining counseling to the client, noticing resistance, avoiding advice, listening for metaphors, and arranging the physical setting appropriately.
Mitchell, E. (Ed.). (2005). *Beyond tears: Living after losing a child*. New York: St. Martin's Griffin.
   Nine mothers share what they have learned with parents experiencing a similar tragedy. Advice, reassurance, and the impact on their lives are some of the topics.
Ramchand, R., Acosta, J., Burns, R. M., Jaycox, L. H., & Pernin, C. G. (2011). *Preventing suicide in the military*. Washington, DC: Rand.
   This book, commissioned by the Center for Military Health Policy Research, reviews the current incidence of suicide in the military, identifies best

practice programs, outlines Department of Defense programs, and accesses the relationship of these programs to best practice.
Richter, D., & Whittington, R. (2010). *Violence in mental health settings: Causes, consequences, management*. New York: Springer Science.
   The authors define violence from the psychological, sociological, and ecological perspectives. They outline what violence looks like within a mental health treatment context and suggest ways of addressing the violence that occurs.
Schein, E. H. (2009). *Helping: How to offer, give, and receive help*. San Francisco: Berrett-Koehler Publishers.
   A well-known organizational development professor analyzes the dynamics of helping relationships, explains why help is often not helpful, and shows what helpers must do to make sure help is actually provided.
Young, M. E. (2012). *Learning the art of helping: Building blocks and techniques* (4th ed.). Upper Saddle River, NJ: Prentice Hall.
   This book introduces both basic and advanced helping techniques for those interested in a counseling career.

Case Study

If you would like to learn more about the application of the concepts discussed in Chapter 7, read about Gloria in Chapter 7 of *Introduction to Human Services: Cases and Applications,* the companion text to *Introduction to Human Services.* Gloria is a Puerto Rican woman who is married and has three children. She has an opportunity to study in the United States. What this means for her immediate and extended families is the dilemma. She consults two helpers, one a pastor and one a counselor. Her experience with these helpers is the focus of the dialogue in Chapter 7.

References

Association for Specialists in Group Work. (2012). *Home.* Retrieved from http://www.asgw.org/

Egan, G. E. (2010). *The skilled helper: A problem management and opportunity development approach to helping* (9th ed.). Pacific Grove, CA: Brooks/Cole.

Ivey, A. E., Ivey, M. B., & Zalaquett, C. P. (2011). *Essentials of intentional interviewing: Counseling in a multicultural world.* Pacific Grove, CA: Brooks/Cole.

Jacobs, E. E., Masson, R. L. L., Harvil, R. L., & Schimmel, C. J. (2012). *Group counseling: Strategies and skill.* Pacific Grove, CA: Cengage.

Levine, J. (2012). *Working with people: The helping process.* Upper Saddle River, NJ: Pearson.

Miller, W. R., & Rollnick, S. (2002). *Motivational interviewing: Preparing people for change.* (2nd ed.). New York: Guildford.

Miller, W. R., & Rollnick, S. (2010). *What's new since MI-2?* Presentation at the International Conference on Motivational Interviewing, Stockholm, June 6, 2010. Retrieved from http:/www.fhi.se/Documents; ICMI/ICMI-2010/Abstract-Program-Book-webb.pdf

Negri, G., & Kramer, A. (1995). Mother Teresa brings message of love. *Boston Globe.* Retrieved from http://www.boston.com/globe/search/stories/nobel/1995/1995q.html

Okun, B. F., & Kantrowitz, R. E. (2008). *Effective helping: Interviewing and counseling techniques* (6th ed.). Pacific Grove, CA: Brooks/Cole.

Rogers, C. (1958). The characteristics of a helping relationship. *Personnel and Guidance Journal,* 37 (1), 6–16.

Russell, J., & Batalova, J. (2012). *Refugees and asylees in the United States.* Retrieved from http://www.migrationinformation.org/USfocus/display.cfm?id=907

Slavin, S., Gulanti, G. A., & Kuo, A. (n.d.) *The 4 C's of culture: A mnemonic for health care professionals.* Retrieved from http://gagalanti.com/articles/The4CsofCulture.pdf

Taylor, C. (1985). *Carl Rogers and client-centered therapy.* Unpublished manuscript. Knoxville, TN.

The History of Alcoholics Anonymous. (2012). *Welcome to Alcoholics Anonymous.* Retrieved from http://www.aa.org/?Media=PlayFlash

The Provider's Guide to Quality and Culture. (n.d.). *Non-verbal communication.* Retrieved from http://erc.msh.org/mainpage.cfm?file=1.0.htm&module=provider&language=english

CHAPTER **8**   # WORKING WITHIN A SYSTEM

Allen Einstein/National Basketball Association/Getty Images

After reading this chapter, you will be able to:

- Describe the agency environment.
- Use the referral process.
- Build an information network.
- Identify the challenges in day-to-day human services.
- Define encapsulation, burnout, and vicarious trauma in human services.
- Summarize methods of promoting change.

Many human services are provided within the context of an agency or organization in a community or a geographic area. This context or environment for human service delivery is important to those who work within its structure and boundaries. It would be difficult to assist clients, deliver effective services, and develop needed policies and services without an understanding of this context. This chapter will introduce the concept of the human service environment and its integral role in the work of human service professionals.

Agencies and organizations set the parameters or boundaries of the work of their employees. Concepts such as mission, structure, funding, and resources influence the world of human service agencies and organizations. Because agencies and organizations do not function in a vacuum, this chapter then introduces the larger environment of the community to help us understand the context in which the agency operates. Knowledge of the available resources in a community is part of the larger context. Some of the daily challenges encountered by human service professionals are also explored. Agencies and communities are dynamic, constantly shifting in response to social, political, and economic change. The chapter concludes by examining the ways in which the human service professional can facilitate change.

THE AGENCY ENVIRONMENT

The world of the human service agency is a complex one. In fact, when we talk about an agency's purpose or structure, it may almost seem like we are using another language. The purpose of this next section is to introduce the concepts that help define an agency. Understanding these concepts will increase your knowledge of human service delivery and the environment in which it occurs.

MISSION AND GOALS

One of the first questions you may have upon learning about an agency is, "What does this agency do?" One document, a certificate of incorporation, defines the legal parameters of an agency's responsibilities and actions. In addition, agency bylaws provide process and procedures for agency action (National Council of Nonprofit Boards, [2012]). In other words, they operationalize agency practice, including the daily activities of the helping professional. Another important document is the agency's written **mission**. This is a statement that communicates the purpose of the agency by summarizing its guiding principles. Generally, it is relatively brief and appears in a prominent place at the agency, such as the entrance or reception area. It is usually included in all agency publications. A mission statement may identify the population served, the broad goals of the agency, sources of funding, the values that influence decision making, the agency structure, and agency priorities (Lewis, Lewis, Packard, & Souflee, 2012). It is also a source of information about an agency's function and direction. An example of a mission statement is that of the National Organization for Human Services that clearly identifies its goals:

Our mission is to strengthen the community of human services by:

- expanding professional development opportunities,
- enhancing internal and external communications,
- nurturing the financial sustainability and growth of the organization,
- promoting professional and organizational identity through certification, and
- advocating and implementing a social policy and agenda (National Organization for Human Services, 2012).

Other documents shed light on the work of an agency by clarifying rules and regulations, the work of the staff, and the standards of practice. These documents include goal statements, job descriptions, and policies and procedures. An example of a goal statement might read like this one from the Social Support Center in Abu Dhabi, United Arab Emirates: "Our goal: A Community without Crimes, A Stable Family, and A Safe Individual" (Social Support Center, 2006; Abu Dhabi Police, 2012). To achieve this goal, Social Support Center staff are guided by the following principles:

- Respect for human rights and dignity of families and individuals
- Preservation and prevalence of law
- Keeping work as well as the parties related to the cases confidential
- Showing initiative and promptness in response, and fruitful work without limits
- Cooperation and coordination with various related parties and institutions, in order to ensure that all concerned categories are being supported
- To be wise and patient, and to discuss and consider carefully before making decisions (Social Support Center, 2006).

Another way to learn about an agency is by reading information about its job openings. When you apply for a position in a human service agency, the first exposure you will have to that position is the advertisement. Generally, it will include a brief job description, the qualifications, and sometimes a salary range or a statement that "salary is commensurate with experience." As you read the following position announcements, think about the questions you would ask if you were applying for one of these jobs.

Respite Counselor—Bachelor's degree in child development, human services, or related field. Minimum of one year experience working with children, youth, and families, and referral sources; good interpersonal skills working with seriously emotionally disturbed youth; flexible hours with occasional weekend work; some travel within a three-county region. Driver's license and safe driving record required.

Case Manager—Provide counseling, prevention services, mentoring, and case management services to adolescents in the community; facilitate parent and adolescent support groups; maintain accurate case records and reports; link youth and families to appropriate community resources; other duties as assigned. Qualifications: High school diploma or GED and five years experience working with youth and families; Associate's degree preferred and previous experience working with abused, neglected, and special needs clients.

Children and Youth Crisis Treatment Team Member—Bachelor's degree in social sciences and one year professional experience working with children and youth preferred. Provide intensive case management services to mentally ill children, adolescents, and their families; work as part of a multidisciplinary team; position requires some flexibility with schedule.

If you want to learn more about a job, one request you might make is to read the official **job description** of the position. This is a written document that defines the duties and responsibilities and is much more extensive than a brief job announcement. For example, it lists the expectations for the person in the position, the job qualifications, and a salary range. Unfortunately, job descriptions are often general in nature, rarely capturing the realities of the day-to-day work. A job description may also change as a result of reorganization, changing client needs, and economic pressures. Still, it remains an important document that offers guidelines about agency expectations. The job description in Box 8.1 is for the case management position advertised. This position is with a nonprofit agency that serves children and families. As you read this job description, what additional information do you now have about the position? What else would you like to know?

Another source of important information is the policies and procedures that guide the work of the agency. An agency policy might detail how its governing board is selected or who the agency accepts for services. The school you are attending has policies about the number of hours you can take each term. An agency procedure reflects accepted standards of practice. For example, the steps necessary to spend agency funds for a client service or the rules regarding the release of client information provide a guide for the human service professional to do his or her job. Procedures at your school tell you how to register for courses or how to withdraw from school. It is important to be familiar with all policies and procedures.

Policies and procedures also influence the **organizational climate** of an agency. This term refers to the conditions of the work environment that affect how people experience their work. The range of responsibility and decision making and the intensity and frequency of supervision are examples of factors that contribute to the organizational climate. For example, is the human service professional free to determine his or her work schedule, make final recommendations for client treatment, or authorize expenditures for client services?

STRUCTURE

Another way to understand a human service agency is to learn about the way it is organized. This is the structure of the agency, and it refers to the relationships among the people who work there and the departments to which they are assigned. There are two helpful concepts that illustrate the structure of an agency. One is the **chain of command**. This refers to the layers of authority in an agency. For example, those at the top of the chain control resources and actions. Lines of authority

---

BOX 8.1   HELP WANTED: A CASE MANAGER

CHILD AND FAMILY SERVICES
Job Description

POSITION TITLE: Case Manager   **Effective Date: April 1**

Program: PARTNERS Teen Pregnancy and Responsible Parents

POSITION OBJECTIVE:
To provide case management services to adolescents, their families, and noncustodial parents. Case managers are advocates for customers and focus on goals that will move participants toward self-sufficiency.

ESSENTIAL FUNCTIONS:
- Provide counseling, mentoring, and case management services to adolescents.
- Emphasize the importance of self-sufficiency to youth and responsibility to all parents.
- Provide prevention services to youth in the community.
- Facilitate parent and adolescent support groups.
- Establish and maintain accurate case records and reports.
- Link youth and families to appropriate community resources.
- Assist with community presentations.
- Assist noncustodial parents, youth, and their families with any barriers that they feel are preventing progress.

- Monitor attendance and measure progress.
- Maintain regular and predictable job attendance.
- Work cooperatively with coworkers and residents.
- Other duties as assigned.

This list of essential functions is not intended to be exhaustive. Child and Family Services reserves the right to revise this job description as needed to comply with actual job requirements.

QUALIFICATIONS:

Required:
- High school diploma or GED
- Five years experience working with youth and families

Preferred:
- Associate's degree in social services-related field
- Previous experience working with abused, neglected, or special needs children and their families

---

emanate from the top in most agencies. For some agencies, the chain of command is hierarchical with defined responsibilities and accountability from top to bottom. Each person is accountable for those under his or her supervision. Other agencies have a flatter chain of command. This means that there are fewer layers of authority from top to bottom so that decision making is more of a shared responsibility.

A second concept that is helpful in understanding the structure of an agency is a diagram known as an **organizational chart** (see Figure 8.1). At a glance, it is easy to see the boxes that represent offices, departments, and sometimes individuals. The organizational chart also illustrates the chain of command. The solid lines that connect the boxes clearly show lines of authority, information flow, and accountability. Often, lines connect vertically to represent departments or individuals that work closely together. The boxes identify different services and represent staff dedicated to providing those services.

FIGURE 8.1 ORGANIZATIONAL CHART

RESOURCES

Another source of information about an agency is its funding sources. These determine if an agency is public or governmental, not-for-profit (voluntary), or for-profit. The distinction between public and not-for-profit agencies is not always clear because not-for-profit agencies are increasingly providing services for public agencies on a contractual basis. The number of for-profit agencies is also increasing due to limited resources for voluntary agencies, reduced governmental spending, and changing political and economic times.

The term *revenue* refers to the money an agency receives from four primary sources of funding: federal, state, and local governments; grants and contracts; fees; and donations. It is not unusual for an agency to receive money from multiple sources. Public or governmental agencies receive funding from the federal, state, regional, county, and municipal governments. State government agencies such as a department of human services or a department of family and children are examples. Not-for-profit agencies such as the American Red Cross and the Children's Defense Fund are funded by individual contributions, fund-raisers, foundation grants, and corporate donations. For-profit agencies are supported by contracts and fees. In some states, the prison system is run by an agency or organization for profit. This arrangement is often referred to as **privatization**.

These concepts are important in order to understand the context in which human services are delivered. They help human service professionals better understand their job responsibilities and how those responsibilities relate to the agency's mission and goals. They also allow human service professionals who operate within agency policies and procedures to provide the services their clients need effectively and efficiently. Finally, much of the planning and service delivery within an agency relates to funding. Staffing, the number of clients served, and the programs and services provided relate directly to funding.

Agencies have a number of other **resources** to use to develop services and provide them to clients. These resources include the obvious ones, such as available funds, buildings, land, staff, and short-term goods like equipment and supplies. An

TABLE 8.1   SUMMARY POINTS: AGENCY TERMS

- The brief mission statement of an agency communicates its purpose by summarizing its guiding principles.
- A job description is a written document that defines the duties and responsibilities of a particular position.
- The chain of command in an agency refers to the layers of authority.
- An organizational chart is a diagram that illustrates agency structure.
- Funding sources determine if an agency is public or governmental, not-for-profit, or for-profit.
- Human service agencies exist within the context of a community that influences operations, services, clients, and professionals.

agency can also use resources that are not so apparent at first glance. One example is the skills and talents of the employees of the organization. These include artistic ability, physical strength, creativity, fund-raising ability, and a talent for advocacy. The skills and talents of patrons of the organization or individuals who volunteer also count as resources. Finding new resources to support agency work helps expand what the agency can do or balances deficits in funding. Homan (2010) suggests that new community resources may be identified by focusing on several aspects of those resources such as identifying major institutions, collecting relevant community information, and making personal connections to resources. Resources have a broader meaning than just staff, budget, and buildings. They include institutions, personal talents, relationships, and influences. See Table 8.1.

THE COMMUNITY CONTEXT

Just as human service professionals operate within the context of an agency or organization, human service agencies exist within the context of a larger framework—the community. For some agencies this may be a housing project or a neighborhood or a county; for other agencies, like state departments of human services or children's services, the community may be an entire state. Whatever the context, studying this larger framework is another way to understand the complexities of human service delivery.

The environments within which agencies exist influence the way they operate, the services provided, the clients served, and the professionals employed. The shared values of the community also influence the agency. The community environment may include other agencies, institutions, the specific missions and philosophies that guide their service delivery, and the specific needs that they address. Other influences include how individuals within these organizations communicate formally and informally with each other.

Community mapping is a strategy that human service professionals and the agencies they represent use to learn about other professionals and agencies. This strategy helps them connect their agencies to the life of the community and its citizens. The people employed by an agency may not be like the clients with whom they work—economically, racially, or ethnically. Yet their clients and the communities in which they live form a critical part of the helper's knowledge base.

How do agencies and their staffs connect with a community? The effective human service agency and its employees will become part of the communities where they are located. This means offering services within the context of client-identified needs; anticipating reactions to differences in race, ethnicity, attitudes, and roles represented by human service professionals; and planning for interactions among clients and helpers. Agencies accomplish this connection in several ways. Some choose to have clients represented on their governing boards or they appoint an advisory committee of clients. Locating the agency within the community is another strategy.

Youth-In-Need, the community organization you read about in Chapter 3, provides support for other agencies with whom it works and has become part of the larger community. Staff work with clients within the community, especially with teens who are homeless. Many staff spend their workdays meeting children and youth on street corners, alleyways, and other street locations. Other agencies also meet clients where they are: home visits to residences in housing projects; intake interviews under bridges, at shelters, or wherever the homeless are found; meetings at residential centers or institutions for substance abuse, education, or mental illness; or even appointments at local fast-food restaurants.

Interacting in the community with residents, clients, and other professionals is another way that agencies connect with the community. This interaction serves two purposes. The first purpose is to make connections; effective human service professionals who know the community know its resources. These include other human service agencies, religious organizations, service clubs, and businesses. And knowing these resources is the first step toward tapping them. The second purpose is to document the strengths of the community: What are the assets of the community? How can the agency support those assets in order to strengthen the community? How can these strengths be used to attack the problems?

Becoming a part of the community they serve should be the goal of human service agencies. However, the work is not over once this is accomplished. Remaining a part of the community requires continuity and interaction. The process is ongoing.

USING AVAILABLE SERVICES

An important part of the human service professional's responsibility is to work within the larger context of the human service delivery system and the client's environment. Knowledge of both agency and community resources is critical to fulfilling this responsibility. To facilitate this work, the professional will benefit from an understanding of the referral process and related issues.

Referral relates directly to the interaction between the human service professional and the environment by making use of the human service **network** during the referral process. In seeking services for a client, the helper often relies on other professionals both within and outside the agency to locate the needed services, negotiate introductions and meeting times, and establish the groundwork for the client to visit another agency. A successful referral results in the delivery of the services needed. The referral process is described in this section. The nature of and relationships among agencies and human service professionals contribute to the success of the referral.

REFERRAL

One of the most important roles of a human service professional is **brokering,** or referring a client to another agency or service. The actual referral involves a two-step process: (1) assessing the client's problems and needs, and (2) providing the link between the client and the needed service. To understand the process of referral, the helper must know when to refer, how to refer, where to refer, and how to develop the referral. Successful brokering requires considerable time and skill. Effective referral occurs when the referring professional knows what the clients may expect from another agency; it also helps the referral process if the professional has developed a cooperative relationship with other agency personnel. The human service professional and the client need to understand the services that are provided by the agency or the professional who is receiving the referral; it is important that their expectations match. Cooperation is another key ingredient in an effective referral. All the helpers involved must keep the client's needs as the primary focus. If difficulties arise, they need to remember that the goal is to serve the client well.

To make a successful referral, the helper must have information about a service or agency. This includes its history, possible legislation that affects it, its purpose or intent, and the specific client services it provides. Once the helper has this information, then an assessment begins to determine if the agency meets client needs. Several considerations about the agency need to be considered by the helper. The following questions may assist the helper determine if the agency under consideration is the correct one for the client.

- Will this agency be able to provide the service that the client needs?
- Does this agency accept referrals from us? Do we have a memorandum of agreement or an informal linkage?
- Is the client going to be able to travel to the agency's location?
- Is the intake process simple or complicated?
- Are the eligibility standards difficult to meet?

In other words, if the services exist but are not readily available to your clients, the agency is not a good referral source.

WHEN TO REFER   A human service professional may send a client to another professional for several reasons. The referral may be client initiated—that is, the client may request a referral. The client may realize that other services would be helpful and thus suggest a specific referral. The client may request that the referral come from the helper in order to give the client more credibility with the new service, speed up the response, or both. In another case, the client may have come to the helper specifically to ask for help in working with other agencies.

Referral may also be appropriate because the helper is not able to provide the assistance necessary to solve the client's problems. The client may present requests or have problems that the helper cannot solve, or the helper may discover that the client has a major problem that must be addressed before the others can be solved and that requires more specialized assistance than the helper can provide. Another reason for referral is that the client may be in serious psychological distress—suicidal or violent—and require intensive therapy or crisis intervention that the professional cannot provide in the human services setting. The helper may also decide to refer the client because of lack of success with that particular client; a different professional would perhaps be more effective.

There are also reasons to consider what might make a referral difficult for the client. First, the client must want to be referred and be willing to accept services from another source. Second, the client must be able to negotiate another agency setting and provide and receive information. If the client is ambivalent about the referral, then the helper must assess if the client can follow-up on his or her own.

HOW TO REFER   Once the helper has decided that the client needs to be referred, the complex process of referral begins. A key word in the referral process is *communication*. The following four-step process provides guidelines for linking the client with another service.

1. *Explain.* The client needs to understand why the referral is taking place. Even if the client initiates the referral, the client must understand that he or she is not just being passed on to the next human service professional. Referral is a thoughtful activity, initiated for the good of the client.
2. *Describe the services.* The client needs to be informed about the referral agency and its services. The more information the helper can provide about the intake process, the services available, the fee structure, and the professionals in the agency, the more comfortable the client will be in making the initial contact.
3. *Know the contact.* Talk to the agency and get the name of the contact person, the telephone number, the address, and directions to the agency. Help the client make the appointment for the initial visit to the agency.
4. *Transmit information.* Send appropriate information about the client to the new service, always considering what that agency needs to know about the client. This will allow the agency to plan. Sometimes information can be sent electronically, which speeds up the flow of information.

WHERE TO REFER   To determine where to refer the client, the human service professional must first identify the client's problems. Then the helper must find services to meet those needs. The helper may use services that are familiar or may investigate other possibilities. Both formal and informal networks (described later in this chapter) are useful in determining what services are available and appropriate to meet the client's needs.

Home health services, a popular alternative today to hospitalization, depend on referral resources. The goals of these services are increasing client independence and minimizing the limitations of illness or disability. In many cases, this means knowing where needed services and products can be located. Home Health Source is an example of this community-based service (see Box 8.2).

BOX 8.2   HOME HEALTH SERVICES

According to the Bureau of Labor Statistics (2010), home health care services include skilled nursing care or medical services, primarily to the elderly, in the home of the patient. This service was created for dual purposes, to provide care to those who cannot travel to care centers and to save financial resources. This was once a small component of the health care system, but its use and availability is increasing rapidly (Bureau of Labor Statistics, 2010).

Home health care services today include in-home nursing care, rehabilitation, and therapy following hospitalization. They also include assistance in daily living for those who cannot provide care to themselves. Specific services include orthopedic-related treatment, fall-related assessment and treatment, cardiopulmonary disease management, rehabilitation services for traumatic brain injury and spinal cord injury, respiratory therapy, hospice, and consultation.

EVALUATING THE REFERRAL   The referral process does not end once the referral has been made; it continues with systematic follow-up. The helper can call the agency to learn whether the client has kept the appointment and can call the client to get the client's evaluation of the service. The helper needs to know if the service was effective and if the help received matched the helper's assessment of the problem. Such follow-up can be very time-consuming for the helper but will be valuable not only for this client, but also for others in the future. It is especially good feedback for the professional and increases the client's faith in the system. The follow-up also reinforces the professional's care for and commitment to the client.

Making referrals is difficult for several reasons. Agencies are constantly changing, and maintaining an accurate picture of an agency, its current staff, and the services it provides is difficult. Sometimes services are not designed to meet the exact needs of the client, and the referring helper cannot guarantee treatment to the client. Each agency must independently assess the client's needs and the agency's ability to meet those needs. The service may not be provided because the client does not meet the eligibility criteria, because the services needed do not exist, or because there is a waiting list for assistance. The agency may not cooperate fully with the referring agency in the referral process or the follow-up. Many agencies also are so understaffed that they simply do not have the staff to provide follow-up. See Table 8.2.

TABLE 8.2   SUMMARY POINTS: REFERRALS

- The agency to which the client is referred must be able and willing to provide the service, be accessible geographically, and have reasonable eligibility criteria.
- A referral may be appropriate when the professional cannot provide the needed service or when the professional believes another helper might be more effective.
- When referring, the helper explains the purpose of the referral, describes the services, talks with the agency to identify a contact person, and sends appropriate client information to the agency receiving the referral.
- It is necessary to identify the client's problem prior to deciding where to refer.
- Follow-up to evaluate the success of the referral completes the referral process.

Internet Exercise

See this text's website at *www.cengagebrain.com* for video exercises. Choose Chapter 8, then Videos.

This video clip demonstrates the referral process. Joel is a licensed professional counselor who is meeting with Susan for the second time. Joel has decided to refer Susan to another helping professional. Watch, listen, and answer the following questions.

1. *Describe Susan's problem.*
2. *Why does Joel refer her to another helping professional?*
3. *What are the mechanics of the referral?*
4. *How did Susan respond to the referral?*
5. *As you think back to Chapter 7 and the knowledge and skills of the helping process, how did Joel use those communication skills in working with Susan and making the referral?*

Next, Joel talks about making a referral. He discusses the four steps in the referral process.

1. *What are the four steps?*
2. *What does Joel do at each step to encourage Susan about the referral?*
3. *Do you think Susan will follow through with the referral to Gloria Johnson? Why or why not?*

Building an Information Network

To make successful referrals, the human service professional must make effective use of all the resources in a community. First, the helper must know what services are available. The beginning professional is at a particular disadvantage because of a lack of experience in the system, a lack of personal contacts with other professionals in the system, and a lack of knowledge about the many problems that clients may have. Therefore, the helper must develop a systematic way of building a file of information about the human service network for referral purposes. The helper must first decide how to categorize the information to be gathered. Whether services are being organized by the physical, social, and emotional needs of the clients, the specific populations served, or one of the other organizational frameworks mentioned, the categories will help the human service professional think about how services are delivered in the community.

The helper can then begin to collect information and record it using computer software, a BlackBerry or other handheld device, a card file, a file box, a loose-leaf notebook, or any other storage device that allows for easy additions and revisions. In reality the helper is building a database. The summary information needed includes a description of the agency or service, the types of clients it serves, the payment required for the service, the telephone number and address, the e-mail address, the URLs for websites, and a contact person. The human service professional may collect information about community services from colleagues, clients, handbooks of agencies, newspapers, professional meetings, the telephone book, the Web, and any community service directories produced by other agencies. The Internet has increased the access to information about other agencies, and e-mail and shared databases have facilitated communication between agencies.

Knowing more detailed information about each agency is helpful, including the purpose of the agency, eligibility requirements for services, its location and hours of operation, organizational patterns of staffing, and the nature of the agency funding. Prior to using an agency for referral, a human service professional should know what services it provides, to whom they are provided (individuals or families), whether it uses case management services, and whether it has a good record as a client advocate. Other helpful information includes the qualifications of the staff, their caseload, and their experience with specific populations. The human service professional will have a better knowledge of the agency after visiting the facility to determine its accessibility and its psychological and physical environment. Also critical is knowing how the agency receives referrals, if there is a waiting list, how long a client must wait for services, and what follow-up procedure is used to inform the referring agency of the disposition of the referred client's case. All this requires a detailed understanding of the organization and represents quite a bit of information to gather, but once you have this information, updates can be made with relative ease.

Understanding that creating the file is only one part of building a network, the helper should also begin to make personal contacts with other human service professionals. The helper should then try to establish communication as a cooperative effort—sharing information with other agencies, following up on referrals, and providing feedback to other agencies that have made referrals. These efforts will begin to build the new helper's credibility as a serious professional interested in building and maintaining networks among agencies.

Network building takes time, but it makes the referral process more effective. The better the helper knows the services available, the more appropriate the referrals will be. A network is difficult to maintain: It is a never-ending project, no matter how long the human service professional has been serving the community, because agencies are constantly in flux.

KNOWING THE FORMAL AND INFORMAL NETWORKS

A network represents informal and formal connections among individuals and agencies within the social service arena. In human service settings, the fabric of the system is formed by the elaborate channels of communication among the agencies and the helping professionals. The connection takes place when both parties confirm that they wish to communicate, engage in two-way communication, and establish channels of communication. Human service delivery is a complex system containing two networks of communication: the formal and the informal. Both must be understood if professionals are to participate fully in the system.

The formal network consists of organizations such as public and private human service agencies, self-help groups, schools, churches, businesses, and federal, state, and local government agencies. To understand this network, the helper must discover the answers to certain questions: What are the politics of these organizations? Who bears the major responsibilities within each? What are the formal ways to "hook up" the client to the services and resources available?

Beyond the formal network is a valuable informal network that is more difficult to recognize. It is not described in agency policy, formal reporting, or organizational diagrams. It is determined by an established history of agencies working together, personal friendships among professionals, and political pressures, and it is maintained by mutual satisfaction and support. The informal network may also include informal helpers such as family and friends who provide needed support. Understanding this informal network is difficult, and accessing it takes time and effort.

There are three types of formal and informal networks: personal, professional, and organizational networks. Personal networks consist of individuals, families, and groups of people who are part of the helper's family or part of his or her social support. Individuals in this context often know the helper very well and can also reach out to a variety of people who can help in the referral process, including those in churches, social clubs, and exercise and other activity-based environments. Professional and organizational networks consist of individuals with whom you work and include colleagues, teachers, and supervisors. Networking with these individuals can help reduce duplication and fragmentation of services and eliminate service gaps.

One example of formal and informal networks that human service professionals find in the client population is the formal human service system that serves Native American communities and the traditional healers who usually work in their local tribal communities. The formal human service system is recognizing the power of traditional healing in dealing with HIV because of the sense of connection it restores between the individual and the tribe and culture. It also promotes spiritual, psychological, emotional, and physical healing (Native American Traditional Healing, 2009). Thus, a human service professional who wants to help Native Americans with HIV would need knowledge of the two networks. A special knowledge of the informal system, particularly the use of traditional healers, allows the helper to build on the services that are already present rather than duplicate or attempt to replace them with formal services. The helper may learn about the special relationships between helpers in the informal and the formal networks by asking the following questions: What formal services are available? How do the informal and formal systems communicate? Who are the key individuals in both networks who provide services effectively or who assist in accessing services?

CHALLENGES IN DAY-TO-DAY HUMAN SERVICE WORK

Human service professionals face many challenges throughout a typical day. They make decisions that affect their work, their clients, and their agencies. How to meet a client's need? What to tell an individual who is ineligible for services? How to stretch resources to cover the needs of three clients rather than one? Whether or not to recommend revocation of parole? At the time, some decisions are serious while others do not seem so serious; they appear to be merely choices about how professionals organize their work and spend their days. Yet, meeting these daily challenges represents survival in the human service world.

Let us examine some of the issues and their potential effects on helping professionals. You will read about the nature of issues such as allocation of resources, paperwork, and turf issues and their impact on human service professionals through the eyes and experiences of Barb LaRosa. She is the human service professional who worked with Almeada and her baby Anne in Chapter 1. She shares her perspective of these challenges and how they impact her work within the human service delivery system. Too many challenges or working with clients experiencing trauma may result in helper encapsulation, burnout, or vicarious trauma; Ms. LaRosa describes her experiences of times when challenges become overwhelming. Professional development is a strategy that helps professionals meet the challenges they encounter.

ALLOCATION OF RESOURCES

Traditionally, administrators and boards of directors are responsible for allocating resources, such as staff, space, and money. It follows then that direct service professionals are solely involved in providing services once administrators have determined which services are to be provided, and where and to whom they are to be provided. In reality, however, human service professionals are also involved in resource allocation. Often they determine how they will spend their time, how much time they will spend with each client, and which services the client needs or is eligible to receive. Since resources are limited and the demands for resources often exceed their availability in many agencies and organizations, some of the decisions made by human service professionals determine the type of services that each client receives.

When you met Ms. LaRosa in Chapter 1, you read about her work with Almeada and were able to appreciate her ability to support Almeada—providing her with information, services, and support during her prenatal care and after the birth of Anne. In that chapter, the view of Ms. LaRosa was that of Almeada's helper. In the following paragraphs, she talks about her own work during the time when Almeada was her client.

Sometimes I think about my job during the time that I met Almeada. I was serving adolescents in the schools and also working with teenage dropouts. In addition, I was providing support for at-home young mothers. I had over 65 girls on my caseload at one time. I tried to keep track of all of them, but it was an impossible task.

I started each day by making a list of everything I had to do. I saw the at-home young mothers weekly for one month, then monthly for six months. Then, I would reevaluate them to see if they could be referred to another service. During that time, the school wanted me to complete an in-depth intake interview with any girl who was pregnant. Then, I would develop a plan and make appropriate referrals.

The school referred about four girls to me each week. I tried to see all four the same week they were referred. Finally, I worked with teenage dropouts in a special program that identified irregular attendees who showed potential. I received about ten referrals a week for this program, both boys and girls. Sometimes I would discover that these girls were pregnant or that the boys were fathers-to-be.

I had two offices, one at the school and one at the welfare agency. I made it a point to begin each day at the school. That way I could check in with the office to see if I could gather any additional information about my clients. Unfortunately, when I began my work at the school, I did not get to hear the early-morning cries for help that I would occasionally receive from my young mothers. I also missed out on the "talk" with my colleagues at the welfare agency. For them, morning was an important time to check in with each other to discuss professional as well as personal business. It was also a good time to check both voice and e-mail. So what I gained in helping my students at the school, I lost in helping my clients at the welfare office.

The day I received the referral about Almeada, I also received seven other referrals. Almeada was the first student on the list. Taking the first person on the list is a technique of mine that I use to structure my day. I would also review the list of referrals and the list of students left from the day before for crisis situations. I would check with the assistant principal to see if he had any information about the students or if there were any problems that I needed to attend to immediately. I was so alarmed when I first talked with Almeada's parents that I became determined to find her. They told me she was pregnant, and they resented this inconvenience. I knew she needed my help; it was obvious that she had no support from her parents. That afternoon, I found Almeada at the grocery store. I canceled an appointment that evening so that I could meet her after work.

As Ms. LaRosa describes her work, it becomes obvious that she is involved in a daily allocation of her own resources. One resource is time. Although technology, like e-mail, texting, and voice mail, are designed to save time, some days they seem to take too much time. Like many other helping professionals, she is not able to spend as much time as she would like with each client. She constantly makes decisions about how she allocates her time. In general, she has decided that the pregnant teens and dropouts are a priority, so she spends the mornings of each day seeking them out and helping them plan for the future. When she began to gather information about Almeada, she discovered a very difficult situation. She determined that Almeada needed her immediate attention. She canceled an appointment with another client so she could begin her work with Almeada. This meant that another client did not receive Ms. LaRosa's services that evening.

Ms. LaRosa also describes some of the resources that Almeada received at the expense of some of her other clients.

If you asked me about the most difficult part of my job, I would tell you it's not being able to give my clients all of the services that they need. So many times I discover programs that can serve my students or dropouts, especially the girls. Often though, the girls are not eligible for the services or there are not enough services for all of the girls who need them. I tried to find several options for Almeada to continue her education. I had a friend who ran an evening program, and she made an exception for me to accept Almeada because she did not really have enough credits to qualify for the night classes. In the end Almeada did not participate in the class, but the favor was granted and now I owe my friend the next favor.

I took Almeada to a family-planning clinic. Before the appointment we stopped at a fast-food restaurant to have a soda and talk about the appointment and what she could expect. The school believes that we should not buy our clients food—it is not a rule but a suggestion. The school personnel think that sharing food constitutes "friendly" relationships with students and is a use of time that cannot be documented. Honestly, Almeada was so worried about the appointment that I thought if we could just sit and talk in a place where she felt comfortable, then she might feel better about going. It worked, but it was not time that I could account for in my records.

TABLE 8.3 SUMMARY POINTS: ALLOCATION OF RESOURCES

- Resources include staff, buildings, and money.
- Human service professionals are involved in resource allocation.
- When human service professionals determine how they will spend their time, they are involved in resource allocation.
- Decisions about implementation of a client plan also involve resource allocation.
- Special favors, extra attention, or concessions to clients also indicate involvement in resource allocation.

It is obvious that Almeada received quite a bit of special treatment from Ms. LaRosa and other professionals. Almeada brought an intensity and interest to the helping process, and many professionals worked hard and "bent their rules" to help her. Again, decisions were made to provide Almeada with resources—resources that could have been provided to someone else. Ms. LaRosa "broke" the school suggestion not to take students out for lunch or a snack. She is aware that she is violating this protocol, but feels that it was absolutely necessary to help Almeada prepare for her appointment at the family-planning clinic. See Table 8.3.

PAPERWORK BLUES

One demand on a human service professional's time is paperwork. It serves many functions, including providing a permanent record for the services received by the client. This is helpful to any agency employee who works with the client. It documents client history in the human service delivery system and is read by professionals who serve the clients at the same time or in the future. A thorough written record includes an intake interview, a social history, and medical, educational, and mental health records. As this information is obtained and carefully read by the helper, it also becomes a vehicle for organizing what is known about the client and what services are needed. In some cases, this organization may lead to possible solutions.

Paperwork involves a record of referrals and case notes of any client–helper contacts. It also documents the time that has been spent by an agency or professional, which is used for billing and accountability audits. Paperwork is becoming increasingly important in this time of strict professional accountability and scarce resources. Work with insurance and managed care companies has not only intensified and complicated the need for paperwork but has also created additional work for each professional who struggles with managing it all. If an agency is receiving state funds or support from a granting foundation, records are used in the evaluation process. Records provide documentation of the benefits of the work to clients and the community.

Clearly, the task of doing the paperwork signifies less time for client contact. Ms. LaRosa struggles with this problem.

I have always liked to do my paperwork. Most of my coworkers do not like it and procrastinate. When I do my paperwork, it gives me a time to think about my clients,

TABLE 8.4   SUMMARY POINTS: THE IMPORTANCE OF PAPERWORK

- Paperwork has a variety of functions that include establishing a permanent client record, documenting client history, writing important assessments and reports, documenting referrals and billing units, and providing a record for accountability purposes.

- Professionals determine how much time and effort will go into their paperwork and report writing.

- Intensive time spent with paperwork means less time with clients.

their problems, and how I can help them. I will admit that some of the paperwork drives me crazy, especially when I have to fill out multiple forms with the same information. Computers make the paperwork easier, although someone still has to enter the information. When I worked with Almeada, the paperwork actually became a nightmare for me because her case was complicated. Since I was working in three programs, I had to keep three sets of records, and all three were different. Sometimes, I would try to complete one form for the right person in the wrong program. I would catch myself before I wasted too much time. Because I had two offices, it was also difficult to always have the information and records that I needed at the right office.

Each professional learns the importance of paperwork. Knowing how to handle it is a skill and a responsibility. Some helpers are very well organized, and they manage their paperwork successfully and still see a large number of clients. For most, the nature of the job, with its crises and unexpected client requests, works against any set time for paperwork. The best plans are often left unfulfilled. There is no doubt that the paperwork takes valuable time that could be used with the client. To solve that problem, human service professionals often take their paperwork home, working long after hours so that they can spend more time with their clients. They then shortchange themselves on time to focus on self, family, and others. Some helpers shorten the time they spend on paperwork, not being as thorough as they might. Incomplete or spotty records do not help the agency or the client in the long run. Still others take the time to keep excellent records and accept this as part of the job, but then they have less client contact. See Table 8.4.

TURF ISSUES

Within the context of the human service delivery system, there is a tension between competition and coalition building among agencies. For the most part, within communities, human service professionals find cooperation and goodwill among agencies as all strive together to meet common goals. This is a positive environment for human service professionals to work together for the good of the client. At times, however, either underlying tension or open conflict exists among organizations.

This tension, commonly referred to as a dispute over "turf," occurs for several reasons. Sometimes an agency operates in a competitive mode and sees other agencies as competing for the same resources and clients. This competition often occurs when more than one for-profit agency competes for clients; each believes there is room for only one or a few human service agencies to prosper. There are also times when an agency sees no real benefit from cooperating with another agency; it may believe there will be a loss of benefits for the organization. Because flexibility with each agency is essential for cooperation, an agency may not be able to cooperate because its mission and goals cannot change fast enough to work collaboratively. Finally, an agency may simply mistrust the intentions of those with whom they are working.

Working together becomes even more difficult when turf issues become turf battles. Strife in the human service sector can erupt over issues of inequality. For example, sometimes collaboration appears to benefit one agency more than another or one organization has access to more resources. Sometimes agencies feel they are dedicated to serving a particular area or a targeted population, and they are unwilling to share that responsibility. Agencies may also believe that the collaborative effort leads them away from their own mission and goals. Other times agencies do not agree on the methods to solve particular social problems. Finally, personality issues among individuals representing different agencies may interfere with the collaborative effort.

Ms. LaRosa has been involved in collaborative work throughout her career. Here she shares some of her experiences.

> For the most part, my experience with other agencies has been positive, since I usually work at the local level. What I mean by that is I contact other professionals for help, and I help them in turn. I consider these people my colleagues. Sometimes we talk with each other every day, and other times we don't have contact for over a year. But usually we are always ready to help one another. Let me give you several examples that we have already talked about. My friend who runs the night classes and I maintain weekly contact. Sometimes I am able to help her with clients, and other times she is able to help me.
>
> I try to avoid the politics at the higher levels of agency work. The family planning clinic is a good example. I know that the superintendent of schools and his assistant tried working with five clinics in town to establish a coalition for teen pregnancy. The effort failed. My friend was able to tell the story from her perspective.
>
> She said that her boss opposed the mission of two of the clinics that were going to be in the collaborative. The first priority for those clinics is to promote adoption. They will not provide information about abortion, even when asked. They have a waiting list of clients who want babies, and they provide adoption services in concert with family planning. Evidently when the five clinics sat around the table, the issues of mission and goals were raised immediately. One director left the meeting early; the remainder continued to meet with the superintendent. At the end of the meeting, those present decided that no collaborative could be formed; each family planning clinic formalized individualized partnerships with the school system.
>
> Of course, I have some really positive examples to share. When I emailed Mr. Alvarez at the Department of Human Services (DHS), he was able to help Almeada right away because of the partnerships his organization had formed with several employers. In fact, they had formed the partnerships under the umbrella of the Chamber of Commerce and the City Development Council. That meant they did not have to form multiple partnerships; the Chamber and the Development Council, representing over 60 businesses, guaranteed cooperation among its members. Mr. Alvarez says that he has been able to provide vocational services much more effectively than ever before.

Ms. LaRosa provides two examples for us, one in which a collaborative effort was undermined by turf issues and one where a partnership was formed for the

TABLE 8.5   SUMMARY POINTS: TURF ISSUES

- Collaboration among agencies benefits clients and the community.
- Turf issues arise among agencies over resources, power, and political issues.
- Turf issues can become turf battles and diminish opportunities for collaboration.
- Collaborative efforts are complex and need attention and continuous communication.

benefit of clients within the city. Agencies and organizations, human service professionals, clients, and the community all benefit when coalitions exist. Because the relationships are complex, continuous communication about goals, methods, and attention to turf issues helps resolve turf issues before they become turf battles.

Often, working within the human service delivery context can be very challenging. Professionals confront difficult issues every day; at times the organizational setting supports the human service work; at other times the bureaucracy contributes to the stress. Let us look at what happens to helpers when they face too many challenges. See Table 8.5.

ENCAPSULATION, BURNOUT, AND VICARIOUS TRAUMA

Working as a human service professional is challenging and rewarding. Unfortunately, the enthusiasm can fade as helpers become disenchanted, experience disequilibrium, and behave in ways that are less than professional. One reaction to the stresses and strains experienced by helping professionals is **encapsulation**—retreating from the engagement of helping and becoming rigid, insensitive, uncaring professionals. Another result of the pressures of the job may be burnout, a syndrome that can result in poor work performance or a decision to leave the profession.

Helpers who become encapsulated may become static in their work as they face the difficulties of working within the human service delivery system. They may feel so threatened and frightened by the difficult tasks they are asked to perform that they quit learning, growing, and trying—thus becoming encapsulated. Such professionals relate to clients in characteristic ways. First, they become rigid and inflexible, believing that there are enduring truths that must be upheld. Such truths can take many forms, such as "The system's rules are always right and just" or "Individuals who are unemployed do not deserve to be helped." If human service professionals are dynamic, their personal and professional experiences continually modify their ideas about clients and the entire delivery system. They grow, learning about the system and how it operates as well as learning about self. Clinging to the "truths" helpers have at the beginning of their professional careers limits what they can learn from their experiences.

Ms. LaRosa talks about a time when she was encapsulated as a helper. She learned a lot during this time and believes that she is now a more committed professional as a result of the experience.

> Earlier I talked about my incredible schedule and workload. What I did not talk about was how much I enjoy my work. Working with adolescents is a great job.

The preceding year, though, was a time of professional crisis for me. At this point I am able to see how much I have grown as a professional. Because I was once fairly rigid, today it is almost impossible to believe that I could have been an effective helper.

I had been working with teenagers in a Boys & Girls Club setting. I was so excited about my work when I began. I would get up and head to work at 7:00 a.m. just to be the first person in the building. By the time the young children arrived at 7:30 a.m., I was ready for them. I became involved in the lives of many of the families of my clients and worried about each and every one of them. I was also absolutely sure about what was best for them. I came from a wonderful family and was raised by loving parents. I was appalled by what I thought was inadequate and sometimes frightening care. Many of the parents were not at home for their children; babies were left with older siblings while parents worked. Single mothers were raising as many as five or six children. Some parents had extreme ways of disciplining their children. I tried to change the behaviors of these parents and became so frustrated when they refused to change.

When I look back now, I think the only thing that saved my relationship with these parents was my absolute dedication to helping them. They knew they could depend upon me, even if I was constantly trying to show them a better way to raise their children. But, by the end of the school year, I really did not like the parents. I was not sure they deserved my attention since they were not changing their ways.

Encapsulated professionals depend only on their own personal experiences and frames of references, which limits their understanding of their clients. Ms. LaRosa illustrates this limited understanding. There are many different types of clients and client situations, and it is difficult to be familiar with all of them. As a result, helping professionals should constantly read, discuss, and observe clients, so they can broaden the base from which they understand clients' experiences. Professionals who do not expand their knowledge remain limited in the ways in which they can serve their clients.

As mentioned, another result of the stress and strain new professionals experience is **burnout**. This condition results from negative changes in attitudes and behavior that are precipitated by job strain (Weiten, Lloyd, Dunn, & Hammer, 2011). Like encapsulation, burnout affects the day-to-day work of the professional and results in behavior that has negative effects on the work environment as well as the helping process. There are identifiable pressures that lead to burnout. Loss of idealism and disappointment in client motivations may result in a loss of commitment to both job and clients. Professionals who experience burnout may also be reacting to a less-than-perfect work setting—one that is too demanding, too frustrating, or too boring.

Some symptoms of burnout are a change in attitude about work, lower expectations of performance, severe emotional detachment from work, reduced psychological involvement with clients, and an intense concern with self. With burnout, helpers are likely to perceive work more negatively, resulting in sick days, tardiness, and clock watching. The syndrome also affects how they perceive clients. They may call them names behind their backs, become angry with them, or feel that they are irresponsible and ungrateful for the help that is given them. These behaviors all impact negatively on the helper's ability to assist the client. They violate many of the basic values of helping, such as tolerance and acceptance of the client. In addition, individuals who are themselves involuntary clients are less likely to respond positively or see helpers in a positive light.

There are also some physical symptoms of burnout, such as chronic fatigue, frequent colds, serious illness, stomach trouble, lower back pain, and perhaps even substance abuse. Burnout may also affect the person's relationships with others outside of work, and the helper may be unable to take up new hobbies or concentrate on anything for long periods of time.

Ms. LaRosa has only experienced periodic burnout, but she has worked with a number of professionals who have severe cases of the syndrome. During the time she was working with Almeada, she had many of the symptoms. It was because she had such a large caseload and worked such long hours. Although she was never late or tardy, she began to resent her work. She would complain about her job to her friends and family, but she never took it out on her clients, or so she thought. Ms. LaRosa had begun to notice little things that denoted signs of burnout. As a result, she tried to adjust her pattern of unrealistic expectations for each workday. It is easy to lose your sense of professionalism when work demands exceed energy and resources.

For human service professionals who help individuals with more severe levels of trauma exposure, such as child abuse, violent crime, natural disasters, or torture, vicarious traumatization may result (Painter, 2012). What happens to helpers who work with victims of trauma? Researchers indicate that **vicarious trauma** may integrate into the helper's worldview; the world no longer seems a safe and secure place (Harrison & Westwood, 2009). As with symptoms of burnout, vicarious trauma may also influence varying aspects of the helper's life such as relationships, physical health, mental health, and faith and hope (Trippany, White Kress, & Wilcoxon, 2004). In addition, similar to burnout, vicarious trauma may affect the helping abilities, resulting in decreased empathic abilities, defensive reactions, and a decreased concern for clients (Trippany et al., 2004).

Burnout and vicarious trauma are not temporary strains but rather patterns of being and thinking that cannot easily be interrupted unless specific efforts are made to alleviate it. They represent not just "poor adjustment" that can be corrected easily. Recovery from burnout and vicarious trauma is a long process that necessitates many changes in the life and work of the professionals affected. See Table 8.6.

PROFESSIONAL DEVELOPMENT

One approach that counters the devastating effects of encapsulation, burnout, and vicarious trauma is professional development. In fact, this is a positive approach to address the challenges that affect the day-to-day work of helpers. A commitment to professional development is a means of keeping positively engaged and well supported while delivering services.

Critical to improving one's professional standing is a commitment to developing new knowledge and skills. The ultimate goal is to be a more effective helper and to be able to respond to each helping opportunity in a way that positively supports the client. If the helper is involved in learning new knowledge about clients, developing and improving skills, and reflecting on current practice, then the services he or she is delivering are more effective. Within the field of human services, new information is always available about the problems of clients' experiences. New methodologies are constantly being developed to help professionals address

TABLE 8.6 SUMMARY POINTS: ENCAPSULATION, BURNOUT, AND VICARIOUS TRAUMA

Encapsulation occurs when:

- professionals become static in their work;

- professionals become rigid and inflexible and uphold their own beliefs or truths;

- professionals support the beliefs of the traditional culture; and

- clients are asked to accept norms of the traditional culture.

Burnout occurs when:

- there are multiple pressures at work over a long period of time;

- professionals have unrealistic expectations about their job outcomes;

- professionals begin to miss work, arrive late, denigrate their clients; and

- the bureaucracy does not support the professional or the client.

Vicarious trauma occurs when:

- there is exposure to clients who experience trauma such as violent crime, natural disasters, or torture;

- trauma becomes part of helper's worldview;

- the world no longer appears to be safe and secure;

- specific aspects of helper's life, social, emotional, and work, become difficult; and

- the ability to help others is diminished.

client needs. As the field of human service delivery constantly changes, professionals need to assess what these changes mean for their work with clients. Professional development means helpers do not serve clients in the same way, year after year, but recognize that their clients' problems change, the world in which they live shifts, and new ways of helping continually emerge.

Both formal and informal approaches to continuing education are important to professional growth. Returning to school for an advanced degree—whether it be an associate's, baccalaureate, master's, doctorate, or specialist degree—is a legitimate way to continue professional education in the human services. Such formal education will also open alternative career paths and allow helpers to increase their qualifications and competence. Workshops and conferences are also available within an organization or within the working radius of the professional to broaden his or her understanding of client needs and the changing times. Other educational opportunities may focus on developing one or two specific skills in greater depth. Ms. LaRosa shares with us her own experiences with professional development.

> I am indebted to a summer educational experience I had when I worked with the Boys & Girls Club. My fellow students allowed me to see the "client experience" from another perspective. As they talked about their work with helpers and their frustrations with the helping process, I felt shame for the way in which I had treated the parents with whom I had worked. But we learned in class how to avoid treating clients in such

a disrespectful way, so I was able to replace one set of thoughts and behaviors with another. Since that summer, I have continued to believe that professional development is a critical part of becoming a professional.

Sometimes it is easy to be involved in professional development. Other times it seems impossible to take the time to attend a workshop, lecture, or class. I know the times that I think I am too busy to go are the very times that I should quit what I am doing and sign up for that seminar or workshop. I am always so glad once I am there. There is an excitement I feel when I am involved in learning. It is also a good way to share ideas with other professionals and to expand my professional network. The last workshop that I attended was three months ago. The focus was substance abuse, which is a common problem among my clients. I learned how the very latest brain research impacts the ways in which we now deliver treatment to this population. Three professionals I met at the workshop volunteered to establish a "group counseling" experience for my pregnant girls.

Commitment to the profession is also a part of professional development. When human service professionals become active in an organization or become active members of the community, they expand their professional associations and their professional awareness. Anytime they study political issues or become deeply involved in solving individual or community problems that are difficult to comprehend, they are expanding their professional understanding. Even the continuous updating of their knowledge of the community, its professionals, and its resources is an informal professional development process.

PROMOTING CHANGE IN A DYNAMIC WORLD

One continuous theme throughout this text is that the world is changing rapidly. We are experiencing the globalization of the economy, increased immigration, the development of new technologies, and the emergence of new methodologies for approaching the problems in this third millennium. For a human service professional to be effective with and responsive to clients, and knowledgeable about and sensitive to community needs, it is increasingly important to function as a change agent. Becoming involved in change is often difficult for the beginning professional.

This section will present three contexts in which professionals can promote change. The first context is within the arena of the local community, becoming involved in developing specific services in response to community needs. The second context is also related to the community, initiating and participating in **community organizing**. The focus on this type of change occurs with the development of a new vision or a new focus for the community. Community organizing occurs when the development of a coalition of individuals and communities is powerful enough to continue to create and promote change. The third context centers around the **empowerment** of a specific population with little previous status or power. The empowerment occurs once the population is identified and a team of professionals and other interested individuals work with that population to build the skills that allow them to advocate for themselves and facilitate their own change. A description and examples of each of these three contexts or approaches follow.

Developing Services in Response to Human Needs

In developing, maintaining, and reevaluating human service delivery, a primary consideration is the response to community needs. The community has a dual role in the causation and resolution of client problems. On one hand, the community is a source of client problems. On the other hand, it provides many of the resources needed for resolving problems. The World Bank announced a project beginning in 2007 to empower women in developing countries as a way of addressing community needs (World Bank, 2012). The project links women's economic power with education, reduction of infant mortality, improved health, and the reduction of HIV/AIDS. Issues identification, advocacy for nonexistent services, and planning based on community needs are integral components of fostering change.

Advocating the establishment of services that are nonexistent is one of the most difficult responsibilities of the human service professional. The **advocate** is one who speaks up for the rights of others and defends those who cannot defend themselves. When helpers discover that their clients have needs that cannot be met through the human service delivery system, they have a responsibility to work with others to develop alternative ways of meeting those needs. To do so requires skills that incorporate working with the individual, agencies, and legal and legislative bodies. Regardless of the type of advocacy, the process is much the same:

- Identify the needs of the individual or the population.
- Determine how to meet the needs.
- Work with a network of individuals or agencies to provide the services.
- Identify the barriers that must be overcome.
- Teach clients about the advocacy process and give them a role.

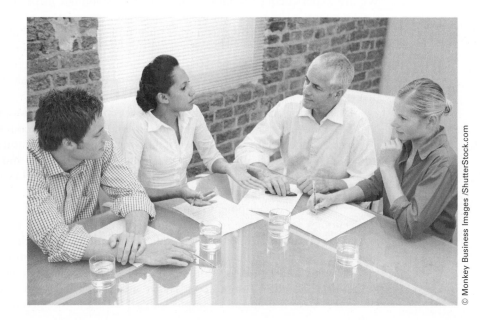

© Monkey Business Images /ShutterStock.com

- Negotiate to meet goals and objectives.
- Develop a framework that continues the success of the advocacy process.

Many professionals are successful in acting as advocates for their individual clients and can use their networking skills to find food where no food services exist, eyeglasses and other special medical needs where resources are unavailable, and housing for those who temporarily need shelter. More difficult is the advocacy that involves developing a political voice for the larger issues that require community, state, or national attention. Moveon.org, an organization that works to bring ordinary people into politics by taking stands on policy issues, advocating for campaign finance reform, and supporting candidates, and the Tea Party Patriots, a community committed to standing together to protect the United States and its Constitution, are two examples of advocacy. NARAL Pro-Choice America is a national organization that advocates for and provides comprehensive information on reproductive rights in the United States. Focus on the Family is a Christian organization that offers practical, biblical advice on marriage, parenting, and life challenges. As you will note, there are many advocacy organizations at all levels that address different stances on issues and concerns from varying perspectives.

A critical component in developing services is knowing both the needs and the characteristics of the populations served. See Box 8.3 for an example. The following case study illustrates the importance of planning for services that address relevant issues. A change project located in Redwood City, California, did just that.

BOX 8.3

INTERNATIONAL FOCUS
WORLD BANK: GENDER EQUITY AS SMART ECONOMICS

The World Bank is working to address the economic needs of women in developing countries. The focus is on working with countries, donors, and other development agencies to further the economic empowerment of women by encouraging women's participation in government and business infrastructures, finance, and agriculture. The project also supports research about the factors that restrict gender equality and those that encourage women's participation in the economic sector. One example that illustrates the power of economic involvement comes from Ethiopia.

A study in Ethiopia by the Gender Equity Project examined a program that issued 20 million land-use certificates to about six million households. The study found that by providing space on the certificate for both spouses' names and photos, women's registration for land ownership increased significantly.

Another example is a project for adolescent girls. The Adolescent Girls Initiative supports the transition from schooling to paid employment for young women through skills training in partnership with governments and the Nike Foundation. Activities are underway in Liberia, Afghanistan, Nepal, Rwanda, and (South) Sudan.

The World Bank believes that programs such as these will reflect the needs of each country. For example, in many countries women are more educated than ever before, but they are still having difficulty finding jobs so they can support themselves. Because there is a strong link between women's economic status and poverty, level of education, health, and infant mortality, the World Bank's directors believe that this project, by creating opportunities for women, will help eradicate poverty in developing countries.

Source: Adapted from the *World Bank and Gender Equity: At a Glance* (2010). Retrieved from http://www.worldbank.org

Community organizers in this mid-size city near San Francisco were interested in improving the lives of youth who lived in their community. They had always worked from a community collaboration model, but when it came to identifying the needs of the youth in their community, they realized that they were not clear what those needs were. Not only did they ask these youth what they needed, they also involved the youth in the data gathering process.

To begin the project, they asked eighth graders to help them collect information about the youth in their city using the research methods that they were learning in their social science classes. The youth would then help design programs and evaluate them. In other words, their involvement would span the entire life of the program. These middle-school students would work with adults from community organizations and schools to develop services and programs to meet the needs identified.

The interviews that the middle-school students collected surprised the adult participants of the project. Instead of just raising youth-related issues, these young interviewers uncovered a concern for broader community issues among their interviewees. For example, the youth talked about the lack of fun in their communities and wished they had some place to just hang out and be with each other. But they also talked about the high cost of food and housing, little access to transportation, and violence.

The middle-school participants were able to contribute to the dialogue about the planning and programming to address the issues identified. And they advocated for services that would help other populations, not just themselves. Specific recommendations included concrete suggestions for improving the community, such as an archway ramp across a busy street so that all members of the neighborhood could cross without harm. They also asked for broader participation in the political process (Fernandez, 2002, pp. 1–8).

Suppose you are a human service professional planning services to reduce youth-related violence in your city or rural area. What needs must be considered? How would you discover what those needs are? What problems might you anticipate in implementing new programs in the community? What actions might you take to ensure successful planning and implementation? In answering these questions, you may realize how difficult planning is. Your responses should consider a variety of viewpoints and take into consideration how the services fit within the context of the current environment.

ORGANIZING TO PROMOTE COMMUNITY CHANGE

Promoting community change relies on the development and use of a network or larger confederation to advance the cause, mobilize individuals and agencies in the community, and create a financial resource base and a willing workforce of professionals and volunteers. Although promoting community change is a broader activity than just creating services, the change that you want to create must be defined, and numerous issues could benefit from the effort and focus. Read any national or local newspaper, listen to conversations between friends, tape dialogues in a teacher's lounge, or monitor the exchanges in a human service agency and organization lounge. In all of these settings you will hear numerous issues

TABLE 8.7 PRINCIPLES OF COMMUNITY ORGANIZING

- Individuals and organizations identify a common goal.
- Like-minded individuals and organizations consolidate themselves to have a more effective voice in the community.
- All individual members of the community are welcome to participate in the effort, including politicians, business leaders, citizens, and others.
- Organizations and agencies are welcome to form a network of the concerned. This network includes schools, financial institutions, social service organizations, political organizations, nonprofit organizations, and others.
- The combined effort of many voices has the power to facilitate change.
- Basic to the work is organizing as a team and gathering information to understand the community and its needs.
- Action plans provide the foundation for community change efforts.

being raised. Unfortunately, most of these communications end with frustration, hopelessness, some humor, but no hope for action. The difficulties seem too challenging to overcome (see Table 8.7).

The process of community action begins with a community action plan (CAP). The Presidents' Summit for America's Future prepared material that outlines the steps in developing a CAP (America's Promise Alliance, 2012). It is during the development of this plan that the concerned coalition answers the question: "How will this initiative be carried out?" To answer that question fully, the following questions are adapted from the America's Promise plans for promoting change:

- What will be the community effort focus?
- Where can we find the resources we need?
- What knowledge and skills do we need to support our effort?
- What offices, technology, and equipment do we need?
- How will we gather support?
- What are the benefits of being in this coalition?
- How do we promote ourselves?

The development of the CAP focuses on meeting the goals and objectives. It begins to bring people together to talk about issues. For the first time, individuals from every corner of the community are talking together. The action plan becomes the forum for the conversation; a strong community network is being built. Not all conversation has to occur when individuals are meeting together. There are new models of community organizing that use technology to bring people together to discuss major issues and develop CAPs. These programs are developed to teach organizers how to effectively use technology to allow individuals in remote areas to participate in the community action process. See Box 8.4.

In summary, work within the community to promote change is an important part of the human service professional's responsibility. It can be a rewarding way to improve client environments and services and can expand the helper's network to include many individuals and organizations outside the human service.

BOX 8.4 WEB SOURCES

Search the Web to find out more about community organizing.

Center for Community Change

Change.org

Community building

Community organizing

World Bank

USING A MODEL OF CLIENT EMPOWERMENT

Throughout this text we have discussed the importance of both advocacy for the client and empowerment of the client. Using a model of client empowerment is another approach to facilitating change, a model that is commonly used in many developing countries. The primary goal of this model is to ultimately place the advocacy and empowerment in the hands and voices of the clients or those in need (See Table 8.8). The basic thrust of this model is to educate and train those in need to organize, establish their agenda, and work for their own cause by organizing campaigns, networking with government and business leaders, proposing legislation, and participating in the political, economic, and social processes of the community. How does an effort like this begin?

One such example is the Women's Bean Project (WBP), a not-for-profit effort begun 16 years ago in Denver, Colorado. It is an on-site packaged food business (Haynes, Ryan, & MacDonald, 2007).

> This project prepares women for the world of work by teaching them basic job skills and basic life skills. Each woman commits to enrollment in the project for at least six months and for as long as a year. Women with backgrounds of chronic poverty and

TABLE 8.8 SUMMARY POINTS: PROMOTING CHANGE

- Promoting change is an important role for the human service professional.
- One way of supporting change is to develop services in response to community needs, including establishing services that are nonexistent.
- The process to promote change involves identifying needs, deciding how needs can best be met, working with a network of individuals or agencies to provide services, identifying barriers that must be overcome, and teaching clients the advocacy process.
- Negotiating the meeting of goals and objectives and developing plans for future services are also part of the process.
- Community involvement to promote change uses a confederation of individuals and organizations committed to the same cause.
- One model of client empowerment focuses almost entirely on supporting clients to develop their own agenda, support structure, plan for change and evaluation, and the recruitment of new members.

unemployment are eligible to enroll. Success stories include Mary, who kicked a two-year-old heroin addiction, left prison, and is now a productive worker and an involved grandparent for the children she wasn't able to care for. Barbara came to the Bean Project when she was living in a homeless shelter and had no job skills to help her obtain employment and has now been employed at the same place for seven years. She owns a home and a car (Haynes et al., 2007).

The Women's Bean Project uses the Results Oriented Management and Accountability (ROMA) method that helps link project goals to outcomes, indicates measures of success, and demands a data collection and data analysis process. In line with the commitment to empowerment and advocacy, the agency itself has changed with its use of ROMA. Successes include participants who focus on improving their lives, an increased graduation rate in the program and an increase in the rate of employment. The program offers women an opportunity to develop skills, stabilize their lives, and in turn begin to help others. (Haynes et al., 2007).

Another example is the work of Disha Kendra described in Box 8.5.

There are many ways the human service professional can become involved in change. You do not have to spearhead a movement or fight single-handedly for your clients. Just look around your neighborhood, city, or organization to find efforts you wish to support to ultimately improve the lives and environments of your clients.

| **BOX 8.5** | INTERNATIONAL FOCUS: *DISHA KENDRA* |

Disha Kendra was established in 1978 by Jagrut Bhaubandhi Sangatana to help village tribal people in India fight their socioeconomic and political oppression. Tribal people are indigenous people who live in remote rural areas in India. Each tribe has a different culture, speaks a unique dialect, and lives according to long-standing traditions.

The first phase of the organization's work (1978–1983) focused on economic and human rights development. One example of this work was the two-year process of breaking the economic hold of the money-lender on the 35-household village of Chadhawadi and substituting a six-year bank-loan program to support local farming efforts. During this initial phase, education was also enhanced with the formation of preschool and adult education programs. From 1983 to 1991—the second and third phases of the organization's history—the effort determined long- and short-term needs of the village and assessed the outcomes of past efforts. In addition, the organization promoted the tribal people's ability to lead their own political organizations as they struggled to increase the availability of water, electricity, and

employment opportunities. The fourth phase of the agency's work is underway and includes strengthening political organization and leadership training, improving community organization, and improving the lives of tribal women. The emphasis is on helping tribal people help themselves.

During the authors' visit to the village, the agency's political action director, Bunsi, conducted a meeting of the village committee, a group of six men from surrounding villages. Their task was to prepare for a meeting the following week with the police superintendent inspector who would rule on a land-access dispute. A wealthy Mumbai businessman had bought a large tract of land near the village and was denying access to their farmland, water supply, and firewood. Bunsi asked those in attendance to decide who would speak for the committee, and he explained the hearing process. They then role-played what the spokesman would say at the hearing.

The agency staff visit the villages weekly or live in the villages themselves. They are available to help with whatever issues arise that affect the rights of tribals as a protected class of people in India.

KEY TERMS

advocate	empowerment	network	referral
brokering	encapsulation	organizational chart	resources
burnout	job description	organizational climate	turf
chain of command	mission	privatization	vicarious trauma
community organizing			

THINGS TO REMEMBER

1. The work of the human service professional occurs within an agency or organization.
2. An agency's written mission statement communicates an agency's purpose by summarizing its guiding principles.
3. Goal statements, job descriptions, and policies and procedures are other agency documents that clarify the work of an agency and its employers.
4. The relationships among the individuals who work in an agency and the departments to which they are assigned describe an agency's structure.
5. A chain of command, often illustrated by an organizational chart, refers to the layers of authority in an agency.
6. Funding sources determine if an agency is public or governmental, not-for-profit (voluntary), or for-profit.
7. Human service agencies exist within the context of a community that influences agency operations, services, clients, and professionals.
8. One of the most important roles of a human service professional is brokering, or referring a client to another agency or service.
9. The referral process involves the professional, the client, and the other agency to which the client is referred.
10. In referral, the beginning human service professional is at a disadvantage because of a lack of experience in the system, a lack of personal contacts with other helpers in the system, and a lack of knowledge about the many problems that clients may have.
11. The beginning professional must develop a systematic way of building a file of information about the human service network for referral purposes.
12. Challenges such as allocation of resources, paperwork, and turf issues influence the work of the human service professional.
13. Responses such as encapsulation, burnout, and vicarious trauma leave professionals unable to be effective helpers.
14. Professional development strategies such as attending workshops and participating in professional organizations help professionals respond to changes in human services.
15. An important responsibility of the human service professional is to be an advocate for change.
16. In developing, maintaining, and reevaluating the delivery of human services, it is important to consider human services as a response to community needs.
17. Empowering clients to advocate for their own change is one model of responding to client needs.

SELF-ASSESSMENT

- Identify ways the professional can learn more about an agency.
- What is a "good" referral?
- Describe the challenges the human service professional faces.

- How can professional development counter these challenges?
- How can human service professionals promote change?

- What are the pitfalls a professional may encounter while developing services in response to community needs?
- Why is the client empowerment model for change an effective one?

WANT TO KNOW MORE?

There are several resources you can access to learn more about human services and the concepts discussed in this chapter.

Additional Readings: Focus on Organizations

Austin, M. J., Brody, R., & Packard, T. R. (2008). *Managing the challenges in human service organizations: A casebook.* Thousand Oaks, CA: Sage. The cases in this book are inspired by real situations and are designed to encourage the reader to think about responses to the dilemmas that are presented.

Bolman, L. G., & Deal, T. E. (2008). *Reframing organizations: Artistry, choice, and leadership.* San Francisco: Jossey-Bass. This book offers practical ways of thinking about today's challenges for leadership.

Gibelman, M. (2012). *Navigating human service organizations: Essential information for thriving and surviving in agencies* (3rd ed.). Chicago: Lyceum Books. This book provides strategies to help practitioners improve their ability to work effectively within human service organizations.

Gitlin, L. N. (2008). *Successful grant writing: Strategies for health and human service professions.* New York: Springer. This author introduces the knowledge and skills to read a funding opportunity, determine its appropriateness to pursue ideas, and the process for applying for funding.

Hasenfeld, Y. (2009). *Human services as complex organizations.* Thousand Oaks, CA: Sage. This is a collection of essays that provide a comprehensive and contemporary perspective on human service organizations.

Mathieu, F. (2011). *The compassion fatigue workbook: Creative tools for transforming compassion fatigue and vicarious traumatization.* New York: Routledge. The author provides practical and insightful exercises for helping professionals to address issues of encapsulation, burnout, and lack of empathy. It addresses the cost of caring.

Sen, R. (2003). *Stir it up: Lessons in community organizing and advocacy.* Hoboken, NJ: Jossey-Bass. This text provides the steps of building a constituency and organizing for social justice. There are multiple case studies to illustrate the concepts presented.

Smith, M. B., Graham, Y., & Guttmacher, S. (2005). *Community-based health organizations: Advocating for improved health.* New Brunswick, NJ: Jossey-Bass. This text presents basic principles to create community-based health organizations. Included is a history of community-based care and a structured outline of developing services in communities.

Case Study

If you would like to know more about the application of the concepts discussed in this chapter, read the case study of Kirkpatrick Mental Health Center in Chapter 8 of *Introduction to Human Services: Cases and Applications*, the companion text to *Introduction to Human Services*. Steve Jackson, the director, and his staff, and Board of Directors face a crisis precipitated by two recent deaths in the community. These losses prompt them to reexamine their work in community-based mental health.

REFERENCES

Abu Dhabi Police. (2012). Social Support Centers in Abu Dhabi and Family Development Discuss Cooperation. Retrieved from http://www.adpolice.gov.ae/en/News/social.suport.tnmia.aspx

America's Promise Alliance. (2012). *Home*. Retrieved from http://www.americaspromise.org/

Bureau of Labor Statistics. (2010). *Career guides to industries, 2010–2011: Healthcare*. Retrieved from http://www.bls.gov/oco/cg/cgs035.htm

Fernandez, M. A. (2002). *Creating community change: Challenges and tensions in community youth research*. Palo Alto, CA: John W. Gardner Center for Youth and Their Communities.

Harrison, R. L., & Westwood, M. J. (2009). Preventing vicarious traumatization of mental health therapists: identifying protective practices. *Psychotherapy Theory, Research, Practice, Training, 46* (2), 203–219.

Haynes, S., Ryan, T., & MacDonald, B. (2007). The Women's Bean Project: Defining the mission and measuring outcomes to better serve the needs of women. *Human Service Education, 27* (1), 39–44.

Homan, M. (2010). *Promoting community change: Making it happen in the real world*. Belmont, CA: Brooks/Cole.

Lewis, J. A., Lewis, M. D., Packard, T., & Souflee, F. (2012). *Management of human service programs* (5th ed.). Belmont, CA: Brooks/Cole.

National Organization for Human Services. (2012). *Home*. Retrieved from http://www.nationalhumanservices.org/

National Center for Nonprofit Boards. (2012). *Effective boards*. Retrieved from http://www.nsba.org/sbot/toolkit/EfBoards.html

Native American Traditional Healing. (2009). *Aidsinfornet*. Retrieved from http://www.aids.org/factSheets/708-Native-American-Traditional-Healer.html

Painter, E. R. (2012). *Trauma work and the impact of vicarious traumatization*. Unpublished paper, Knoxville, Tennessee.

Social Support Center. (2006). *Community policing department*. Abu Dhabi, United Arab Emirates Ministry of Interior, Abu Dhabi Police G. H. Q.

Trippany, R. L., White Kress, V. E., & Wilcoxon, S. A. (2004). Preventing vicarious trauma: What counselors should know when working with trauma survivors. *Journal of Counseling and Development, 82*, 31–37.

Weiten, W., Lloyd, M., Dunn, D. S., & Hammer, E. Y. (2011). *Psychology applied to modern life: Adjustment in the 21st century*. Belmont, CA: Wadsworth.

World Bank. (2012). *World development report 2012: Gender equality and development*. Retrieved from http://hdl.handle.net/10986/4391

HUMAN SERVICES AND
ETHICAL PRACTICE

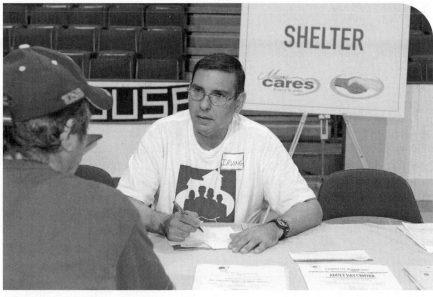

CHAPTER 9

Jeff Greenberg/PhotoEdit

After reading this chapter, you will be able to:

• State the purpose and limitations of codes of ethics.
• Summarize the influence of law, diversity, and technology on codes of ethics.
• Write vignettes to illustrate the concerns of competence, responsibility, confidentiality, and client's rights.
• List the steps in the ethical decision-making model.
• Apply the ethical decision-making model to an ethical dilemma.

This final chapter focuses on the ethics of human service practice. The helper is continually faced with ethical decisions. Sometimes these issues arise between the professional and the client; other times there are multiple individuals and even agencies with a stake in the decisions made. The helper's responsibilities are not simply to recognize an ethical situation and make the "right" decision. In fact, ethical practice and decision making require that the helping professional consider the situation from all points of view, develop a list of issues that represent multiple viewpoints, generate possible decisions, and weigh carefully the consequences of each decision. This type of ethical practice demands that the helper have knowledge of the professional code of ethics, critical thinking skills, an understanding of human behavior, good communication skills, the ability to establish rapport, and decision-making skills.

In this chapter, you will use your knowledge of the history of human services, the work of the professional, and the nature of clients and settings to imagine yourself in the role of the helper. The chapter includes an introduction to codes of ethics, definitions of competence and responsibility, a discussion of confidentiality, a description of the client's rights, ethical standards of human service professionals, and a model for ethical decision making.

ETHICAL CONSIDERATIONS

As you deliver human services, situations will arise in which you may be unsure about the appropriate action to take. A third party requests information about a client; you observe a colleague joking about a client in the break room at work; a client requests information about obtaining an abortion, but your agency opposes providing this type of information. These situations represent **ethical dilemmas** for the human service professional. Even though education and training in human services emphasize the values of confidentiality, acceptance, individualism, self-determination, and tolerance, situations will inevitably occur in which simply possessing these values will not be enough to determine the right course of action.

The foundation of ethical behavior is based upon principles that are shared by members of the profession. Professions such as medicine, nursing, psychology, counseling, health, and human services adhere to similar principles that underlie practice. These principles focus on the way in which professional helpers work with clients. They include autonomy, nonmaleficence, beneficence, justice, fidelity, and veracity.

> *Autonomy* represents the commitment to respect a client's right to define his or her own problems, help choose interventions, and help evaluate successes and satisfactions. Helpers who provide the client with autonomy foster self-determination and support client independence.

Nonmaleficence essentially means that the professional will not harm the client. This means that human service professionals will not take risks that might, in the short or long run, hurt the client.

Beneficence defines an act that is in someone's best interest. Helpers guided by this principle provide services or serve as advocates with what the client needs in mind. At times, family considerations or agency rules and regulations clash with perceived client needs.

Justice as a principle means that the human service professional works tirelessly to promote equality of access for clients, is fair in all interactions, and is obligated to adhering to the principles of nondiscrimination.

Fidelity is respecting the trust that clients place in their helpers and guarding against an erosion of that trust. Helpers are careful to fulfill their responsibilities, keep promises, and be honest in their interactions with clients.

Veracity means being honest with clients. Human service professionals commit to providing clients with all of the information that they need and to providing fair and honest feedback.

In the past decade, increased public awareness of professional behavior, coupled with the passage of federal and state legislation controlling the helping professions, has underscored the importance of ethical concerns in service delivery. The Family Educational Rights and Privacy Act of 1974, state legislation requiring the reporting of child abuse, and *Tarasoff v. Regents of the University of California* (1976), which imposed a duty to warn potential victims, are examples of government action that directly affects the ethics of service provision. A more recent example is the Health Insurance Portability and Accountability Act (HIPAA) that went into effect in 2003 and has greatly impacted informed consent practices. The human service professional must both obey the law and also be cognizant of the implications of the law.

An exploration of codes of ethics or statements of standards of behavior as guides for professional behavior begins the next section. Some major areas of ethical concern for the human service professional follow. Then we describe an ethical decision-making model that can be applied to dilemmas for which there is no relevant guideline. Vignettes are used to illustrate the range of dilemmas that may arise.

CODES OF ETHICS

Professionals have responded to the dilemmas of service provision by developing codes of ethics, or statements of ethical standards of behavior for the members of their profession. Codes of ethics or ethical standards reflect professional concerns and define the guiding principles of professional activities. As an aid to ethical decision making in dilemmas arising in service delivery, such standards or codes help clarify the professional's responsibilities to clients, to the agency, and to society. Typically, a **code of ethics** includes items that state the goals or aims of the profession, that protect the client, that provide guidance to professional behavior, and that contribute to a professional identity for the helper. A complete understanding of a code of ethics or ethical standards requires knowledge of the code's strengths and purposes as well as its limitations.

PURPOSES AND LIMITATIONS   The primary functions of a code of ethics or ethical standards are to establish guidelines for professional behavior and to assist members of the profession in establishing a professional identity. Other purposes include providing criteria for evaluating the ethics of a professional's practice and serving as a benchmark in the enforcement of ethical standards.

Ethical codes do have limitations; they cannot cover every situation. They do, however, present a framework for ethical behavior, although their exact interpretation will depend on the situation to which they are being applied. As a result of this vagueness, codes may have a limited range, and some codes of ethics will likely conflict with others regarding some standard of behavior. Such conflicts pose problems for professionals who are members of more than one professional organization.

Other entities that set standards may also issue ethical standards that conflict. For example, a code may not include a statement relating to the duty to warn, but the California Supreme Court has ruled in *Tarasoff* (1976) that there is a duty to warn potential victims of danger. Members who are bound by a code of ethics must be alert to the possibility that other forums may reach conclusions that differ from their code. Of course, this is especially critical when the other forum is a court of law or a legislative body.

Some other limitations of codes of ethics are beyond the scope of this text; however, human service professionals must be aware that such limitations exist. The professional must develop ethical reasoning skills to help resolve ethical dilemmas that may arise. A first step in this process is differentiating ethical dilemmas from situations in which the guidelines are clear. For resolving problem situations for which there are no specific guidelines, an ethical decision-making model is presented later in this chapter.

ETHICS AND THE PROFESSION   A code of ethics is binding only on the members of the group or organization that adopts it. Several organizations in human services have issued codes of behavior expected of their membership—organizations such as the National Organization for Human Services, the American Counseling Association, the National Council for Social Work Education, and others in the fields of corrections, mental health, gerontology, and education. Most codes of ethics stipulate that the helper's first responsibility is to enhance and protect the client's welfare. Codes also give guidance about the helper's responsibilities to employers, to colleagues in the profession and other fields, and to society in general.

Ethical codes adopted by a professional association are usually based on the premise that a profession polices itself. Members of helping professions are assumed to be responsible, sensitive persons who are accountable for their behavior

---

BOX 9.1   WEB SOURCES

Check out the following organizations to learn more about codes of ethics of major professional helping organizations.

American Counseling Association

American Psychological Association

National Board of Certified Counselors

National Organization for Human Services

and the behavior of their colleagues. Self-regulation involves two types of discipline: informal and formal. Informal discipline is seen in the subtle and not-so-subtle pressure that colleagues exert on one another in the form of consultations, client referrals, and informal and formal discussions. Formal discipline occurs when professional associations publicly criticize or censure their members—in extreme cases, barring them from membership.

CODES OF ETHICS AND THE LAW   The law is generally supportive of, or at least neutral toward, ethical codes and standards. It is supportive in that it enforces minimum standards for practitioners through licensing requirements and generally protects the confidentiality of statements and records provided by clients during service provision. It is neutral in that it allows each profession to police itself and govern the helper's relations with clients and fellow professionals. The law intervenes and overrides professional codes of ethics only when necessary to protect the public's health, safety, and welfare. One instance of legal intervention occurs when the profession's standards of confidentiality (deemed necessary to ensure effective treatment) call for the suppression of information that government authorities require to be disclosed to prevent harm to others.

The California Supreme Court's ruling in the case of *Tarasoff* (1976) legally supported a duty to warn possible victims of clients once counselors have this information. The Court stated that

> when a therapist determines, or pursuant to the standards of his profession should determine, that his patient presents a serious danger of violence to another, he incurs an obligation to use reasonable care to protect the intended victim against such danger.
> The discharge of this duty may require the therapist to take one or more steps, depending on the nature of the case. Thus, it may call for him or her to warn the intended victim or others likely to apprise the victim of the danger, to notify the police, or to take whatever other steps are reasonably necessary under the circumstances. (p. 340)

ETHICS AND DIVERSITY   Ethical concerns in providing human services in a diverse society occur on two levels. One is at the individual level. The unintentional bias of a human service professional may encompass hidden beliefs and attitudes that can be a harmful influence on the helping relationship. Sometimes human service professionals may even consciously endorse prejudiced beliefs and attitudes. Behaving in such a way is unethical.

On a more general level, the basic tenets or underlying principles of some codes of ethics may not always apply to all cultures. For example, the United States is recognized as an individualist culture where the focus is on the individual or the self. Think of the words in English that begin with self: *self-actualization, self-disclosure, self-concept, self-acceptance, self-esteem, self-control*, and so forth. Other cultures are collectivist in nature, emphasizing the importance of the family, the extended family, or even a larger group. These associations take precedence over the individual. In practical terms, one illustration of this difference is the health and well-being of the individual versus the health and well-being of the group. In the past, failure to take culture into account and to acknowledge individual differences within cultures has contributed to the ineffectiveness of human service delivery with diverse groups.

Today, codes of ethics emphasize cultural competence that encompasses three broad dimensions: awareness, understanding, and skill (Sue & Sue, 2012). Later in this chapter you will read the *Ethical Standards of Human Service Professionals*. The preamble of this document recognizes "an appreciation of human beings in all their diversity." Specific standards address the "respect, acceptance, and dignity" due each client (#2), the need to be advocates (for the rights of all members of society, particularly those who are members of minorities and groups at which discriminatory practices have historically been directed) (#16), and the provision of services "without discrimination or preference based on age, ethnicity, culture, race, disability, gender, religion, sexual orientation, or socioeconomic status" (#17). Human service professionals are also "knowledgeable about the cultures and communities within which they practice" (#18), and they are "aware of their own cultural backgrounds, beliefs, and values" (#19). Other professional helping associations and organizations have indicated that helpers who work with other cultures without culture-specific awareness about those cultures are behaving in an unethical manner (Pedersen, 2000).

But ethics in a multicultural society are more complex. For example, self-disclosure, encouraged in European-American culture and often considered necessary for understanding by the helper, is taboo in other cultures. Asian Americans, American Indians, and Hispanic Americans do not value self-disclosure and believe that it reflects negatively not only on the individual but also on the family. Also prized in Western culture are eye contact and directness. Other non-Western cultures perceive these actions as signs of rudeness that should be avoided. A final example is the express prohibition of dual relationships in the ethical standards of many helping organizations, as for example statements 6 and 7 in the *Ethical Standards of Human Service Professionals* found later in this chapter. In some cultures like India, for instance, it is likely that dual relationships may be more normal and acceptable (Nagpal, 2001). For example, meetings with clients at their homes rather than an office may be expected. Clients may also be people who are known to the helper through relatives or friends, and it is these very associations that make it acceptable for the client to seek help from the helping professional.

How do human service professionals provide human services ethically in a diverse culture? Here are several guidelines (Corey, Corey, & Callanan, 2010; Sue & Sue, 2012; Welfel, 2012):

- Develop an attitude of openness, respect, and appreciation toward other cultural views; expand your comfort zone with cultural differences.
- Acquire knowledge of specific cultures other than your own.

TABLE 9.1   SUMMARY POINTS: CODES OF ETHICS

- Reflect professional concerns
- Define guiding principles of professional activities
- Clarify responsibilities to clients, the agency, and society
- Do not address every situation
- Are binding only on members of the group that adopts it

- Learn to modify interventions so that they are appropriate and effective with other cultures.
- Develop a tolerance for ambiguity and divergent philosophies, worldviews, and problem-solving behaviors that may be different from your own.

ETHICS AND TECHNOLOGY   The rapidly changing world of technology and its impact on human service delivery have created a number of concerns for both professionals and constituents. These concerns include access to personal information, online instruction, the electronic transmission of records, Internet use, Web counseling, and teleconferencing. Faxes, answering machines, voice mail, and e-mail also raise issues regarding privacy, confidentiality, and security. These concerns have prompted professional associations to respond through revisions of ethical codes, statements, or guidelines, such as the following:

- American Counseling Association: Ethical Standards for Internet On-Line Counseling
- ACES Guidelines for Online Instruction in Counselor Education
- National Board for Certified Counselors: The Practice of Internet Counseling
- APA Statement on Services by Telephone, Teleconferencing, and Internet
- NCDA Guidelines for the Use of the Internet for Provision of Career Information and Planning Services

As indicated by these professional organizational responses, using technology in the human service arena means focusing on several concerns such as a lack of confidentiality, limited training, and at times, unequal access to technology and its accompanying resources. As mentioned in Chapter 3, privacy is not guaranteed when individuals and organizations use listservs, e-mail, and the Web. This means that client information, related treatment documents, agency records, and correspondence may become more public than is warranted in service delivery. At best, the professional must make every effort to secure information and communication between professionals and those being helped. Clients should be warned of the potential for violation of privacy. They should also be informed of the steps that they can take to increase the likelihood of privacy from their end of the electronic communication.

Human service professionals are encouraged to help within their own scope of expertise. If helpers are to use technology to implement treatment strategies, gather data, record data, or make assessments, then they will need training to use technology in service delivery. Technology continues to change so rapidly that training needs to be ongoing. As helpers integrate computers into their work, they need to be encouraged to try new approaches and new ideas.

Because helpers are ethically obligated to provide quality services or use best practice, they need to study the effectiveness of the use of these new technologies. Also, helpers need to be sensitive to their clients' comfort with technology and client access to the Internet. For some clients, access is not possible, or at best, difficult. Maintaining this sensitivity will help human service professionals use technology to actually support clients and not to create additional barriers for them.

COMPETENCE AND RESPONSIBILITY

Before any involvement with clients, helpers must concern themselves with two areas: their competence as professionals and their responsibility to the individuals, groups, or organizations with whom they are affiliated, or with whom they serve as clients. Ethical concerns of competence and responsibility pervade all areas of professional practice.

Competence is a difficult concept to define from an ethical standpoint. One way to define it is by identifying the standards for practice within the profession. Most codes of ethics in helping professions include statements about academic training, practical training, or supervised experience and areas of specialization in which the helper is most knowledgeable or competent. During their training, human service professionals must acquire knowledge about the helping process, professional ethics, the limits of professional practice, and the pertinent legislation that governs practice.

In addition to the competence acquired through preparation to be a professional, the human service professional in practice also has an obligation to ensure that available services meet acceptable standards. Helpers have a further obligation to improve services and skills through activities such as involvement in ongoing research and study, participation in peer consultation, and review of the current professional literature. All these activities contribute to the competence of the helper.

The second concept that pervades all phases of service delivery is **responsibility**. This means that the helping professional is committed to helping clients develop to the best of their abilities and to protect them from harm. Helpers also have obligations to support the profession. Furthermore, human service professionals value their work within a social service environment that promotes social justice for society as a whole. The idea that helpers have obligations to others in addition to the client may present dilemmas for the helper in cases of conflict. It is important for the helper to understand the nature of the conflict and be able to explain to the client how this may limit the client–helper relationship. To fulfill their commitment to being responsible, helpers must know the ethical and legal procedures that are pertinent to their service delivery functions. These include the profession's code of ethics, its standards of behavior, and the consequences of failure to conform to codes and standards.

In many instances, ethical standards of competence and responsibility are compatible. For example, human service professionals are obligated to provide high-quality service to their clients. Discharging this obligation relies to a certain extent on the competence of the worker, as the helper is expected to provide only those

TABLE 9.2   SUMMARY POINTS: COMPETENCE

Standards for professional practice include:

- Academic training
- Supervised experience
- Areas of specialization
- Obligation to improve services and skills

---

services he or she is trained and qualified to deliver. If the client has needs beyond the competence of the professional, then he or she has a duty, according to codes and standards of professional behavior, to locate alternative services from a coworker or another agency. In this situation, the competence of the human service professional is reflected in an awareness of available services and knowledge of how those services relate to the client's problems.

The responsibility of the helper extends beyond client contact. The helper is also concerned with having sufficient time to work with a client and the resources necessary for effective practice. Should these not be present, the helper is responsible for locating or developing resources such as grants for additional funding or increased staff for specialized caseloads. The overriding concern, of course, is the obligation and commitment to provide good quality services to whomever needs those services.

The vignettes that follow illustrate some of the dilemmas that a helper might face while working with human service clients. The primary issues in these vignettes are competence and responsibility.

CASE 1

Sue is a night counselor for a cerebral palsy group home. She works four nights a week, arriving at 5:00 pm and staying until 5:00 am the next morning. Right now the group home is in the process of hiring three new staff members: a van driver, an evening visiting nurse, and a day teacher/counselor. Until these professionals are hired, much of the responsibility falls to Sue. She does not mind doing all that she can for the group home and the clients, but she feels that she is not qualified to do some of the things asked of her.

CASE 2

George is a case worker for a mental health outpatient service. He provides individual and group counseling for adult clients. One of his clients, Kim, is having trouble relating to her husband, her son, and her father. George suggests to Kim that she practice various forms of sexual intimacy with him as a part of her therapy to improve her relationships with men.

CASE 3

Natalia is a social service worker in a health care facility for the elderly. She is in a dilemma because several of her clients are requesting that she provide them with cigarettes even though smoking has been discouraged by the doctor. Natalia's colleague, Betty, laughs when she tells her of her dilemma. She tells her that there is no dilemma. She has provided cigarettes for patients for the past three years.

TABLE 9.3   SUMMARY POINTS: RESPONSIBILITY

Helpers must know the ethical and legal procedures, including:

- Profession's code of ethics
- Standards of behavior
- Consequences of failure to uphold codes of ethics and ethical standards

---

| BOX 9.2 | ETHICAL PRINCIPLES OF PSYCHOLOGISTS: *AMERICAN PSYCHOLOGICAL ASSOCIATION* |

Competence

2.01 Boundaries of Competence

a. Psychologists provide services, teach, and conduct research with populations and in areas only within the boundaries of their competence, based on their education, training, supervised experience, consultation, study, or professional experience.

b. Where scientific or professional knowledge in the discipline of psychology establishes that an understanding of factors associated with age, gender, gender identity, race, ethnicity, culture, national origin, religion, sexual orientation, disability, language, or socioeconomic status is essential for effective implementation of their services or research, psychologists have or obtain the training, experience, consultation, or supervision necessary to ensure the competence of their services, or they make appropriate referrals, except as provided in Standard 2.02, Providing Services in Emergencies.

c. Psychologists planning to provide services, teach, or conduct research involving populations, areas, techniques, or technologies new to them undertake relevant education, training, supervised experience, consultation, or study.

d. When psychologists are asked to provide services to individuals for whom appropriate mental health services are not available and for which psychologists have not obtained the competence necessary, psychologists with closely related prior training or experience may provide such services in order to ensure that services are not denied if they make a reasonable effort to obtain the competence required by using relevant research, training, consultation, or study.

e. In those emerging areas in which generally recognized standards for preparatory training do not yet exist, psychologists nevertheless take reasonable steps to ensure the competence of their work and to protect clients/patients, students, supervisees, research participants, organizational clients, and others from harm.

f. When assuming forensic roles, psychologists are, or become reasonably familiar with, the judicial or administrative rules governing their roles.

Source: Material from "Ethical Principles of Psychologists and Code of Conduct." Copyright © 2002 by the American Psychological Association, Inc.

CASE 4

Jim, the sports program director for the Millerville Home for Boys, walks by a group of new workers who are discussing their recent orientation session. They mention the newest rule that prohibits workers from transporting a client in a private car. Jim had heard about the new rule, but so far he has ignored it, hoping to plead ignorance if someone challenges his behavior. Many of the relationships he forms with the children are established during one-on-one private outings to the mall, movies, and out to dinner. He hates to give them up.

CASE 5

Bradley's job as coordinator of the hospice program in a local hospital is very demanding. His hours are 8:00 a.m. to 5:00 p.m., Monday through Friday, but the needs of the clients do not follow these regular hours. He is operating the program with little help: one half-time secretary to answer the telephone and respond to e-mails. He often works 15 to 18 hours a day. He feels committed to his work but is often so tired that he is afraid he cannot be effective.

CASE 6

Susan is a traveling health department worker in a rural area. She is the only worker serving clients in 12 counties. Once every two weeks, she meets with other health department officials from the district, but for the most part she has limited contact with other professionals. She read her last professional magazine two years ago, and she has attended only one in-service meeting in the past five years.

CASE 7

Luis works for an outpatient AIDS clinic whose major goals include prevention and therapeutic counseling. Luis feels that meeting the demands of his clients is the most important service he provides, and he has difficulty ignoring the clients. Consequently, he is booked solid each day, seeing individual AIDS victims and their families. The director thinks he should spend more time on preventive efforts to promote the agency's other main goal.

CASE 8

Enrique has a new client with a psychiatric diagnosis that is new to him. Even though the agency has a *Physician's Desk Reference*, Enrique searches the Internet for information and finds a site on herbal remedies that he believes will be helpful to both him and the client.

In each of these situations, the helper faces a dilemma regarding worker competence and responsibility for which there is no easy solution. Competence is a

---

BOX 9.3	ETHICAL STANDARDS FOR SOCIAL WORKERS

Code of Ethics of the National Association of Social Workers

5. Social Worker's Ethical Responsibilities to the Social Work Profession
   5.01 Integrity of the Profession
      a. Social workers should work toward the maintenance and promotion of high standards of practice.
      b. Social workers should uphold and advance the values, ethics, knowledge, and mission of the profession. Social workers should protect, enhance, and improve the integrity of the profession through appropriate study and research, active discussion, and responsible criticism of the profession.
      c. Social workers should contribute time and professional expertise to activities that promote respect for the value, integrity, and competence of the social work profession. These activities may include teaching, research, consultation, service, legislative testimony, presentations in the community, and participation in their professional organizations.
      d. Social workers should contribute to the knowledge base of social work and share with colleagues their knowledge related to practice, research, and ethics. Social workers should seek to contribute to the profession's literature and to share their knowledge at professional meetings and conferences.
      e. Social workers should act to prevent the unauthorized and unqualified practice of social work.

Source: Material from "Code of Ethics of the National Association of Social Workers." Copyright 2006 NASW. Revised by the 2008 NASW Delegate Assembly.

personal issue that demands professional self-assessment and then commitment to professional development. Responsibility involves the interpersonal relationships the helper has with individual clients or groups and human service agencies. The common ground between responsibility and competence is the helper's primary commitment to serving the client.

CONFIDENTIALITY

Confidentiality is the helper's assurance that information the client divulges will remain between the two of them. If information is to be shared, it will be shared only with those designated by the client. These two statements regarding the concept of confidentiality provide only general guidelines for the helper. In some situations, laws require confidentiality to be breached: Parents have the legal right to information about their offspring in most circumstances. Courts may require the disclosure of information that would otherwise be confidential; and helpers have a duty to alert authorities if they suspect child abuse (Remley & Herlihy, 2009). The concept is a complex one. This section provides an introduction to confidentiality and gives examples of the complex situations helpers may encounter in human service practice.

Confidentiality is a complex concept. For example, a term often associated with confidentiality is **privileged communication**. Both terms address the commitment to keep a client's identity and communications secret. There is a basic difference. *Confidentiality* is a moral obligation grounded in values and ethics (Welfel, 2012); *privileged communication* is a legal term that allows practitioners to legally refuse to release certain information in response to a subpoena. The term *legally* is used because privileged communication is a right granted to a group of professionals by state lawmaking bodies. Examples of situations in which helpers are ethically or legally obligated to breach confidentiality include, but are not limited to, the following:

1. When the client is dangerous to self or others.
2. When there is suspicion of abuse or neglect.
3. When the client brings charges against the counselor.
4. When the client has already introduced privileged material into litigation.

Another example of the complexity of confidentiality is a type often called **relative confidentiality**. This term refers to the informal sharing of information that occurs in an agency or organizational setting among coworkers or treatment team members and supervisors. The client's permission is not required for this type of exchange to take place. Typically, agency policy will also guide this sharing by determining who has access to confidential information. The Federal Privacy Act of 1974, which governs confidentiality in federally funded and administered programs such as the Department of Veterans Affairs and the Social Security Administration, states that clients have access to their records and establishes procedures for this to occur. It also supports the concept of relative confidentiality by providing for the sharing of information among those professionals within the agency who need the information in the performance of their duties.

An issue that has recently emerged is maintaining confidentiality within the technological environment. One concern is the safety of records that exist in large management information systems. Organizations and agencies that maintain their records in networks adopt policies and software to ensure limited access. In other words, no one has access to the client files without a security clearance, a password, and the need to know. Personal communication with clients via e-mail must also be regarded as confidential exchanges. Helpers take care to ensure the security of their e-mail systems. Several professional organizations have adopted guidelines for technology-related helping. These guidelines include password-protecting information stored on a computer, storing information on a secure server, maintaining confidentiality when workspaces are open or shared, and asking individuals to limit the types of information they share on a nonsecure e-mail system.

In summary, privileged communication and relative confidentiality illustrate the complexity of confidentiality. Privileged communication rarely exists for the beginning human service professional, but relative confidentiality is a concept that deserves the worker's attention. Agency guidelines, the profession's code of ethics, and the laws of the state in which one practices are important considerations in the delivery of services. A professional should be familiar with all three as guides to circumstances that may arise. Communication via the Internet brings an additional set of issues regarding confidentiality. The following vignettes provide examples of confidentiality dilemmas that you may face as a beginning human service professional.

CASE 1

Sue works for the Department of Human Services in Child Protective Services and visits families once a week to review the status of the home environment. Yesterday she received a subpoena and will be required to testify in court that the father in one of the families in her caseload was not at home the last two times she visited. He is charged with armed robbery and states in his defense that he was at home during the time of the crime. That time coincides with her visit.

CASE 2

Joe works in a small agency that provides educational services to children with developmental disabilities. He promises clients that his records are confidential and is very careful not to divulge the names of the clients or the nature of their problems. The mother of one of his young clients reports to him that "someone at her church" had heard that her child was receiving his services. If it was not Joe who breached confidentiality, it might be the secretary who answers the telephones or the typist who keeps the records.

CASE 3

Faye is a counselor and recreation specialist working in an after-school recreation facility. One of her favorite teenagers has just told her "in confidence" that she is pregnant. Should she keep this information confidential?

CASE 4

Betsy needs to reschedule an appointment she has with a new client tomorrow. When she called the client at home, she got her voice mail. Knowing that anyone can access messages left on voice mail, Betsy decides not to leave a message; instead she e-mails the client at her workplace.

CASE 5

Ezra is a recovering alcoholic and has not had a drink in the last two years. He understands and practices confidentiality in his human service work, but he cannot help but wonder how well he would do in this regard if he were to go on a drinking binge.

CASE 6

Cynthia works in a high-stress hospice program. Working with the dying patient and family and friends is emotionally draining, and she often "takes her work home." Many of her clients communicate with her via e-mail, since clients and care-givers are homebound. How does she ensure confidentiality?

CASE 7

Jefferson works with adults on probation and has just heard one of his clients tell how she punishes her six-month-old child which seems excessive to him. Does he report this information? To whom does he report it?

CASE 8

Raphael is a vocational rehabilitation counselor working with a veteran who has returned from service in Iraq. His client has been very depressed during the last month, and during his last individual conference with Raphael, he talked of "ending all the agony." Raphael wonders what he should do and whom he should tell.

These are just a few examples of the many conflicts that can arise over the issue of confidentiality. Many of the troublesome dilemmas result from the constant tension among worker responsibilities, agency policies, and client needs. Privileged communication and relative confidentiality are difficult principles to follow. The preceding cases illustrate the problems helpers may encounter as they translate their values into action in the workplace. An equally complex issue that human service professionals encounter concerns clients' rights.

CLIENTS' RIGHTS

Clients are first and foremost citizens of a democratic society; as such, they have certain rights and privileges. In a helping situation, the client's trust in the helper is important for the development of the helping relationship. In exchange for the trust of the client, the helper is ethically obligated to protect the rights of the client. Two examples of clients' rights are the right to privacy and informed consent.

Clients have the right to share whatever information they wish with a helper. They also have the right to withhold information they do not want to share. The helper is ethically bound to respect clients' **right to privacy** by not pressuring them to reveal things they do not wish to reveal.

Informed consent is another example of the rights of clients involved in the helping process. It is the client's right to know about the qualifications of the helper, treatment procedures, costs of services, confidentiality, and access to records. The concept of informed consent extends beyond simply telling the client about such matters. The client must comprehend this information and consent voluntarily. In some cases, the helper must educate the client about his or her rights with regard to consent.

Informed consent is a particularly critical aspect of client rights with respect to decision making. In the helping process, the client is an active participant who has a voice in what is happening. In the absence of informed consent, the client's right to self-determination is compromised. The helper has an ethical obligation to ensure that clients receive and understand the appropriate information.

One way the client can become informed about the helper is for the helper to write and to share with the client a **professional disclosure statement**. This form should include information about the worker and the worker's credentials, which will allow the client to make an informed assessment of the worker's competence. In addition to name, business address, and telephone number, other information may include education and training competency areas, and the name, address, and telephone number of the state government agency that regulates human service delivery.

Developing a personal professional disclosure statement has several benefits. As the helper shares the statement with the client, it promotes the development of a helping relationship. Not only does it signal to the client that this relationship is different from informal helping relationships, but it also acquaints the client with the person in whom the client will soon place his or her trust. While working out the statement, the helper has an opportunity to think about and put into words exactly who he or she is as a human service professional. It also allows the helper to define himself or herself as a professional and links the individual to the common knowledge, skills, and values of the profession.

The following sample professional disclosure statement was written by Carmen Rodriguez, the vocational evaluator introduced in Chapter 6.

CARMEN RODRIGUEZ

My name is Carmen Rodriguez, and I am a case manager. Specifically, my job is to assist people in preparing for and finding gainful employment, housing, and support. I want my clients to understand who they are and what they can do to make their lives more satisfying.

Once a client meets the eligibility requirements established by the agency, there is no charge for my services. I have worked for this agency for four years. I graduated from college with a major in human services and frequently attend workshops to update my knowledge.

I may work with an individual from two weeks to six weeks. It really depends on the client and his or her situation. Sometimes it is necessary to refer my clients to other team members in my agency or to other professionals in the community. The clients I see usually have such complex problems that I cannot address them all by myself, so I work with a team. Because my agency uses this team approach, I may share

TABLE 9.4   SUMMARY POINTS: PROFESSIONAL DISCLOSURE STATEMENTS

- Introduces the helper to the client
- Provides opportunity for the helper to clarify his or her professional identity
- Promotes the development of a helping relationship

BOX 9.4   Code of Professional Ethics for Rehabilitation Counselors: *Confidentiality*

SECTION B: CONFIDENTIALITY, PRIVILEGED COMUNICATION, AND PRIVACY

B.1. RESPECTING CLIENT RIGHTS

   a. CULTURAL DIVERSITY CONSIDERA-
       TIONS. Rehabilitation counselors main-
       tain beliefs, attitudes, knowledge, and
       skills regarding cultural meanings of con-
       fidentiality and privacy. Rehabilitation
       counselors hold ongoing discussions with
       clients as to how, when, and with whom
       information is to be shared.

   b. RESPECT FOR PRIVACY. Rehabilitation
       counselors respect privacy rights of
       clients. Rehabilitation counselors solicit
       private information from clients only

when it is beneficial to the counseling
process.

   c. RESPECT FOR CONFIDENTIALITY.
       Rehabilitation counselors do not share
       confidential information without consent
       from clients or without sound legal or
       ethical justification.

   d. EXPLANATION OF LIMITATIONS. At
       initiation and throughout the counseling
       process, rehabilitation counselors inform
       clients of the limitations of confidentiality
       and seek to identify foreseeable situations
       in which confidentiality must be breached.

Source: Material from "Code of Professional Ethics for Rehabilitation Counselors," adopted June 2009, effective January 1, 2010.

information about clients with coworkers within the agency but not with outsiders or other clients. The agency has strict guidelines about how information is shared and prohibits communicating any client information via voice mail, answering machines, cellular phones, faxes, and e-mail.

Now that you have read Carmen's statement, can you write one of your own? It may be easier to write such a statement if you imagine that you work in a specific agency with a well-defined population.

Protection is another of the helper's obligations to clients. Clients have the right to expect the helper to protect them from harm. It is the helper's responsibility to be sensitive to situations in which the client risks economic or physical harm, and, if possible, to prevent harm from occurring. If there is a clear and imminent danger to a third party, the helper has a duty to take action to protect the individual at risk. Determining when a situation warrants action may be difficult for the human service professional; when questionable occasions arise, consultation with colleagues or supervisors will be helpful in deciding on a course of action.

The following cases provide examples of dilemmas that a human service professional may encounter in relation to clients' rights. Several of the cases present ethical situations in which the human service professional is confronted with a difficult decision about what action to take. In other cases, the dilemma is one over which the worker has little or no control.

CASE 1

Susan and her client, Mr. Rodriguez, have agreed on what referral information should be sent to a local educational reading clinic. The clinic, however, wants more information. Specifically, they want to know whether Mr. Rodriguez is a veteran, but he feels they will treat him "special" if they know that he fought in Vietnam. Susan has agreed that the file to be sent should include a short note explaining why he does not want to answer that particular question.

| **BOX 9.5** | AMERICAN COUNSELING ASSOCIATION CODE OF ETHICS AND STANDARDS OF PRACTICE |

B.1. Respecting Client Rights

  B.1.a. Multicultural/Diversity Considerations

  Counselors maintain awareness and sensitivity regarding cultural meanings of confidentiality and privacy. Counselors respect differing views toward disclosure of information. Counselors hold ongoing discussions with clients as to how, when, and with whom information is to be shared.

  B.1.b. Respect for Privacy

  Counselors respect client rights to privacy. Counselors solicit private information from clients only when it is beneficial to the counseling process.

  B.1.c. Respect for Confidentiality

  Counselors do not share confidential information without client consent or without sound legal or ethical justification.

  B.1.d Explanation of Limitations

  At initiation and throughout the counseling process, counselors inform clients of the limitation of confidentiality and seek to identify foreseeable situations in which confidentiality must be breached. (See A.2.b.)

Source: Material from "American Counseling Association Code of Ethics and Standards of Practice." Reprinted by permission of the American Counseling Association. Approved by the ACA Governing Council 2005.

CASE 2

Once a week, the staff members at the battered women's shelter discuss the cases in which they are involved. One client, age 56, told the helper "in confidence" that she had an abortion when she was 13. She asked the helper not to tell the other staff members.

CASE 3

The local mental health institution has a new professional staff member, the patient advocate, who has been hired by the mental health association to protect the rights of the clients in the institution. The patient advocate explains to each patient his or her rights when he or she enters the institution, but many patients forget or are unable to comprehend how they might use the services of the advocate. Sometimes Ron, a social worker on a treatment team serving the men's locked ward, sees clients' rights being abused, but to recommend that a client see the advocate might cause trouble for the treatment team to which Ron belongs.

CASE 4

Youvella is a patient in a health care facility. She wants to see her medical records before they are examined by the team of specialists who will decide what protocol to prescribe for the treatment of her pancreatic cancer. Although Youvella is entitled to review these records, the nurse questions the wisdom of this decision because of Youvella's emotional instability. The nurse requests assistance from the hospital social service worker in this dilemma.

CASE 5

Emile is a human service field student with a rehabilitation services agency. For the next two weeks, he will be administering vocational aptitude tests to new clients. He is unsure whether he should tell his clients that he is a student. Emile wants them to trust him and have confidence in him, as they would if he were a seasoned worker.

CASE 6

The adoption agency is reviewing the files of a young couple considering adoption. Unfortunately, the adoption counselor has received some damaging information from the couple's landlord of 10 years ago that will make it impossible for the agency to consider them suitable as parents. The counselor really respects this couple and believes that they would make wonderful parents, but she also knows that the information cannot be withheld. The adoption counselor must tell the couple of the agency's decision not to consider them "fit" to adopt and must tell them of the negative recommendation.

CASE 7

The Annas are involved in marital therapy; the stated purpose of the counseling is to "save the marriage." They receive individual counseling once a week, and once a month they participate in counseling sessions together. Ms. Anna has recently told the counselor of her desire to harm Mr. Anna. The counselor wonders how to handle this information, since it was given in confidence and also may jeopardize the goal of saving the marriage.

In clients' rights issues, the helper's judgment and the agency's judgment are often not the only considerations. Legal rulings must also be taken into account. Sometimes legal pronouncements, ethical standards, and personal commitments conflict, presenting a difficult dilemma for the worker. The professional must then decide what action is most ethical.

ETHICAL STANDARDS OF HUMAN SERVICE PROFESSIONALS

In 1995, the National Organization for Human Service Education (NOHSE) approved ethical standards for human service professionals (see Box 9.6 at the end of the chapter). Previously, students and graduates were guided by the codes of ethics or ethical standards of various other professions, some of which have been excerpted in this chapter. These codes did not reflect the unique history or philosophy of the human service profession. In response to the changing context in which human service delivery occurs, the National Organization of Human Services committed to revising its code of ethics. The revision is underway at this time.

As you read these ethical standards, you will note that they address the topics discussed at the beginning of this chapter. The preamble introduces the goals or aims of the profession. The ethical standards then divide professional responsibilities into six areas: to clients, to the community and society, to colleagues, to the profession, to employers, and to self.

These ethical standards and those in other helping professions provide guidelines only. They do not provide answers to all ethical dilemmas. The ethical decision making that follows the ethical standards is helpful when these situations arise.

ETHICAL DECISION MAKING

Clearly, no code of ethics or statement of standards can provide a course of action for every situation that might arise in the practice of human services. What does the human service professional do in situations for which there are no guidelines

| BOX 9.6 | ETHICAL STANDARDS OF HUMAN SERVICE PROFESSIONALS |

National Organization for Human Service Education Council for Standards in Human Service Education

Preamble

Human services is a profession developing in response to and in anticipation of the direction of human needs and human problems in the late twentieth century. Characterized particularly by an appreciation of human beings in all of their diversity, human services offer assistance to its clients within the context of their community and environment. Human service professionals and those who educate them, regardless of whether they are students, faculty or practitioners, promote and encourage the unique values and characteristics of human services. In so doing, human service professionals and educators uphold the integrity and ethics of the profession, partake in constructive criticism of the profession, promote client and community well-being, and enhance their own professional growth.

The ethical guidelines presented are a set of standards of conduct which the human service professionals and educators consider in ethical and professional decision making. It is hoped that these guidelines will be of assistance when human service professionals and educators are challenged by difficult ethical dilemmas. Although ethical codes are not legal documents, they may be used to assist in the adjudication of issues related to ethical human service behavior.

Section I—Standards of Human Service Professionals

Human service professionals function in many ways and carry out many roles. They enter into professional-client relationships with individuals, families, groups and communities who are all referred to as "clients" in these standards. Among their roles are caregiver, case manager, broker, teacher/educator, behavior changer, consultant, outreach professional, mobilizer, advocate, community planner, community change organizer, evaluator and administrator (SREB, 1967). The following standards are written with these multifaceted roles in mind.

The Human Service Professional's Responsibility to Clients

STATEMENT 1 Human service professionals negotiate with clients the purpose, goals, and nature of the helping relationship prior to its onset as well as inform clients of the limitations of the proposed relationship.

STATEMENT 2 Human service professionals respect the integrity and welfare of the client at all times. Each client is treated with respect, acceptance, and dignity.

STATEMENT 3 Human service professionals protect the client's right to privacy and confidentiality except when such confidentiality would cause harm to the client or others, when agency guidelines state otherwise, or under other stated conditions (e.g., local, state, or federal laws). Professionals inform clients of the limits of confidentiality prior to the onset of the helping relationship.

STATEMENT 4 If it is suspected that danger or harm may occur to the client or to others as a result of a client's behavior, the human service professional acts in an appropriate and professional manner to protect the safety of those individuals. This may involve seeking consultation, supervision, and/or breaking the confidentiality of the relationship.

STATEMENT 5 Human service professionals protect the integrity, safety, and security of client records. All written client information that is shared with other professionals, except in the course of professional supervision, must have the client's prior written consent.

STATEMENT 6 Human service professionals are aware that in their relationships with clients power and status are unequal. Therefore, they recognize that dual or multiple relationships may increase the risk of harm to, or exploitation of, clients, and may impair their professional judgment. However, in some communities and situations it may not be feasible to avoid social or other nonprofessional contact with clients. Human service professionals support the trust implicit in the helping relationship by avoiding dual relationships that may impair professional judgment, increase the risk of harm to clients or lead to exploitation.

STATEMENT 7 Sexual relationships with current clients are not considered to be in the best interest of the client and are prohibited. Sexual relationships with previous clients are considered dual relationships and are addressed in Statement 6 (above).

continued

BOX 9.6   ETHICAL STANDARDS OF HUMAN SERVICE PROFESSIONALS *continued*

STATEMENT 8 The client's right to self-determination is protected by human service professionals. They recognize the client's right to receive or refuse services.

STATEMENT 9 Human service professionals recognize and build on client strengths.

The Human Service Professional's Responsibility to the Community and Society

STATEMENT 10 Human service professionals are aware of local, state, and federal laws. They advocate for change in regulations and statutes when such legislation conflicts with ethical guidelines and/or client rights. Where laws are harmful to individuals, groups or communities, human service professionals consider the conflict between the values of obeying the law and the values of serving people and may decide to initiate social action.

STATEMENT 11 Human service professionals keep informed about current social issues as they affect the client and the community. They share that information with clients, groups, and community as part of their work.

STATEMENT 12 Human service professionals understand the complex interaction between individuals, their families, the communities in which they live, and society.

STATEMENT 13 Human service professionals act as advocates in addressing unmet client and community needs. Human service professionals provide a mechanism for identifying unmet client needs, calling attention to these needs, and assisting in planning and mobilizing to advocate for those needs at the local community level.

STATEMENT 14 Human service professionals represent their qualifications to the public accurately.

STATEMENT 15 Human service professionals describe the effectiveness of programs, treatments, and/or techniques accurately.

STATEMENT 16 Human service professionals advocate for the rights of all members of society, particularly those who are members of minorities and groups at which discriminatory practices have historically been directed.

STATEMENT 17 Human service professionals provide services without discrimination or preference based on age, ethnicity, culture, race, disability, gender, religion, sexual orientation, or socioeconomic status.

STATEMENT 18 Human service professionals are knowledgeable about the cultures and communities within which they practice. They are aware of multiculturalism in society and its impact on the community as well as individuals within the community. They respect individuals and groups, their cultures and beliefs.

STATEMENT 19 Human service professionals are aware of their own cultural backgrounds, beliefs, and values, recognizing the potential for impact on their relationships with others.

STATEMENT 20 Human service professionals are aware of sociopolitical issues that differentially affect clients from diverse backgrounds.

STATEMENT 21 Human service professionals seek the training, experience, education, and supervision necessary to ensure their effectiveness in working with culturally diverse client populations.

The Human Service Professional's Responsibility to Colleagues

STATEMENT 22 Human service professionals avoid duplicating another professional's helping relationship with a client. They consult with other professionals who are assisting the client in a different type of relationship when it is in the best interest of the client to do so.

STATEMENT 23 When a human service professional has a conflict with a colleague, he or she first seeks out the colleague in an attempt to manage the problem. If necessary, the professional then seeks the assistance of supervisors, consultants, or other professionals in efforts to manage the problem.

STATEMENT 24 Human service professionals respond appropriately to unethical behavior of colleagues. Usually this means initially talking directly with the colleague and, if no resolution is forthcoming, reporting the colleague's behavior to supervisory or administrative staff and/or to the professional organization(s) to which the colleague belongs.

STATEMENT 25 All consultations between human service professionals are kept confidential unless to do so would result in harm to clients or communities.

The Human Service Professional's Responsibility to the Profession

STATEMENT 26 Human service professionals know the limit and scope of their professional

continued

knowledge and offer services only within their knowledge and skill base.

STATEMENT 27 Human service professionals seek appropriate consultation and supervision to assist in decision making when there are legal, ethical, or other dilemmas.

STATEMENT 28 Human service professionals act with integrity, honesty, genuineness, and objectivity.

STATEMENT 29 Human service professionals promote cooperation among related disciplines (e.g., psychology, counseling, social work, nursing, family and consumer sciences, medicine, education) to foster professional growth and interests within the various fields.

STATEMENT 30 Human service professionals promote the continuing development of their profession. They encourage membership in professional associations, support research endeavors, foster educational advancement, advocate for appropriate legislative actions, and participate in other related professional activities.

STATEMENT 31 Human service professionals continually seek out new and effective approaches to enhance their professional abilities.

The Human Service Professional's Responsibility to Employers

STATEMENT 32 Human service professionals adhere to commitments made to their employers.

STATEMENT 33 Human service professionals participate in efforts to establish and maintain employment conditions which are conducive to high-quality client services. They assist in evaluating the effectiveness of the agency through reliable and valid assessment measures.

STATEMENT 34 When a conflict arises between fulfilling the responsibility to the employer and the responsibility to the client, human service professionals advise both of the conflict and work conjointly with all involved to manage the conflict.

The Human Service Professional's Responsibility to Self

STATEMENT 35 Human service professionals strive to personify those characteristics typically associated with the profession (e.g., accountability, respect for others, genuineness, empathy, pragmatism).

STATEMENT 36 Human service professionals foster self-awareness and personal growth in themselves. They recognize that when professionals are aware of

their own values, attitudes, cultural background, and personal needs, the process of helping others is less likely to be negatively impacted by those factors.

STATEMENT 37 Human service professionals recognize a commitment to lifelong learning and continually upgrade knowledge and skills to serve the populations better.

Section II—Standards for Human Service Educators

Human service educators are familiar with, informed by, and accountable to the standards of professional conduct put forth by their institutions of higher learning; their professional disciplines, for example, American Association of University Professors (AAUP), American Counseling Association (ACA), Academy of Criminal Justice (ACJS), American Psychological Association (APA), American Sociological Association (ASA), National Association of Social Workers (NASW), National Board of Certified Counselors (NBCC), National Education Association (NEA), and the National Organization for Human Services (NOHS).

STATEMENT 38 Human service educators uphold the principle of liberal education and embrace the essence of academic freedom, abstaining from inflicting their own personal views/morals on students, and allowing students the freedom to express their views without penalty, censure or ridicule, and to engage in critical thinking.

STATEMENT 39 Human service educators provide students with readily available and explicit program policies and criteria regarding program goals and objectives, recruitment, admission, course requirements, evaluations, retention, and dismissal in accordance with due process procedures.

STATEMENT 40 Human service educators demonstrate high standards of scholarship in content areas and of pedagogy by staying current with developments in the field of human services and in teaching effectiveness, for example, learning styles and teaching styles.

STATEMENT 41 Human service educators monitor students' field experiences to ensure the quality of the placement site, supervisory experience, and learning experience towards the goals of professional identity and skill development.

STATEMENT 42 Human service educators participate actively in the selection of required readings and use them with care, based strictly on the merits of

continued

BOX 9.6   ETHICAL STANDARDS OF HUMAN SERVICE PROFESSIONALS *continued*

the material's content, and present relevant information accurately, objectively, and fully.

STATEMENT 43 Human service educators, at the onset of courses, inform students if sensitive/controversial issues or experiential/affective content or process are part of the course design; ensure that students are offered opportunities to discuss in structured ways their reactions to sensitive or controversial class content; ensure that the presentation of such material is justified on pedagogical grounds directly related to the course; and differentiate between information based on scientific data, anecdotal data, and personal opinion.

STATEMENT 44 Human service educators develop and demonstrate culturally sensitive knowledge, awareness, and teaching methodology.

STATEMENT 45 Human service educators demonstrate full commitment to their appointed responsibilities, and are enthusiastic about and encouraging of students' learning.

STATEMENT 46 Human service educators model the personal attributes, values, and skills of the human service professional, including but not limited to, the willingness to seek and respond to feedback from students.

STATEMENT 47 Human service educators establish and uphold appropriate guidelines concerning self-disclosure or student-disclosure of sensitive/personal information.

STATEMENT 48 Human service educators establish an appropriate and timely process for providing clear and objective feedback to students about their performance on relevant and established course/program academic and personal competence requirements and their suitability for the field.

STATEMENT 49 Human service educators are aware that in their relationships with students, power and status are unequal; therefore, human service educators are responsible to clearly define and maintain ethical and professional relationships with students, and avoid conduct that is demeaning, embarrassing, or exploitative of students, and to treat students fairly, equally, and without discrimination.

STATEMENT 50 Human service educators recognize and acknowledge the contributions of students to their work, for example, in case material, workshops, research, and publications.

STATEMENT 51 Human service educators demonstrate professional standards of conduct in managing personal or professional differences with colleagues, for example, not disclosing such differences and/or affirming a student's negative opinion of a faculty/program.

STATEMENT 52 Human service educators ensure that students are familiar with, informed by, and accountable to the ethical standards and policies put forth by their program/department, the course syllabus/instructor, their advisor(s), and the Ethical Standards of Human Service Professionals.

STATEMENT 53 Human service educators are aware of all relevant curriculum standards, including those of the Council for Standards in Human Service Education (CSHSE), the Community Support Skills Standards, and state/local standards; and take them into consideration in designing the curriculum.

STATEMENT 54 Human service educators create a learning context in which students can achieve the knowledge, skills, values, and attitudes of the academic program.

Source: Ethical Standards of Human Service Professionals. (2000). *Human Service Education, 20*(1), 61–68. Reprinted with permission of National Organization of Human Service Education.

or there are guidelines that conflict? In such ethical dilemmas, the conflict is in determining the right thing to do regarding obligations to two or more constituencies: situations when a choice exists between contradictory directives or standards or an undesirable outcome for one or more persons results no matter the alternative (Dolgoff, Harrington, & Loewenberg, 2011). The areas of confidentiality, role conflict, and counselor competence frequently present ethical dilemmas. Rather than attempt to provide possible solutions to every situation that comes to mind, this subsection will introduce steps for ethical decision making that can be applied to many dilemmas to determine a course of action.

Determining the best action under the circumstances and with the individuals involved is at the crux of ethical decision making. To accomplish this, the helper must assume an attitude of **moral responsibility**. This should be distinguished from the kind of responsibility discussed earlier in this chapter. That responsibility is imposed by some higher authority, such as the profession or the government; it may be interpreted as one's duty. Moral responsibleness, on the other hand, comes from within the individual, who assumes that there is a course of action that is morally right. A commitment to rational thinking and knowledge of moral principles are necessary components of moral reasoning.

A number of ethical decision-making models exist. Although the process is not necessarily linear in that some steps may need to be repeated, there are steps that many models share:

1. *Identify the problem.* This may involve gathering additional information; considering the legal, ethical, moral, and professional perspectives; and determining the issues involved. It is also prudent to think about relevant cultural factors and, of course, to review ethical standards.
2. *Consult with colleagues or experts.* Legal counsel, coworkers, and supervisors are some of the resources who can be tapped to obtain different perspectives about the dilemma. In addition, consultation is also evidence that a helper has acted in good faith if there is a legal challenge to the decision.
3. *Identify and explore options.* Both brainstorming and consulting are techniques that increase the numbers and types of options worth consideration. An important part of this step is thinking about the desired outcomes and the advantages and disadvantages or risks and benefits of each option.
4. *Choose a course of action and act.* Then evaluate both the process and the choice.

We have discussed dilemmas that involve competency and responsibility, confidentiality, and clients' rights and have presented brief cases to illustrate problems that might arise in actual practice. As you consider how you would respond to each case, review the steps in the previous paragraph and follow them as you deliberate. The following questions may be useful as you consider how you would respond to each case.

1. State the dilemma clearly. There may be more than one; if so, please think of all that you can.
2. What options are available?
3. What are the disadvantages and advantages of each option?
4. What action do you choose?
5. What factor most influenced your decision?

Another place to use the ethical decision-making model is with dilemmas that are unique to a specific setting, for it provides a purposeful way of thinking about them. Human services in a correctional setting provides examples of such ethical conflicts.

The dilemmas that correctional professionals face illustrate the conflict among human service professionals' responsibilities to the client, to the agency, and to

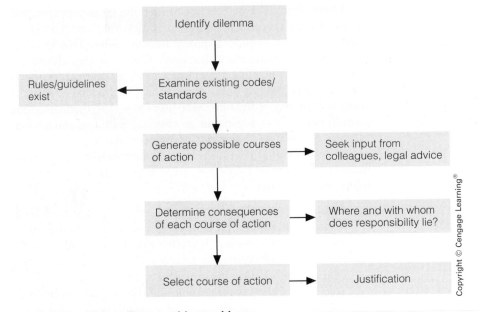

FIGURE 9.1   ETHICAL DECISION-MAKING MODEL

society. As an officer of the court, the corrections worker has the primary role of ensuring that clients do not break the law or injure others. This role places the professional in the position of judge, evaluator, and reporter, making establishing and maintaining helping relationships difficult. The following two dilemmas arise from a conflict between this primary role of the corrections worker and the human service professional's overriding concern for the welfare of the client.

One dilemma may arise when the courts mandate counseling sessions for public offenders. The fact that counseling is imposed will probably impede the helping relationship. The second dilemma, which further complicates the relationship, occurs when the helper explains what confidentiality means in the corrections setting. If a client has violated an institution's rules or any state or federal law and tells the helper of the violations, the professional is expected to report this information to the appropriate authorities. Many clients never develop the trust needed for a good helping relationship, refusing to share problems with the helper. Other clients may be reluctant to disclose real problems they are experiencing, as the worker is often in a position to provide information and make recommendations about clients. Thus, clients may tell the helper only good news in hopes of securing a positive recommendation.

In situations like these, the professional should begin by identifying exactly what the conflict is. After reviewing ethical guidelines, the helper then considers possible courses of action and the consequences of each. It may be helpful at this point to ask coworkers for input and clarification as the professional explores what each course of action will mean to the client, to the agency, and to the helper. At some point, the helper will have to select a course of action. This ethical decision-making model provides only a structure for thinking about a dilemma; selecting a course of action may still be difficult.

PeterHvizdak/TheImageWorks

INTERNET EXERCISE

See this text's website at *www.cengagebrain.com* for video exercises. Choose Chapter 9, then Videos.

Working with people is often fraught with ethical dilemmas. Human service professionals encounter these situations on a daily basis. Watch and listen as three human service professionals describe dilemmas they have experienced. Then, answer the following questions.

1. *Identify the ethical dilemma for each human service professional.*
2. *Using the decision-making model, what alternatives can you identify and what are the consequences of each?*
3. *Are there any legal considerations that you should think about?*
4. *Who would you consult about a course of action?*
5. *In the end, what would you do about each situation?*

You can follow-up your work with the video related to ethical dilemmas that human service professionals encounter by reading about other issues. Similar to the videos, the situations that follow are actual dilemmas that human service professionals encountered. During interviews with human service professionals in urban multicultural areas in the United States, ethical dilemmas were often mentioned as one of the most difficult challenges that they face day to day. As you read these situations, apply what you have learned about ethical decision making. What steps would you take to resolve each one?

Situation 1 Our agency was built on volunteers. Many of our clients come into care, love their experience with case management, and then they want to volunteer. In a volunteer role, they may participate in some of our groups, so they may get some privileged information about other clients. They all sign confidentiality statements but signing a statement for some people does not necessarily mean that they adhere to policies or standards.

Situation 2 A problem we often encounter is illegal aliens. In our area, many are industrial workers or food service workers. We don't have migrants who work in agriculture. I guess we should pick up the telephone and call the INS but we don't. It comes up when they want benefits and need a social security number. There is actually a black market in social security numbers. We don't advocate that; on the other hand, though, if they have a social security number and documentation, we trust it is correct.

Situation 3 I live and work in a small rural community. Most people have lived here for generations, so everyone knows everyone else's business. This is particularly difficult for me as a human service worker, a member of the largest church in town, and president of the PTO. Sometimes it's hard to separate what I know as a person in this community from what I learn about clients as a professional.

In this chapter we explored many of the ethical issues and dilemmas that human service professionals encounter. Professionals use codes of ethics, state statutes and regulations, judicial rulings, and agency policies and procedures as guides as they determine their responses to these issues. After exploring the issue and, at times, using the ethical decision-making model, the human service professional acts, ultimately guided by the principle of moral responsibility.

KEY TERMS

code of ethics	informed consent	professional disclosure statement	relative confidentiality
competence	moral responsibility	protection	responsibility
confidentiality	privileged communication		right to privacy
ethical dilemmas			

THINGS TO REMEMBER

1. In the course of delivering human services, the professional may encounter numerous ethical dilemmas; for some of these, the helper may be unsure of the appropriate action to take.
2. Professionals have responded to the dilemmas of service provision by developing codes of ethics or statements of ethical standards of behavior for the members of their profession. Items are included that state the goals or aims of the profession, protect the client, provide guidance as to professional behavior, and contribute to a professional identity for the helper.
3. Most codes of ethics indicate that the helper's first responsibility is to enhance and protect the client's welfare.
4. The California Tarasoff case establishes the professional's responsibility to warn others if a client threatens harm to self or others.

5. The human service professional has an ethical obligation to respect, understand, and use knowledge of the culture of the client in defining problems and developing treatment plans.
6. Most codes of ethics emphasize that the helper must have adequate knowledge, values, and skills to address the client's needs.
7. Human service professionals have the responsibility to help clients develop their potential and to keep them from harm.
8. Belonging to professional organizations and participating in professional development are ways the helping professional keeps abreast of current trends and develops new methods of helping.
9. Privileged communication is a legal concept that protects the confidentiality between client and helper.
10. Human service professionals write professional disclosure statements that include training, theoretical framework, and experience. They share this information with their clients early in the helping process.
11. Human service professionals have a code of ethics that articulates guidelines for professional behavior.
12. An ethical decision-making model delineates steps that human service professionals can use to consider ethical issues.

SELF-ASSESSMENT

• Identify the purposes and limitations of codes of ethics.
• Why are competence and responsibility ethical issues? How will each influence a human service professional's relationship with a client?
• Describe the components of the *Ethical Standards of Human Service Professionals*.

• What is difficult about the practice of confidentiality? Why is it important?
• What rights do clients have?
• How do professionals make ethical decisions?
• How might a human service professional use the model for ethical decision making?

WANT TO KNOW MORE?

There are several resources you can check to learn more about ethics and some of the other concepts introduced in this chapter.

Additional Readings: Focus on Ethics

Barker, P. (Ed). (2010). *Mental health ethics: The human context*. New York: Routledge.
This book encourages readers to heighten their awareness of the issues in contemporary mental health practice.
Corey, G., Corey, M. S., & Callanan, P. (2010). *Issues and ethics in the helping professions*. Belmont, CA: Brooks/Cole.
This best-selling practical text helps future and current professionals deal with the ethical issues they may encounter in their practice.
Crowell, W. (2006, September 1). Ethics and technology in human services. *Policy and Practice*, 64(3), 30.
A digital document from *Policy and Practice*, a journal published by Thomson Gale, this article addresses the intensifying trend of using technology; its implications for security, privacy, and acceptable use; and the changes in doing business.
Kennedy, R., Richards, J., & Leiman, T. (2012). *Integrating human service law, ethics, and practice* (3rd ed.). New York: Oxford University Press.
This text explores the place of law in Australian human service work and discusses the relationship between law and ethics.
Pack-Brown, S. P., & Williams, C. B. (2003). *Ethics in a multicultural context*. Beverly Hills, CA: Sage.

This book identifies culturally troublesome issues, encourages culturally appropriate interpretations of existing ethical guidelines, and promotes ethical behavior in multicultural contexts. Extensive case studies explore ethical dilemmas, critical decision making, and cultural competency.

Sajoo, A. B. (2009). *Muslim ethics: Emerging vistas.* Montreal: Institute for Islamic Studies.
This is one of a series of papers that explores Muslim ethics and the challenges presented by recent political and social events and advances in science and technology.

Skovholt, T. M. (2010). *The resilient practitioner.* Florence, KY: Routledge.
The author identifies and explains practitioner stress and provides remedies for self-care.

Wilcoxon, A., Remley, T., Gladding, S. T., & Huber, C. H. (2006). *Ethical, legal, and professional issues in the practice of marriage and family therapy.* Upper Saddle River, NJ: Prentice Hall.
This text examines the cultural, ethical, legal, and professional issues using values as a starting point.

REFERENCES

Corey, G., Corey, M. S., & Callanan, P. (2010). *Issues and ethics in the helping professions.* Belmont, CA: Thomson Brooks/Cole.

Dolgoff, R., Harrington, D., & Loewenberg, F. M. (2011). *Brooks/Cole Empowerment Series: Ethical dimensions for social work practice.* Belmont, CA: Brooks/Cole.

Nagpal, S. (2001). Through the cultural looking glass. *Counseling Today, 42.*

Pedersen, P. (2000). *A handbook for developing multicultural awareness.* Alexandria, VA: American Counseling Association.

Remley, T. P. Jr., & Herlihy, B. (2009). *Ethical, legal, and professional issues in counseling.* Upper Saddle River, NJ: Pearson Merrill Prentice Hall.

Sue, D. W., & Sue, D. (2012). *Counseling the culturally diverse: Theory and practice.* Boston: John Wiley.

Tarasoff v. Regents of the University of California. (1976). *Pacific Reporter,* 2nd Series, 551, 340.

Welfel, E. R. (2012). *Ethics in counseling and psychotherapy: Standards, research, & emerging issues.* Pacific Grove, CA: Brooks/Cole.

GLOSSARY

acceptance The ability of the helper to be receptive to the client regardless of factors such as dress or behavior.

administrator A human service professional whose primary responsibilities are planning and organizing services.

advocacy Speaking out on behalf of clients who cannot speak for themselves.

advocate A human service role that involves speaking on the client's behalf.

AFDC A federally funded public assistance program, titled Aid to Families with Dependent Children, that was replaced in 1996 as a result of welfare reform.

almshouses Workhouses for the mentally ill, the elderly, children, able-bodied poor, criminals, and other groups of people who needed care.

Americans with Disabilities Act Legislation passed in 1990 to enable people with disabilities to have equal access to goods, services, and employment.

antianxiety drugs Psychotropic medications prescribed to relieve anxiety, fear, or tension.

antidepressant drugs Psychotropic medications that relieve depression.

antipsychotic drugs Psychotropic medications that are effective in managing psychotic disorders.

assisted living Residential living that matches level of care to individual need.

asylums Institutions for the mentally ill.

attending behavior Verbal and nonverbal components that describe listening: eye contact, vocal qualities, verbal tracking, and body language.

barriers Factors or experiences that prevent clients from seeking help.

brokering Linking clients with needed services through a referral process.

burnout Physical or mental symptoms that result from overworking or stressful work.

case management The activities of planning and coordinating and, in some cases, delivering treatment strategies.

Centers for Faith-based and Community Initiatives (CFBCI) Created by President George W. Bush to strengthen the partnership between faith-based social services initiatives and the federal government and to provide financial support for these activities.

297

chain of command Layers of authority in an agency.

client An individual, small group, or larger population that needs help.

client strengths An approach to human service delivery that incorporates a client's positive attributes and those of his or her environment.

code of ethics A statement of ethical standards of behavior.

community-based services Services available in the community that enable clients to interact with their environments in the least restrictive setting in which they can function.

community caretakers Individuals who reside in the community and provide assistance and support to those in need without the benefit of education or training.

community mental health centers Multiservice centers established to provide a variety of community-based services for the mentally ill, including inpatient and outpatient care, emergency services, assistance to the courts, and services for the mental health of children and the elderly.

community organizing Activity based on like-minded people joining together to promote change.

competence Knowledge and skills that meet established professional standards.

confidentiality The helper's assurance to clients that their cases will not be discussed with others.

consumer A term that designates the recipient of human services.

counselors Individuals who help people deal with a variety of problems, including personal, social, educational, and career concerns.

crisis intervention The skills and strategies that helpers use to provide immediate help for a person in trouble.

cultural broker A helping professional who commits to help clients negotiate the cultural divide that influences access and effective use of services.

deinstitutionalization The movement that promoted the transfer of patients from institutions to the community for outpatient care.

developmental process The process of engaging in certain tasks or activities that occur at different life stages.

diversity Refers to many demographic variables, including age, color, disabilities, gender, national origin, race, religion, and sexual orientation.

effective communication The result when the receiver interprets a message the way the sender intended.

electroshock therapy The administration of electricity to the brain to diminish problem behaviors.

e-mail A convenient communication mode that allows for the transfer of messages via the Internet.

empathy Acceptance of the client that allows the helper to see the situation or understand feelings from the client's perspective.

employee assistance programs Programs that address the needs of workers and are available to the employees of companies and corporations.

empowerment Providing services based on client strengths and moving clients to self-sufficiency.

encapsulation When a human service helper retreats from the engagement of helping and becomes rigid, insensitive, and uncaring.

environment The client's surroundings, which include both the physical and the interpersonal (other people).

e-therapy Counseling and other support services provided online.

ethical dilemmas Situations with two or more values in conflict.

ethical standards Guidelines for the behavior of human service professionals.

ethnicity A common culture, heritage, and shared meaning.

evidence-based practice A growing trend in the human services to provide services to clients based upon knowledge about their effectiveness.

external reviews Ways that managed care organizations influence human service delivery, including authorization for services and continuous review.

Facebook A social networking website that allows individuals, organizations, and communities to communicate with each other.

fee-for-service The standard charge for a specific service.

flexibility Multifaceted trait that allows human service professionals to shift their perspectives of helping, clients, problems, and interventions.

frontline helper A human service professional who focuses on direct services to the client.

gang Two or more individuals who form a group that engages in illegal activities.

gatekeeping One method used in managed care to control patient or client access to services.

generalist A human service professional with diverse skills and functions that are applicable in a number of settings with a variety of client groups.

generic focus General helping knowledge and skills to serve individuals with a variety of problems in different settings.

gentrification Urban renewal to revitalize the downtown area of cities.

group A number of individuals who interact with each other, sharing values, a social structure, and cohesiveness.

health care reform A prominent issue of several past presidential campaigns that is a major focus of the Obama administration.

helping relationship The medium through which help occurs.

hierarchy of needs A pyramid of the needs of individuals that identifies lower-order needs such as food, clothing, and safety and higher-order needs such as social relationships and self-esteem.

homelessness An urban and rural problem that describes single men, women, children, and families who are without the basics of shelter, food, and clothing.

HS-BCP Human Service-Board Certified Practitioner certification indicates that the individual meets 11 core human service content areas.

human service model A treatment approach that utilizes problem solving to work with clients and their problems within the context of the environment.

human service professional An educated and trained individual who provides services to individual, families, groups, and communities in need.

human service system The combination of several parts of the social welfare system, including resources, policies, programs, and knowledge.

individualism The belief that hard work by any individual is the way to success.

individuality The qualities or characteristics that make each person unique and distinctive from all other people.

informed consent The client's right to know about the helper and the helping process.

involuntary clients Individuals who do not freely choose the services they are receiving.

job description A written document that defines the duties and responsibilities of a particular position.

laissez-faire An economic concept that advocated a society or government with little responsibility to those in need.

managed care A set of tools or methods designed to manage resources and deliver human services, especially in the areas of health care and mental health.

Medicaid An amendment (Title 19) to the Social Security Act that provides grants to states to assist them in helping medically indigent citizens receive medical and hospital care.

medical model A system of treatment that suggests that mental disorders are diseases or illnesses that impair an individual's ability to function.

Medicare An amendment (Title 18) to the Social Security Act that provides health insurance for those over age 65.

Medicare Prescription Drug, Improvement, and Modernization Act of 2003 (MMA) Provides outpatient prescription drug benefits for individuals on Medicare.

mission The purpose of an agency as summarized by its guiding principles.

moral responsibility A commitment to rational thinking and an orientation to moral principles.

motivational interviewing Provides a methodology to encourage behavior change.

multiracial A term that refers to individuals with mixed ancestry.

National Institute of Mental Health (NIMH) A federal agency created in 1946 to help states develop programs for increased training, research, and practice.

network Channels of communication among human service agencies and professionals.

networking Establishing links among human service professionals and agencies to deliver quality services.

neurosis A disorder of the mind or emotions.

New Federalism An approach advocated by the Nixon administration to limit federal spending and human services.

nonprofessional helpers Individuals who engage in helping with little training and agency responsibility.

nonverbal messages Behaviors or body language.

organizational chart A diagram illustrating an agency's structure.

organizational climate Conditions of the work environment.

paraphrase A helper statement that is interchangeable with the client's statement.

partisanship Approaching issues and challenges with one philosophical stance.

partnerships When two or more human service organizations work together to better serve the client.

patient Recipient of services in the medical model.

Patient Protection and Affordable Care Act Expands health care coverage to millions of Americans previously uninsured.

Personal Responsibility and Work Opportunity Reconciliation Act (PRWORA) The primary welfare reform legislation that ended the welfare system created by the Social Security Act of 1935.

physicians Medical doctors who perform medical examinations, diagnose illnesses, treat injured or diseased people, and advise patients on maintaining good health.

poor relief Food and protection for the poor provided by the church.

prevention A component of the public health model to improve the present and future quality of life and to alleviate health problems.

privatization Arrangement in which an agency or organization provides a human service function for profit.

privileged communication The legal right of some professionals to refuse to release certain information.

probation Term of supervision given to individuals who break the law but are not incarcerated.

problem solving A five-step approach to solving problems that focuses on the present.

problems Situations, events, or conditions that are troublesome for the client.

problems in living The term used to describe problems that focus on the client, the environment, and the interaction between them.

profession An occupation that is important to society, is based on academic training, and is bound by ethical standards.

professional disclosure statement A form that includes information about the helper and the helper's credentials.

protection A helper's ethical obligation to prevent harm to clients.

psychiatrist Physician concerned with the diagnosis, treatment, and prevention of mental illness.

psychiatry A medical specialty that diagnoses and treats mental, emotional, and behavioral disorders.

psychiatric drugs Psychiatric drugs are now among the most widely used treatments for mental disorders.

psychoanalytic method A method of therapy for investigating unconscious mental processes and neuroses.

psychologists Helping professionals who have advanced degrees in the study of human behavior and who provide counseling, perform assessments, and conduct research in that field.

psychopharmacology The study of the effects of drugs upon mental health.

psychotherapy Often used interchangeably with the term *counseling* to describe professional helping services.

public health model A service delivery model that extends health care beyond the medical model, applies a multicausal approach to studying the causes or origins of problems, and emphasizes a preventive approach.

questioning A common verbal technique used to elicit information.

referral Important role where professionals link clients to another service.

rehabilitation The process of returning an individual to a prior state of functioning.

relative confidentiality The informal sharing of information that occurs in an agency or organization among coworkers or treatment team members and supervisors.

reluctance Hesitancy to seek help.

resistance Behavior that can occur at any time in the helping process with a client who is unwilling to participate in the helping process.

resolution-focused brief therapy A counseling intervention that is focused on specific outcomes in a short time.

resources The funding, personnel, volunteers, buildings, and other assets at an agency's disposal.

responsibility The obligation to promote and safeguard the dignity, well-being, and growth of clients, colleagues, the profession, and society.

responsive or active listening The behaviors of helpers as they attend to the words and behaviors of their clients.

right to privacy An individual's right to withhold information he or she does not wish to share.

self-awareness The process of learning about one's self.

self-determination The act of deciding for one's self a course of action or resolution to a problem.

self-help groups Numbers of like-minded individuals facing similar challenges that meet together to support each other.

self-sufficiency The ability to care for one's self.

settlement house A large house in a slum area that serves as a community center, sponsoring classes, vocational training, and child care.

situational problems Difficulties individuals experience that occur without any predictability and may result in both short-term and long-term problems.

social care Assistance to clients in meeting their social needs, especially those clients who either temporarily or long-term cannot care for themselves.

social control Assistance for those individuals who could provide for themselves but have failed to do so or have done so in a manner that deviates from society's norms for appropriate behavior.

Social Darwinism The belief that the fittest of society would survive through the process of natural selection.

Social Security Public assistance to those in need that was provided as part of the American welfare state created by Roosevelt's New Deal legislation, the Social Security Act of 1935.

social workers Professionals with training in social welfare, human behavior, and the social environment who work with individuals, families, and groups.

societal change A state when individuals experience problems as a result of the breakdown of many traditional forms of society.

strengths-based approach An approach to interventions that focuses on the positive attributes of the client and the client's environment.

systems of care Delivery systems that provide a comprehensive approach to assistance.

TANF (Temporary Assistance to Needy Families) Federal funding that was available to states in block grants to replace the federal AFDC program.

teaming Working together in groups or units to provide efficient and effective client services.

teleconferencing A way in which human service professionals in different locations can communicate with each other.

termination The final stage of the helping process.

tolerance The helper's ability to be patient and fair with each client.

turf The clients, services, and resources that an agency or organization believes it controls or serves.

Twitter Communication delivery system via the Web that focuses on short messages and interactions.

urbanization A long-term global trend that describes population movement from rural areas to cities.

values Statement of beliefs about what guides behavior and provides direction to people's lives.

verbal messages Words spoken by a person.

vicarious trauma An emotional response that human service professionals who help individuals with more severe levels of trauma exposure, such as child abuse, violent crime, natural disasters, or torture, may develop.

volunteers Individuals who provide a service to others without expectation of pay or financial benefit.

war on poverty Program initiated by President Lyndon Johnson in 1964 to eradicate poverty by providing means for the poor to improve their economic situation.

Web logs Sites where individuals can post their diaries, journals, thoughts, and opinions.

welfare reform Legislation passed in 1996 to end the federal government's six-decade guarantee of aid to the poor.

whole person The many components of a person, such as psychological, social, physical, financial, and vocational, that comprise the total individual.

World Wide Web (or Web) Online method of expanding communication and information about individuals and organizations through the use of Web pages.

wraparound services Focus on individualized treatment plans within the context of community-based service.

INDEX